THE AMERICAN ACADEMY OF ORTHOPAEDIC SURGEONS

Instructional Course Lectures

Volume XIX 1970

THE AMERICAN ACADEMY OF ORTHOPAEDIC SURGEONS

Instructional Course Lectures

Volume XIX 1970

With 436 illustrations

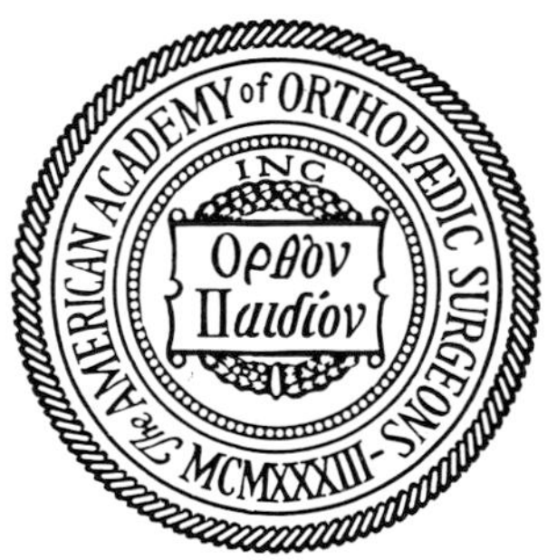

Saint Louis

THE C. V. MOSBY COMPANY

1970

Second printing

Printed in the United States of America

Standard Book Number 8016-0008-1

Library of Congress Catalog Card Number 43-17054

Distributed in Great Britain by Henry Kimpton, London

Contributors

HENRY H. BANKS, M.D.

Chief of Orthopaedic Surgery, Peter Bent Brigham Hospital; Assistant Professor of Orthopaedic Surgery, Harvard Medical School, Boston, Massachusetts

BURR H. CURTIS, M.D.

Medical and Executive Director, Newington Children's Hospital, Newington, Connecticut; Associate Clinical Professor of Orthopaedics, Yale University School of Medicine, New Haven, Connecticut

JOSEPH H. DIMON, III, M.D.

Instructor in Orthopaedic Surgery, Emory University School of Medicine; Staff, Piedmont Hospital and St. Joseph's Infirmary, Atlanta, Georgia

MARY E. GRAY, Ph.D.

Assistant Professor of Experimental Pathology, Vanderbilt University School of Medicine, Nashville, Tennessee

PAUL P. GRIFFIN, M.D.

Professor of Orthopaedics, George Washington University School of Medicine; Chairman, Department of Orthopaedics, Children's Hospital of District of Columbia, Washington, D. C.

CHARLES M. HAMILTON, M.D.

Clinical Instructor in Orthopaedics, Vanderbilt University School of Medicine; Chief of Orthopaedic Service, Midstate Baptist Hospital, Nashville, Tennessee

WILLIAM H. HARRIS, M.D.

Associate Clinical Professor of Orthopedic Surgery, Harvard Medical School; Visiting Orthopedic Surgeon, Massachusetts General Hospital; Orthopedic Surgeon, New England Baptist Hospital, Boston, Massachusetts

MICHAEL HARTY, M.A., M.B., M.Ch., F.R.C.S.

Associate Professor, Department of Graduate Anatomy, School of Medicine and School of Allied Medical Professions, University of Pennsylvania, Philadelphia, Pennsylvania

WILLIAM F. HEJNA, M.D., F.A.C.S., A.A.O.S.

Associate Attending Orthopaedic Surgeon and Assistant Chairman, Rush Presbyterian–St. Luke's Medical Center; Clinical Assistant Professor of Orthopaedic Surgery, University of Illinois, Chicago, Illinois

ARTHUR J. HELFET, B.Sc. (Capetown), M.D., M.Ch. Orth. (Liverpool), F.R.C.S. (Eng.), F.A.C.S.

Professor and Director, Division of Orthopaedic Surgery, Albert Einstein College of Medicine, Yeshiva University, Bronx, New York

J. WILLIAM HILLMAN, M.D.

Professor of Orthopedic Surgery and Head of the Department, Vanderbilt University School of Medicine, Nashville, Tennessee (Deceased)

EARL P. HOLT, JR., M.D., F.A.C.S.

Assistant Clinical Professor, Department of Orthopedic Surgery, Washington University School of Medicine, St. Louis, Missouri

JACK C. HUGHSTON, M.D.

Orthopaedic Consultant, Auburn University and Ft. Benning Army Hospital, Ft. Benning, Georgia; Staff, Columbus Medical Center, Columbus, Georgia

JOHN J. JOYCE, M.D.

Assistant Professor of Orthopaedic Surgery, Graduate Department, School of Medicine, University of Pennsylvania; Chief of Orthopaedic Services, Germantown Hospital; Director of Orthopaedics, The Episcopal Hospital, Philadelphia, Pennsylvania

KRISTAPS J. KEGGI, M.D.

Assistant Clinical Professor of Orthopaedic Surgery, Yale University School of Medicine, New Haven, Connecticut; Associate Attending in Orthopaedic Surgery, Waterbury Hospital, Waterbury, Connecticut

VIRGIL S. LeQUIRE, M.D.

Professor of Experimental Pathology and Professor of Anatomy, Vanderbilt University School of Medicine, Nashville, Tennessee

HENRY J. MANKIN, M.D.

Director of Orthopaedics, Hospital for Joint Diseases; Professor of Orthopaedics, The Mt. Sinai School of Medicine, New York, New York

JACQUELIN PERRY, M.D.

Chief, Kinesiology Service, Rancho Los Amigos Hospital, Downey, California; Associate Clinical Professor of Orthopaedic Surgery, University of Southern California School of Medicine, Los Angeles, California; Associate Clinical Professor of Orthopedic Surgery, University of California School of Medicine, San Francisco, California

THOMAS B. QUIGLEY, M.D.

Clinical Professor of Surgery, Harvard Medical School; Surgeon, Peter Bent Brigham Hospital; Surgeon, Harvard University Health Services, Boston, Massachusetts

ROBERT T. SNOWDEN, M.D.

Surgical House Staff, Johns Hopkins Hospital, Baltimore, Maryland

WAYNE O. SOUTHWICK, M.D.

Professor and Chief, Orthopaedic Surgery, Yale University School of Medicine, New Haven, Connecticut

HERBERT H. STARK, M.D.

Associate Clinical Professor of Surgery (Orthopaedics), University of Southern California School of Medicine; Attending Orthopaedic Surgeon, California Hospital, The Orthopaedic Hospital, and the Hospital of the Good Samaritan, Los Angeles, California

Preface

Volume XIX of *Instructional Course Lectures* is the fourth to be published by The C. V. Mosby Company. The appearance of this volume marks a departure from the practice, since 1961, of publishing material from certain selected courses in the *Journal of Bone and Joint Surgery.*

This volume contains information gleaned largely from the instructional courses given at the annual meeting of the American Academy of Orthopaedic Surgeons in New York City in January, 1969. A faculty of over 200 gave 110 courses of instruction to more than 3,000 orthopaedic surgeons.

The problem of education is first to know and then to speak. In this volume appropriately edited utterances of many able authors are compiled to add to our continuing education.

The decade of the 1960's saw great advances in the science of medicine, and, hopefully, in the art. But the 1970's promise to bring changes in the ways and means of getting the benefits of these advances to all the people in a more efficient and economical manner. One important facet of the problem of delivery of care is to communicate swiftly to practicing physicians the distillate of observations and experiences of their peers and teachers in a readily available medium. Toward this noble end the volume is dedicated.

The availability of the courses in one volume is highly desirable, especially for the physician in training and for the young orthopaedist just entering practice. Review articles, so necessary for teaching and for good patient care and yet not wholly suited to the *Journal of Bone and Joint Surgery,* find a place in this separate volume.

The publication of yearly volumes will provide orthopaedic surgeons with current information in a readily accessible manner. The specialty of orthopaedic surgery will reap continuing benefits therefrom.

The various authors provided contributions of a high level of quality, and each is commended and thanked.

The true order of learning is: first, what is necessary; second, what is useful; and third, what is ornamental. Despite the attractiveness of the volume, it is not an ornament. The contents are both necessary and useful to all of us concerned with giving our patients the best possible care and with teaching our students and residents the safest, surest, and most effective way to treat the sick and injured.

"Education is the apprenticeship of life."—Willmott

Committee on Instructional Courses

John C. Wilson, Jr., *Chairman*
Rocco A. Calandruccio
Wood W. Lovell
William R. MacAusland, Jr.
Warren G. Stamp

Contents

THE AMERICAN ACADEMY OF ORTHOPAEDIC SURGEONS

Instructional Course Lectures

Volume XIX 1970

Chapter 1

Surgical anatomy and exposures of the foot and ankle

JOHN J. JOYCE, M.D., and MICHAEL HARTY, M.A., M.B., M.Ch.
Philadelphia, Pennsylvania

Perhaps because of its distal location and sometimes unsightly appearance, the foot often receives cursory coverage by books devoted to surgical approaches. Of his entire anatomic makeup, man's foot is his most distinctly human structure. The hemidomed arch with its multiple articulations acts as a shock-absorbing mechanism in such activities as running or descending stairs.

Although varied anatomic nomenclature has previously been a source of confusion to both the anatomist and the clinician since the introduction of the *Basle Nomina Anatomica* (B.N.A.) in 1895, it is hoped that the terms for ankle movements recommended by the American Academy of Orthopaedic Surgeons in 1966 and by the International Congress of Anatomists in 1960 will reduce the chaos. More senior clinicians are familiar with the terms "plantar flexion" for the flexion motion and "dorsiflexion" for the extension motion (Fig. 1-1).

ANATOMY

The visible and palpable bony prominences provide constant landmarks to maintain the accurate orientation so necessary during surgical exposures. The tibia, which transmits the body weight to the foot, may be palpated beneath the skin from its proximal end to the medial malleolus. On the medial aspect of the foot, the head and neck of the talus is more obvious on eversion; the navicular tuberosity is more evident on inversion; the base, shaft, and head of the first metatarsal are further helpful bony landmarks. The posterior margin of the navicular marks the medial end of the midtarsal joint (Fig. 1-2).

Laterally the fibula becomes subcutaneous and forms the lateral malleolus. This easily accessible landmark of the outer aspect of the ankle joint extends 1 to 2 cm. further distally than the medial malleolus, and its tip helps to identify the proximal margin of the subtalar joint. The styloid process, shaft, and head of the fifth metatarsal, as well as the phalanges of the little toe, provide additional palpable bony landmarks on the lateral side of the forefoot (Fig. 1-3). Beneath the overlying fibrofatty tissue of the heel, the calcaneus may be felt. Lying in the depression anterior and distal to the lateral malleolus, the sinus tarsi outlines the lateral end of the subtalar joint, and the muscle belly of the extensor digitorum brevis may be palpated along its inferior margin. The bony sinus contains the strong talocalcaneal ligaments and a fat pad.

Midway between the lateral malleolus and the base of the styloid process of the fifth metatarsal lies the calcaneocuboid joint, marking the lateral component of the entire midtarsal joint. The peroneal tendons cross the calcaneus as they pass from the lateral malleolus to the base of the fifth metatarsal. The peroneal tubercle of the calcaneus, located about 3 cm. distal to the tip of the lateral malleolus, is occasionally missing.

The talar dome, which is wider distally, is wedged firmly between the medial and lateral malleoli. In ankle extension the malleoli are forced apart 1 to 2 mm. by the talus, whereas in flexion they are drawn together by contraction of the elastic fibers in the inferior tibiofibular joint (Fig. 1-4). Thus the malleoli maintain continuity with the collateral articular facets of the talus. The

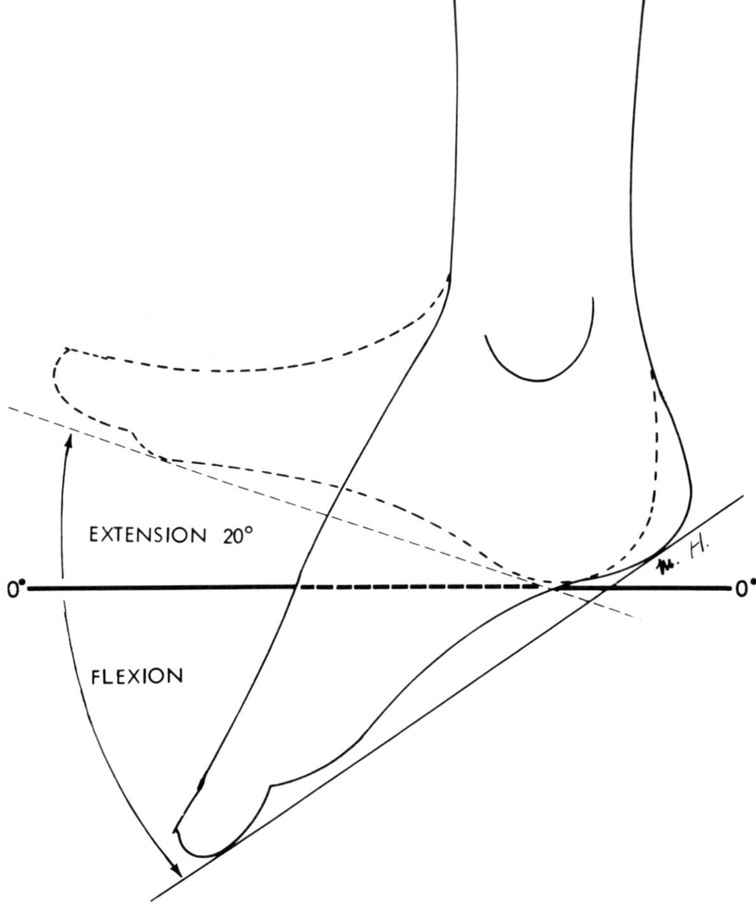

Fig. 1-1. Ankle movement. Flexion or plantar flexion and extension or dorsiflexion.

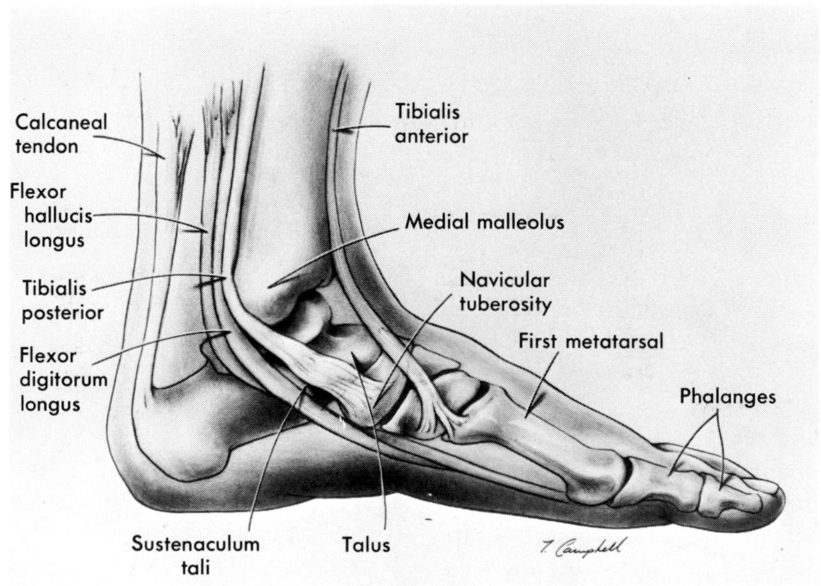

Fig. 1-2. Major palpable features on medial aspect of left foot. (From Giannestras, N. J.: Foot disorders, Philadelphia, 1967, Lea & Febiger.)

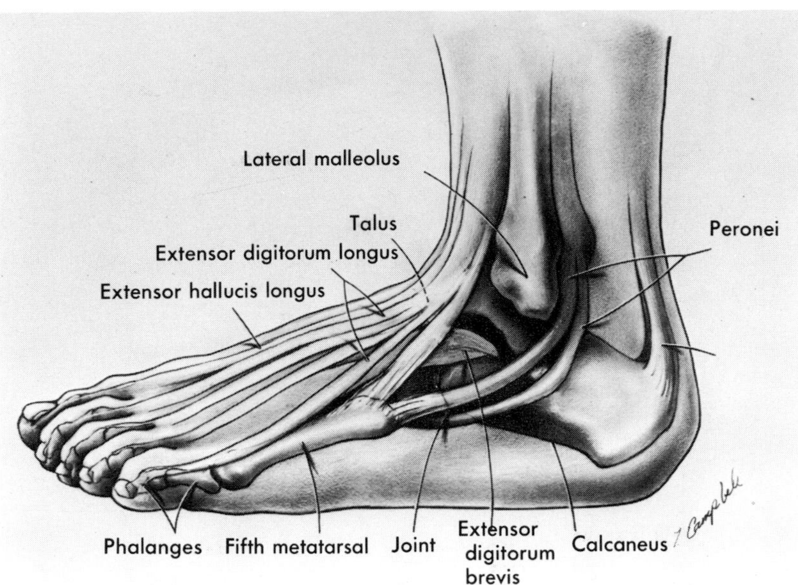

Fig. 1-3. Lateral side of the left foot. The extensor digitorum brevis is at the inferior margin of the sinus tarsi. (From Giannestras, N. J.: Foot disorders, Philadelphia, 1967, Lea & Febiger.)

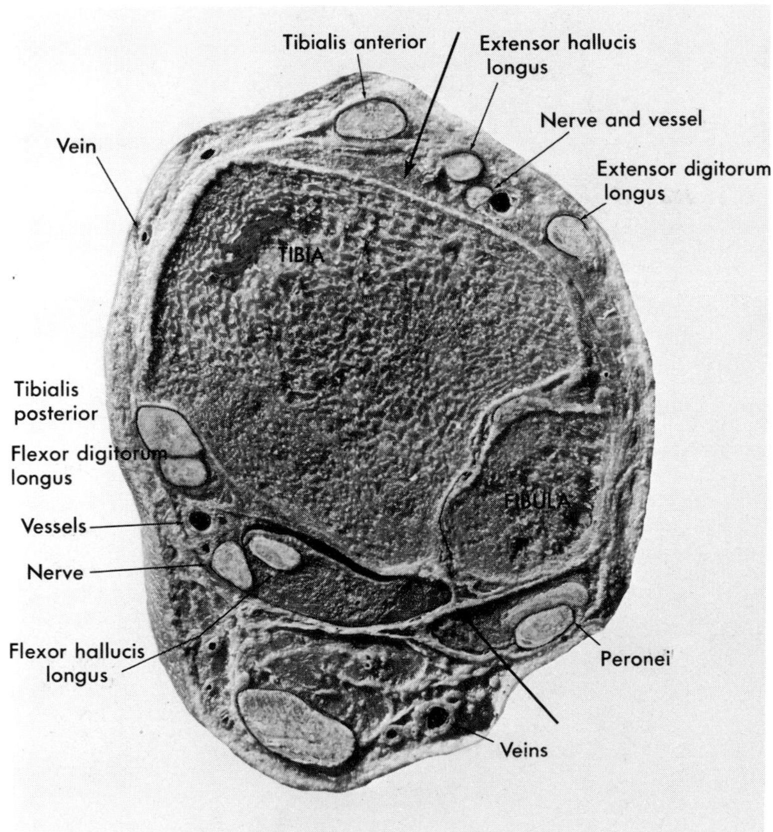

Fig. 1-4. Transverse section through right inferior tibiofibular joint. Heavy arrows indicate the site of the anterior and the posterolateral exposures.

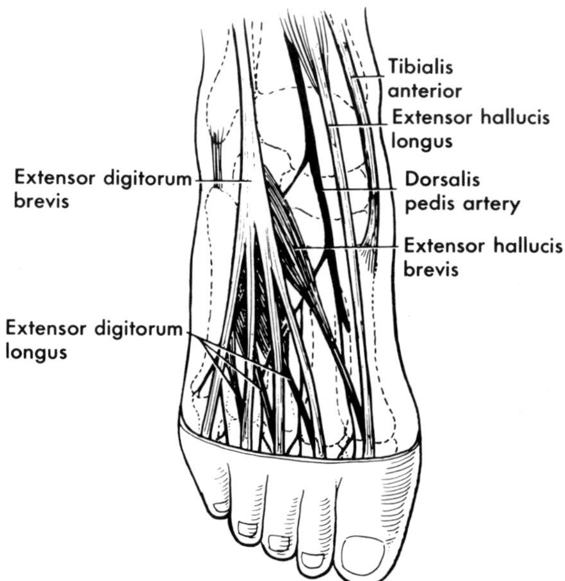

Fig. 1-5. Dorsal aspect of right foot. Extensor digitorum tendon is retracted laterally. (From Joyce, J. J., III, and Harty, M.: Orthopaedic approaches, Baltimore, 1961, The Williams & Wilkins Co.)

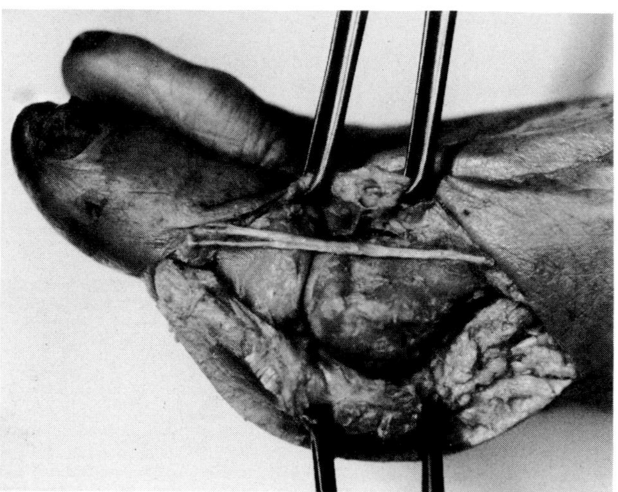

Fig. 1-6. Exposed right metatarsophalangeal joint. Medial capsule is reflected plantarward. Note cutaneous nerve.

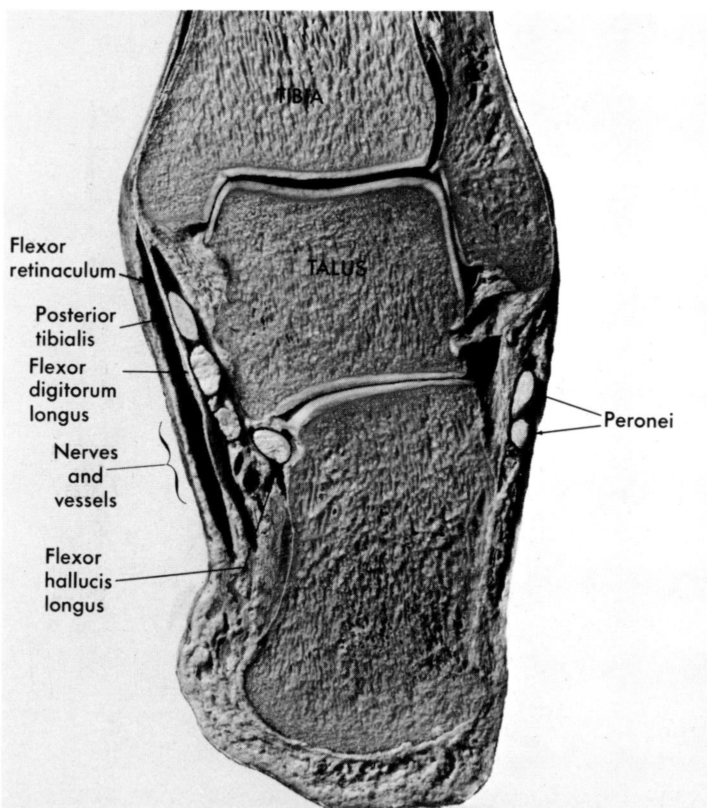

Fig. 1-7. Coronal section of right ankle in full extension or dorsiflexion. The tarsal tunnel is deep to the flexor retinaculum and conveys the long flexor tendons and neurovascular bundle to the sole.

long extensor tendons are readily palpable over the anterior aspect of the ankle joint (Fig. 1-5). At the level of the ankle the dorsalis pedis artery lies between the tendons of the extensor hallucis longus and the extensor digitorum longus. Because the extensor hallucis tendon arises from the lateral aspect of the leg, it crosses the anterior neurovascular bundle as the tendon reaches the great toe. The metatarsophalangeal joints may be easily felt beneath the extensor tendons (Fig. 1-5). Although the extensor tendon is easily displaced medially during an exposure of the first metatarsophalangeal joint, the digital branches of the superficial peroneal nerve should also be identified and protected (Fig. 1-6).

Although fascia is often regarded as the "packing material" of the animal organism, its multiple planes and septa provide the channels of the body for the passage of vessels and nerves, permit movement, between adjacent structures, restrict and retain many specialized structures, and in the foot, especially, give additional attachments for muscles and tendons.

The tarsal tunnel

The long flexor tendons and major neurovascular supply lie behind the medial malleolus in the tarsal tunnel bounded by the deltoid ligament with its tarsal attachments and the more superficial flexor retinaculum (Fig. 1-7). Not only does the tunnel provide an easy connection between sole and lower leg, allowing infection to pass proximally from the foot, but the more constricted proximal portion of this passageway may also be the site of nerve compression. Since this side contributes the principal nerve and blood supply to the skin of the heel, horizontal incisions may jeopardize the viability and sensation in the area.

BASIC PRINCIPLES OF SURGICAL EXPOSURES

Surgical exposures are based on some well-established principles, which include the following:

1. Complete orientation is essential at all stages of the procedures.
2. The position and draping of the patient must allow easy access to the operative site and free mobility of the limb.
3. By paralleling the skin creases, by avoiding bony prominences, and by making an incision of adequate length, forced retraction and subsequent maceration of the skin edges are minimized.
4. Careful control of bleeding is necessary, by tourniquet when feasible, by selection of a dry route, by ligation of the larger vessels, and by electrocautery of the smaller ones. Postoperative elevation, adequate splintage, and compression dressings also help to reduce the incidence of hemorrhage.
5. Protection of vital structures at the operative site is achieved either by placing the approach at a safe distance from these vital structures or by identifying and gently retracting them from the danger zone.
6. By placing the skin incision in a nonweight-bearing area, avoiding bony prominences and sites that may be irritated by footwear, many annoying sequelae may be obviated.
7. Preservation of the neurovascular apparatus to the foot and toes is indispensable for successful foot surgery.

The ankle joint, the subtalar region, the metatarsophalangeal joints, and the medial or lateral margin of the foot and the calcaneus are the areas more commonly requiring surgical visualization. The exposures will be discussed under the general headings of indications, limitations, position of patient and limb, anatomic landmarks, danger points, and technique.

SURGICAL EXPOSURES OF THE ANKLE JOINT

As an essential weight-bearing and complex joint, the importance of the ankle is well recognized. Recently the greater number of transportation accidents, the physical fitness drive, and athletic emphasis have produced an increase in the incidence of complicated ankle injuries requiring surgical repair. The correct selection of the surgical approach plays an important part in the results achieved by a given operation. The anterior, the lateral, the posterior, and the medial exposures of the ankle joint provide ample access for the usual required procedures.

Anterior approach to the ankle joint

Indications. The usual indications for employing this route are stabilization of certain fractures, arthrodesis, astragalectomy, or arthrotomy to drain or explore the ankle joint.

Limitation. The greatest limitation in this approach is lack of accessibility to the posterior compartment of the ankle joint.

Position of patient. By placing the patient in a supine position with the foot on a low support and somewhat plantar-flexed, the anterior ankle compartment is easily exposed. Draping of the extremity should permit free maneuverability of the leg and foot.

Landmarks. The tibial crest, the malleoli, the talar head, the navicular tubercle, and the extensor tendons provide the better landmarks to assist in correctly placing the skin incision. Beneath the skin, the extensor tendons and the dorsalis pedis vessels provide additional guideposts for a safer and more accurate continuation of the exposure.

Danger points. Throughout the procedure care must be taken to protect the anterior tibial nerve with its vessels and the extensor tendons.

Technique. The skin cut starts about three inches proximal to the ankle joint, one fingerbreadth lateral to the tibial crest, and extends distally beyond the joint for the same distance. Immediately beneath the skin, terminal branches of the superficial peroneal nerve should be sought and protected. To expose the neurovascular bundle, the interval between the extensor hallucis longus and the extensor digitorum longus tendon is developed. Lateral retraction of the long digital extensors with the neurovascular pedicle and medial displacement of the extensor hallucis tendon usually provide a dry route to the joint capsule (Fig. 1-8). Some surgeons prefer to displace the hallucis tendon laterally and so use it as a guardian for the vessels and nerves. Occasionally a medial malleolar arterial branch may require ligation. A longitudinal cut through the capsule and periosteal reflection provide a wide exposure of the anterior ankle joint and adjacent bony region.

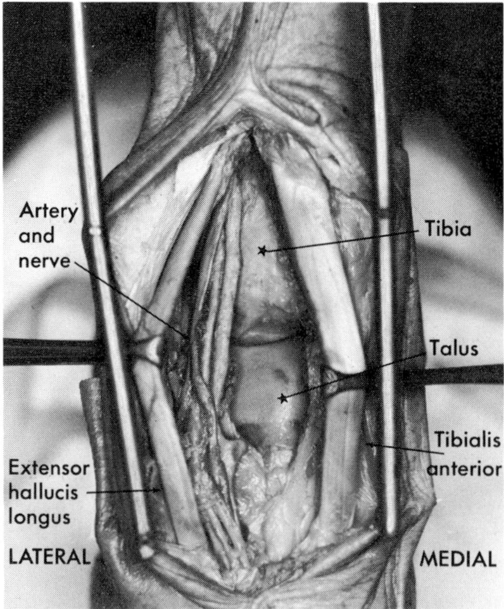

Fig. 1-8. Anterior exposure of right ankle region.

Posterolateral approach

A safe, adequate view of the back of the ankle may be obtained through the posterolateral route.

Indications. Open reduction of fractures, removal of loose bodies from the posterior ankle compartment, tendon transfers, and bone block procedures may be performed through this approach.

Limitations. Although plantar flexion of the ankle permits wider retraction, exposure is limited to the distal and posterior aspect of the tibia, fibula, and ankle joint.

Position of patient. Although the patient is usually placed in a prone position with the extremity draped so as to permit free mobility of the limb, some procedures are more readily performed with the patient lying on his sound side and resting the foot on a sandbag.

Landmarks. At the skin level, the easily palpable tendocalcaneus, the lateral malleolus, and the calcaneus serve as landmarks in accurate placement of the incision (Fig. 1-9, *A*).

Danger points. In the subcutaneous tissue the sural nerve and short saphenous vein are often found and should be preserved (Fig. 1-10). At the deep fascia the tendons of the peronei and lateral malleolus are more in evidence. About 5 cm. proximal to the lateral malleolus, the flexor hallucis longus swings medially from the peroneal tendons to reveal the strategic triangle of Henry and the depression between the lower tibia and fibula, which may be occupied by the peroneal artery (Fig. 1-10).

Technique. A hockey stick incision about one inch behind the lateral malleolus exposes the nerve and vein. Division of the deep fascia exposes the peroneal tendons, which are retracted laterally; medial displacement of the flexor hallucis longus displays the lower tibia and joint capsule. This intertendinous interval is more readily located distally at the ankle level and developed in a proxi-

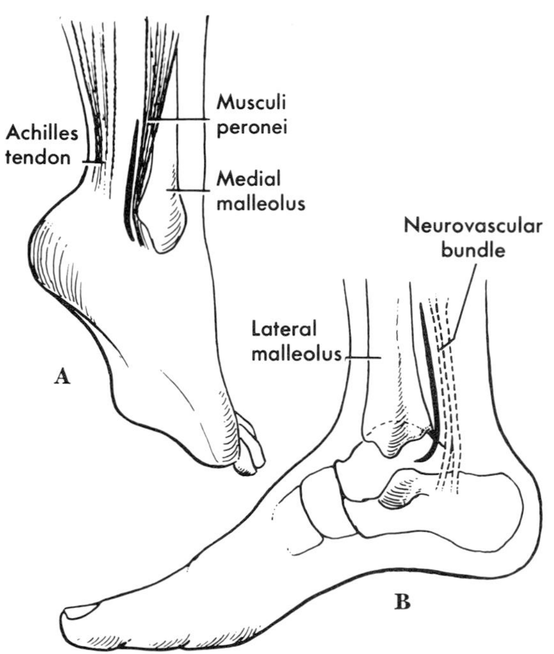

Fig. 1-9. A, Lateral. **B,** Medial postmalleolar incision. (From Joyce, J. J., III, and Harty, M.: Orthopaedic approaches, Baltimore, 1961, The Williams & Wilkins Co.)

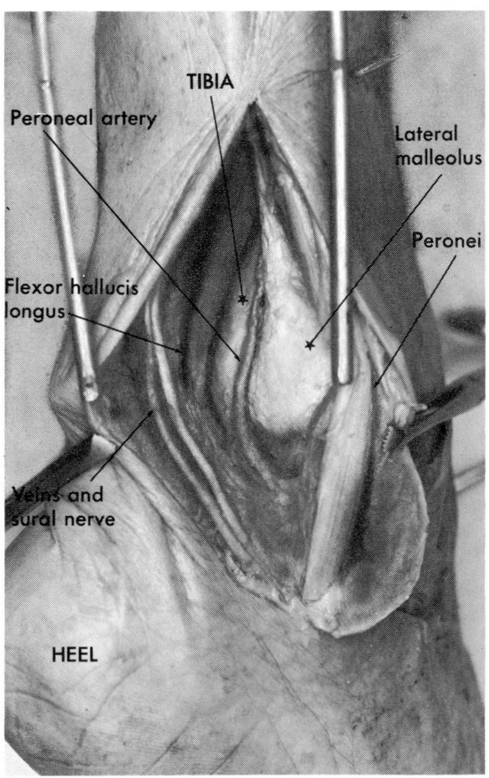

Fig. 1-10. Posterolateral exposure of right ankle joint.

mal direction. Subperiosteal reflection and division of the capsule expose the joint and region of the third malleolus. The posterior overhang of the lateral malleolus often conceals the peroneal artery or even the lower tibia.

Lateral approach

The lateral approach is the most versatile of all ankle exposures because wide visualization of the ankle joint is possible with few vital structures intervening.

Indications. The usual indications for employing the lateral exposure of the ankle joint are recent injuries such as fractures and dislocations requiring reconstruction, ununited fibular fractures, ankle arthrodesis, certain ligamentous repairs or tendon transfers, and removal of loose bodies.

Limitations. Although the entire lateral compartment is fully available and most of the anterior and posterior portions of the tibiotalar joint may be seen, the lateral exposure does not provide access to the medial portion of the ankle.

Position of patient. Placing a sandbag beneath the buttock of the side for operation and flexion of the knee usually make the lateral ankle area available.

Landmarks. The tendocalcaneus, the lateral malleolus, the calcaneus, and the talus guide the surgeon in the correct placement of the skin incision. After the skin is opened, the fibula, the peroneal tendons, the anterior tibiofibular ligament, and the sinus tarsi serve as deeper guideposts (Fig. 1-3).

Danger points. An annoying cicatrix may complicate skin incisions placed directly over the lateral malleolus. Damage to the peroneal tendons or superficial peroneal nerve must also be avoided, and the articular surfaces of the talotibial joint should be protected unless arthrodesis is anticipated.

Technique. The skin incision usually follows the anterior or posterior border of the fibula to reach a handbreadth proximal to the tip of the lateral malleolus (Fig. 1-9, *A*). Subperiosteal separation at the anterior fibular margin affords protection of the peroneal tendons and adjacent nerves. Osteotomy of the fibula is performed approximately four fingerbreadths proximal to the tip of the lateral malleolus. Usually the distal fragment is separated from everything except the posterior tibiofibular ligament on which it is hinged backward. Alternatively the distal fibular ligaments are retained, and the bone is detached completely from the tibia and rotated distally.

Approach to the medial malleolus

Ankle injuries frequently require operative repair of the deltoid ligament or of the medial aspect of the ankle joint. The intimate relationships between the neurovascular bundle and tendons passing behind and beyond the medial malleolus demand surgical care and anatomic precision in the area (Fig. 1-7).

Indications. The commoner indications for exposure of the medial ankle are open repair of recent or ununited medial malleolar fractures, defects in the deltoid ligament, and, occasionally, exposure of the medial aspect of the talus.

Limitations. Vital nerves, vessels, and tendons limit posterior prolongation of the approach. Only the medial aspects of the talus, including its dome, are available through osteotomy of the medial malleolus. Careful repositioning of the malleolus and repair of the deltoid ligament are essential for the preservation of ankle stability and function.

Position of patient. With the patient supine, a sandbag under the buttock of the sound side, the extremity for operation in external rotation, and the knee joint partly flexed, the medial side of the ankle joint is easily available. Because both the medial and lateral sides of the ankle may require simultaneous exposure at the same operation, draping must permit free mobility of the limb.

Landmarks. Convenient landmarks in placing the skin incision are provided by the medial malleolus, navicular tuberosity, sustentaculum tali, and tibial borders (Fig. 1-2). Beneath the skin the medial malleolus and posterior and anterior tibial tendon sheaths provide guideposts to the medial ankle.

Danger points. The long saphenous vein and the saphenous nerve lie immediately beneath the skin at the anterior margin of the medial malleolus (Fig. 1-4). When the deep fascia is opened, the tendinous and neurovascular structures passing closely behind the medial malleolus must be adequately protected (Figs. 1-4 and 1-7).

Technique. The skin incision may follow either the anterior or posterior tibial border. Immediately beneath the skin the medial malleolus, covered by the deep fascia of the leg and the flexor retinaculum, is encountered. Division of this retinaculum exposes the deltoid ligament (Fig. 1-7). Subperiosteal elevation and distal reflection of the deltoid ligament permit visualization of the medial malleolus and the medial aspect of the talar head and neck (Fig. 1-2). Osteotomy of the medial malleolus displays the medial body and dome of the talus.

FOOT EXPOSURES

Subtalar joint

Indications. The usual indications for visualization of the subtalar joint are reconstruction procedures to correct deformities due to trauma, congenital deformities (clubfoot, with severe pronation or equinus), correction of the sequelae of certain neurologic disorders, and removal of loose bodies (bony or foreign).

Limitations. Only the talocalcaneal, calcaneocuboid, and talonavicular joints are available through the subtalar route. Difficulties are invited by excessive retraction of the wound edges or extending the incision beyond the limits planned.

Position of the patient. By placing a support beneath the buttock of the side on which surgery is anticipated, the patient is tilted toward his sound side. Easy access to the subtalar area is further facilitated by draping the leg for free mobility of the extremity. The foot for operation should be supported on its medial side by a roll of sterile linen or small sandbag.

Guideposts. At the skin level the guide to the accurate position of the incision may be determined by locating the lateral malleolus, the peroneal tendons, and the sinus tarsi with the head and neck of the talus. Subcutaneously the fat pad in the sinus tarsi, the tendons of the peronei posteriorly, as well as the extensor longus and peroneus tertius on the dorsolateral portion of the foot are further factors in determining the limitations of the cut. The ligaments between the components of the triple joint, the extensor brevis attachments, and the joints themselves can be identified by instrument palpation after the talocalcaneal joint has been precisely located.

Danger points. Not only does the misplaced skin incision often result in a painful area due to rubbing of the shoe on a cicatrix placed over a bony prominence, but also skin necrosis may result from zealous retraction performed to force additional exposure of the area. Pressure on the wound edges must be scrupulously avoided at all times. Beneath the skin, the three peroneal and extensor longus tendons, as well as the dorsalis pedis vessels, are vulnerable to the assault of the unwary surgeon.

Inadvertent opening of the ankle joint adds two major problems: the traction needed to open the subtalar joint is now lost, and the blood supply to the talus is even more precarious than ever. Needless to add, the adequacy of the foot circulation must be evaluated prior to employing the subtalar approach.

Technique. After the sinus tarsi, the talonavicular, the talocalcaneal, and the calcaneocuboid joints have been identified, the incision is made from a point at the edge of the peroneus tertius tendon to end at approximately a fingerbreadth below the lateral malleolus. The cut should be directly over the talocalcaneal joint (Fig. 1-3). By preserving the subcutaneous skin attachments, the blood supply to the skin flaps is protected. Visualization and maintenance of the fat pad in the sinus tarsi aid in filling this dead space at the time of wound closure. Mobilization of the peronei, if needed, can be obtained by additional careful posterior and proximal extension of the wound.

Subperiosteal detachment of the extensor digitorum brevis and division of the talocalcaneal attachments exposes the sinus tarsi. This is facilitated by gentle inversion of the foot. Meticulous removal of all soft parts permits good visualization of the talocalcaneal, the calcaneocuboid, and the talonavicular joints (Fig. 1-12). Careful protection of the blood supply to the skin flaps, avoidance of pressure on the wound edges by forceful heavy retraction, and meticulous preservation of the subcutaneous skin attachments are helpful in avoiding the complication of wound necrosis.

FOREFOOT APPROACHES

Poorly planned incisions about the foot may result in painful scars, painful neuromas, or a failure of good wound healing. Because of the frequency of operations on the first metatarsophalangeal joint, a discussion of this exposure is included.

First metatarsophalangeal joint

Indications. The indications for this approach are reconstruction of the first metatarsophalangeal joint for hallux valgus, hallux rigidus, correction of deformities due to injuries or neurologic disorders, removal of exostoses, certain tendon transfers, trauma, and arthritic problems. Only the great toe, the first metatarsophalangeal joint, and the first metatarsal are available through this route.

Position of patient. The patient is usually placed in a supine position with the limb in external rotation.

Guideposts. At the skin level the guideposts aiding in the correct placement of the incision are the joint, the great toe, and the dorsomedial aspect of the first metatarsal. Beneath the skin the joint becomes more obvious, the extensor tendons are easily located, and the sensory nerves should be identified (Fig. 1-6). At the bone level the proximal phalanx of the great toe, the first metatarsal, and the metatarsophalangeal joint are easily available.

Danger points. Misplacement of the skin incision too far dorsally, on the plantar aspect of the foot or on the direct medial aspect, often results in an exposed and easily irritated painful scar. Beneath the skin inadvertent division of the extensor tendon or digital nerve produces a "dead toe" or a chronically flexed toe with callus formation on the tip or dorsum. Within the joint, injury to the cartilage of the metatarsal head or to the long or short flexor tendons usually causes a poorly functioning toe.

Technique. Placement of the skin cut on the dorsomedial aspect of the first metatarsal avoids an area subject to shoe pressure and is well away from important structures beneath the skin (Figs. 1-6 and 1-11). The incision begins about three fingerbreadths proximal to the joint line, curves

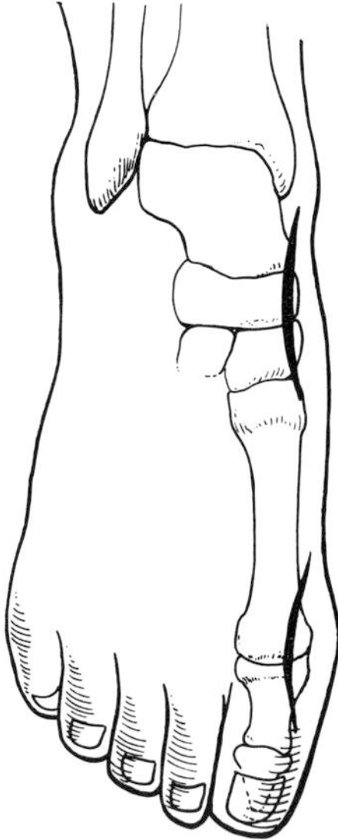

Fig. 1-11. Skin incisions for exposures of the medial tarsal and metatarsophalangeal joints. (From Joyce, J. J., III, and Harty, M.: Orthopaedic approaches, Baltimore, 1961, The Williams & Wilkins Co.)

slightly dorsally at the joint, and ends at the interphalangeal joint. Careful undermining of the skin permits visualization of the nerve. The capsule is easily identified. The extensor tendons may be retracted to one side. After the tip of the knife has been inserted into the joint, the blade is turned so that its flat side parallels the bone shaft. By cutting proximally and distally away from the joint, the capsule is dissected from its osseous attachments (Fig. 1-6). Resection of the proximal third of the proximal phalanx allows good visualization of the flexor tendon and sesamoids. Meticulous dissection and careful wound edge approximation are important to good wound healing.

Approach to metatarsals

By placing the skin incision in the interspaces between the bones, the metatarsals may be easily exposed, and a painful scar over a bony prominence is avoided (Fig. 1-5). In spite of the ready availability of the metatarsals, protection of the long extensors from division or adhesion is essential for good postoperative foot function.

Indications. The indications for this approach are severely deformed or open fractures that cannot be reduced by closed means or that require debridement, correction of congenital anomalies requiring osteotomy or excision of accessory metatarsals, removal of bone tumors, procurement of tendons for grafts, or drainage of infections. The bases and heads of the metatarsals, as well as the intervening soft parts, are available through this route.

Guideposts. Guideposts are usually readily available. The toes and metatarsal shafts are both visible and palpable. Beneath the skin the extensor tendons, nerves, and major blood vessels can usually be identified, so that the danger of injury to those structures should be minimal (Fig. 1-5).

Technique. The skin incision is made in the interspace parallel to the metatarsal shaft. Skin reflection displays the extensor tendons. Gentle retraction of the soft parts gives an unimpeded view of the shafts, which are approached by periosteal elevation.

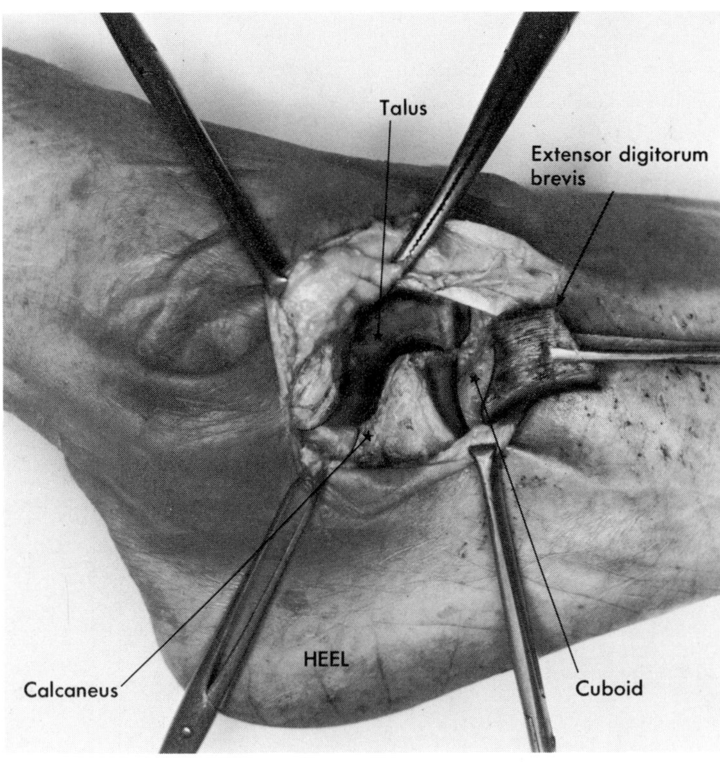

Fig. 1-12. Left subtalar joint exposed. The extensor digitorum brevis is reflected off the calcaneal beak.

Medial tarsal exposure

Indications. Reconstructions such as proximal or distal fusions of the medial cuneiform, tendon transplants, drainage of infection, or removal of foreign bodies may be performed by this approach. Plantar dissection is limited by the long flexor tendons, and the anterior tibial tendon commonly crosses the wound (Fig. 1-2).

Guideposts. Guideposts are the navicular tuberosity, the first metatarsal, and the medial cuneiform. Subcutaneously the termination of the saphenous nerve and vein may be encountered and should be preserved.

Technique. The skin incision extends from the neck of the talus to the base of the first metatarsal (Fig. 1-12). The tendons of tibialis anterior and posterior must be sought before any attempt is made to open the dorsomedial aspect of the capsule.

SUMMARY

Some of the salient features of the applied anatomy of the foot and ankle are illustrated, and the parts they play in the surgical exposures are discussed.

REFERENCES

1. Gianestras, N. J.: Foot disorders, medical and surgical management, Philadelphia, 1967, Lea & Febiger.
2. Goss, C. M., editor: Gray's anatomy, Philadelphia, 1966, Lea & Febiger, ed. 28.
3. Henry, A. K.: Extensile exposures, Baltimore, 1957, The Williams & Wilkins Co.
4. Joyce, J. J., III, and Harty, M.: Orthopaedic approaches, Section I, Lower limb, Baltimore, 1961, The Williams & Wilkins Co.

Chapter 2

Clinical and pathologic studies of fat embolism*

VIRGIL S. LeQUIRE, M.D., J. WILLIAM HILLMAN, M.D., and MARY E. GRAY, Ph.D.
Nashville, Tennessee

ROBERT T. SNOWDEN, M.D.
Baltimore, Maryland

INTRODUCTION

For over a century, vascular impaction by fat has intrigued pathologists and clinicians alike as an unpredictable complication of trauma. With the use of fat stains, embolic fat in pulmonary vessels (though variable in amount and clinical significance) has been found almost routinely at necropsy following all types of tissue injury. Rarely, the clinical syndrome of fat embolism develops that, paradoxically, has emerged as a major complication of trauma.

The prevalent concept of pathogenesis has been that globular fat from ruptured fat cells gains entry into torn venous channels and impacts subsequent capillary beds, especially in the lungs. This concept has been supported by the occasional association of bone marrow cellular elements and even spicules of bone with embolic fat. Any surgeon familiar with an open operation on bone has been impressed by the globular fat that floats to the surface of the operative site, and, therefore, it is easily reasoned that pulmonary or cerebral embolic fat has its origin from traumatized depot fat.†

This rationale is so straightforward that little attention has been given to reports of fat embolism complicating clinical situations in which trauma has not been a factor; for example, in such diverse conditions as diabetes mellitus,[52] sickle cell crisis,* bacterial infections,[25] alcoholism,[57] decompression to altitude,[56] certain types of poisoning,[22] and immunosuppressive therapy.[23,51]

We suggest that a common denominator in all these conditions is cellular injury, whether inflicted by an automobile, a burn, anoxia, steroid imbalance, bacteria, or some poisonous agent, and that cellular injury is accompanied by profound alterations in cellular metabolism. In fact, it has been demonstrated and generally accepted that trauma and surgical stress[64,68] cause remarkable alterations in protein and carbohydrate metabolism. We propose to demonstrate that normal lipid metabolism is also altered by these factors.

PATHOLOGIC ANATOMY

The gross and microscopic appearance of tissue in which fat embolism is a prominent feature is extremely variable and is primarily dependent upon duration from time of onset as well as superimposed complications such as infection or contusion. In general, the pathology seen can be at-

*Supported in part by U.S.P.H.S. Research Grants HE 01570 and HE 10197.

†For the most recent reviews see reference 33, 85, and 95.

*See references 32, 70, 79, and 86.

tributed to anoxic occlusion of small blood vessels and right heart failure. These manifestations have been described in detail by many investigators.* They resemble microembolization by fibrin, and, indeed, this is a fairly common associated finding. Frequently, there is no distinguishing feature on gross examination to alert the prosector that embolic fat is present (Fig. 2-1).

The unit lesion may be described as an occluded vessel, an arteriole, capillary, or venule, which is markedly dilated by fat and surrounded by congested edematous tissue in which hemorrhage may or may not be prominent (Fig. 2-2, *A-C*). On the skin or serosal surfaces, the lesion is marked by petechial or purpuric hemorrhages in some cases. The amount of embolic fat is not generally appreciated unless fat stains are made.

The lungs are the most prominently involved visceral organ. They present a mottled or patchy congested appearance. They may not collapse upon opening the pleural cavities. They weigh more than normal and may float poorly in water. Lower lobe atelectasis, with or without pleural effusion, may be present. On cut surface (Fig. 2-1, *B*), the patchy involvement is again apparent, and a frothy bronchial exudate is frequently a prominent feature. Microscopic examination reveals the focal nature of the involvement characterized by perivascular, perilymphatic, and peribronchial edema or hemorrhage (Fig. 2-2, *C*). Infarction is rare. The alveolar walls appear thickened, and a proteinaceous material typical of pulmonary edema, together with erythrocytes, is present (Fig. 2-2, *B* and *C*). Fibrin and leukocytes may be seen within blood vessels between globules of embolic fat (Fig. 2-2, *B*). Other areas of the lung may be normal in appearance or with minimal involvement (Fig. 2-2, *A*). Bone marrow fragments with adipose tissue cells, hematopoietic tissue including megakaryocytes, and even spicules of bone are occasionally seen (Fig. 2-3). In our experience, these are found most often in patients in whom vigorous resuscitative measures have been performed, with resultant rib fracture.

*For the most recent review see reference 85.

By the use of polarization microscopy on frozen sections, birefringent crystals may be seen in association with embolic fat (Fig. 2-4). Long acidular crystals, presumably fatty acids, are most frequently seen, and these disappear with heating the slide to 40° C. Short rhomboid crystals may also be seen that are characteristic of cholesterol crystals. The

A

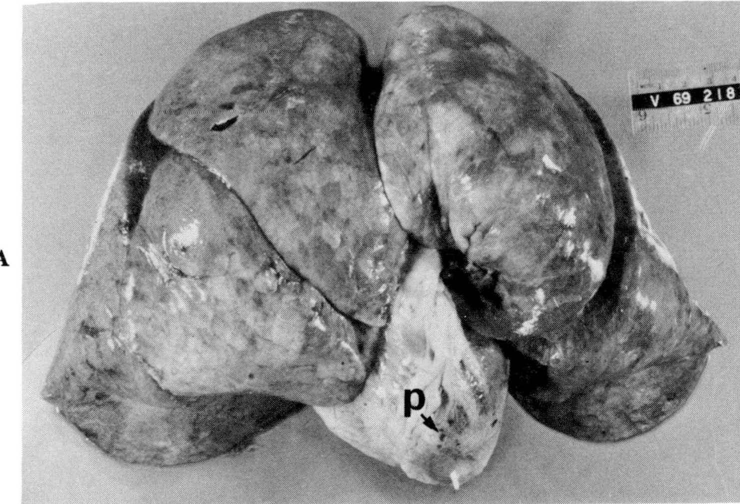

B

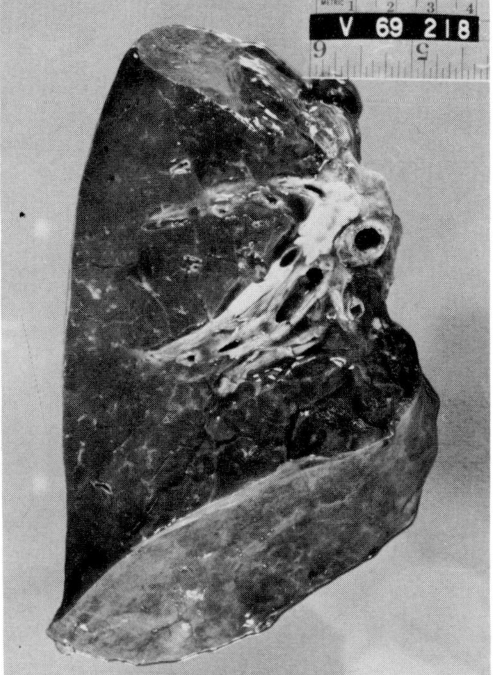

Fig. 2-1. A, The gross appearance of the lungs from a patient with 4+ fat embolism. The heavy, congested, noncollapsing character is not specific for fat embolism and is compatible with massive circulatory overload as well as nonspecific microembolization. Note the patchy distribution of increased congestion. Note petechiae, **P,** on visceral pericardium. **B,** Cut surface of left lower lobe of lungs shown in **A.**

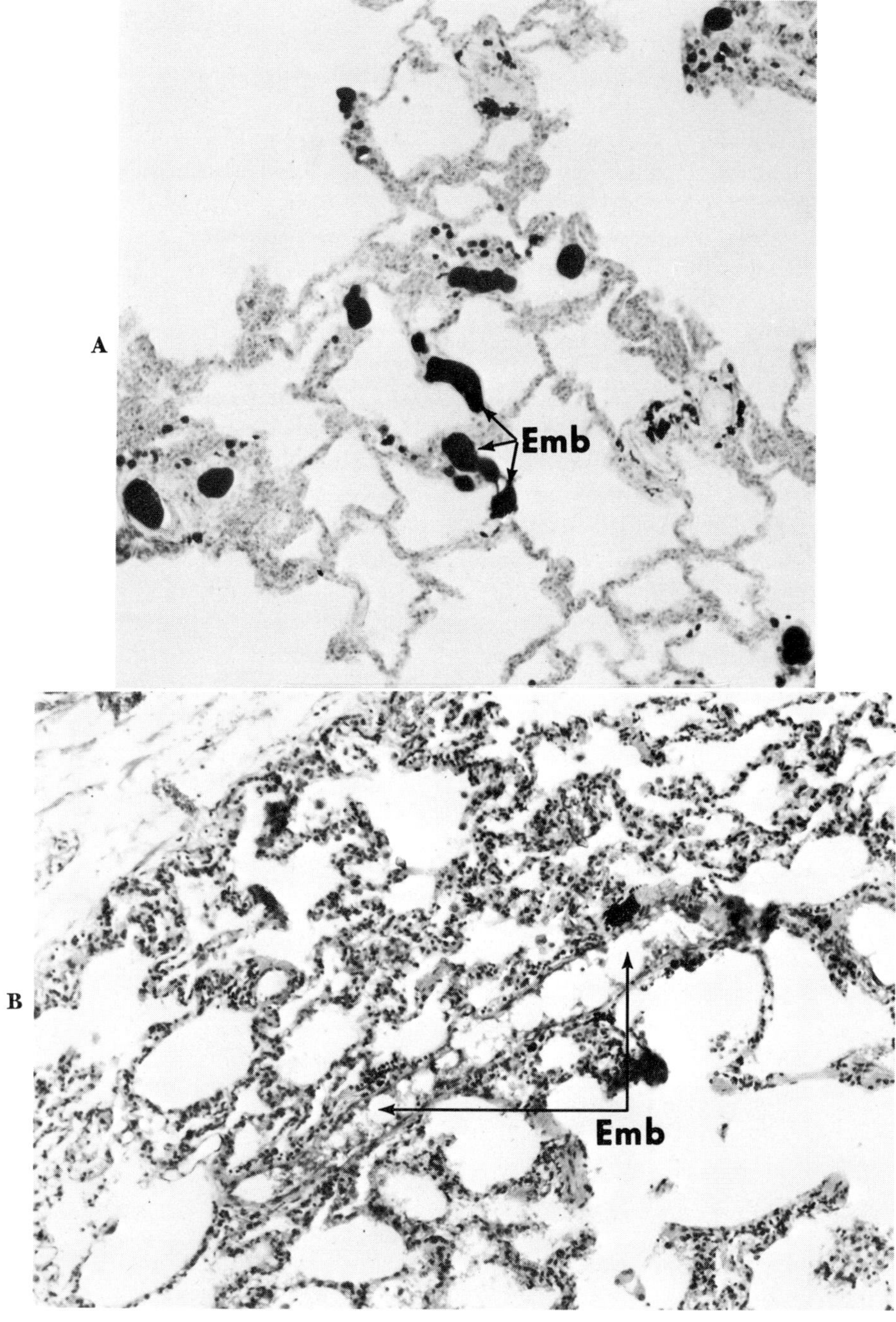

Fig. 2-2. A, Lung from patient dying 8 hours after sustaining multiple fractures in an automobile accident. This lung was ranked 4+ for fat embolism, using the classification of Kent.[52] Note the aneurysmal dilatation of many segments of the pulmonary vasculature. **Emb,** Emboli. (Fat Red 7 B stain; ×138.) **B,** Lung from patient dying 16 hours after sustaining multiple fractures in an automobile accident. A small muscular artery is impacted with globules of fat, **Emb.** Except for a few small areas of edema, the surrounding tissue is relatively normal. (Hematoxylin and eosin stain; ×173.)

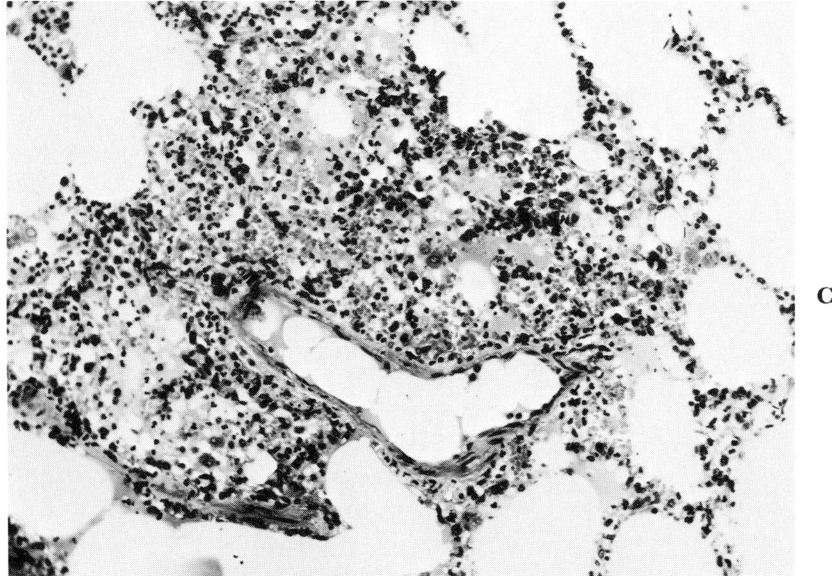

Fig. 2-2, cont'd. **C,** Lung from patient dying 16 hours after sustaining multiple fractures in an automobile accident. A small muscular artery is impacted with globules of fat. The tissue in the immediate vicinity is edematous, and there are areas of hemorrhage. (Hematoxylin and eosin stain; ×275.)

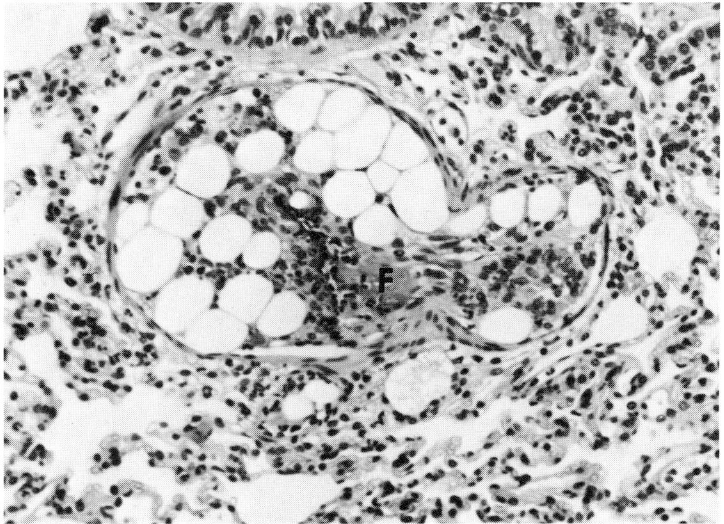

Fig. 2-3. Pulmonary arteriole impacted with hematopoietic and adipose tissue. Note fibrin, **F,** incorporated into the embolus. (×375.)

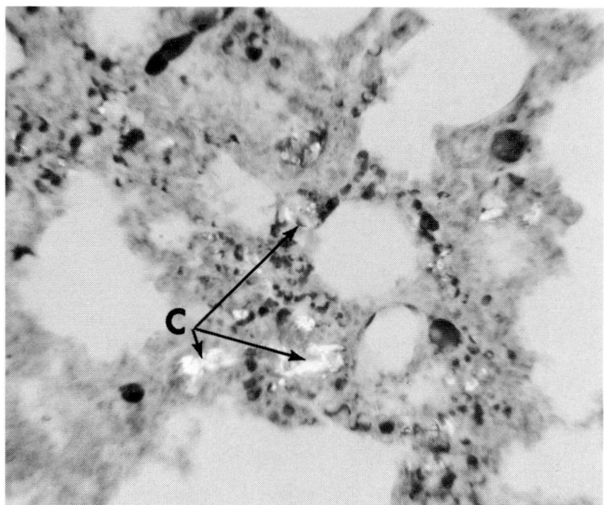

Fig. 2-4. Partial polarization microscopy of lung with embolic fat showing birefringent crystals, **C.** (×200.)

Schultz histochemical reaction for cholesterol may be positive in some cases.

If the patient survives several days, small granular fat may be found in macrophages as well as free in the alveoli. There is surprisingly little inflammatory reaction in the tissue immediately surrounding embolic fat. By electron microscopy the vascular endothelial cells are vesiculated, or markedly compressed by the embolus (Fig. 2-5, *A*). Intracellular details are lost, and the nuclei have condensed chromatin. There is usually evidence of interstitial edema with collagen dispersal, and on occasion markedly swollen cells resembling fibroblasts are seen (Fig. 2-5, *B*). Fat globules within endothelial cells and in interstitial macrophages are seen in the vicinity of fat emboli. Fibrin strands and leukocytes may be seen intravascularly (Figs. 2-2, *B* and 2-3).

If one can interpolate from animal experiments in which embolization was caused by injecting triolein, the lack of a cellular inflammatory reaction would be expected, and the evidence of macrophage phagocytosis is seen by 3 to 5 days. The latter, in addition to the acidular fatty acid crystals in embolic fat, may represent triglyceride hydrolysis by tissue lipase present in the walls of blood vessels. As shown with isotope-labeled triolein, the majority of pulmonary embolic fat is removed within 7 to 10 days, whereas the same lipid injected subcutaneously remains in situ for more than 1 month.[13] This strongly suggests a more active lipolytic mechanism in the pulmonary parenchyma than that present in subcutaneous tissues. However, it is possible that considerable fat may extrude through defects in anoxic alveolar walls to be hydrolyzed by bronchial epithelium or eliminated in bronchial secretions. Granular lipid in bronchial epithelium and fat globules in sputum[69] support this possibility.

Right heart dilatation with liver congestion is a frequent necropsy finding, especially in patients dying within a few hours after the onset of fat embolism, and this is consistent with mechanical obstruction of the pulmonary vascular bed. This is not as marked with prolonged survival; however, congestion of parenchymous organs is a constant observation. Embolic fat in myocardial vessels is usually found with searching. A granular lipid infiltrate in the myocardial fibers may be found. This is not related to fat embolism per se but is a reflection of metabolic alterations.

The brain is usually edematous, with fairly marked vascular congestion. The precise morphology of embolic fat is more difficult to determine in brain tissue, due primarily to perivascular macrophages. These cells are frequently filled with granular fat and may give the appearance of embolic fat to the casual observer (Fig. 2-6, *A*). They do not appear exclusively in response to embolic fat, and their fat cannot be interpreted as having been phagocytosed from embolic fat alone. They are present normally and fill with fat globules in response to an alimentary lipemia, much as do phagocytic cells in the lung and spleen, or the lipocytes in liver. Embolic fat in the brain is more frequently seen in the gray matter rather than in the white matter (Fig. 2-6, *B*) and may be associated with perivascular edema, hemorrhage, and ischemic necrosis.

Embolic fat may be seen in the portal and sinusoidal vessels of the liver on occasion. However, when found, it is difficult to ascribe definitive morphologic changes to the embolic fat per se. More characteristic is a finely granular or small globular infiltrate of the parenchymal cells most prominent near the sinusoidal walls of a periportal distribution. This is characteristic of the fatty liver induced by metabolic changes. There is usually evidence of central congestion and, at times, necrosis.

The kidneys are usually congested, with some decrease in lines of demarcation on cut surface. Microscopically, embolic fat has been seen in arcuate, afferent, and efferent arterioles, but characteristically in the glomerular capillary loops (Fig.

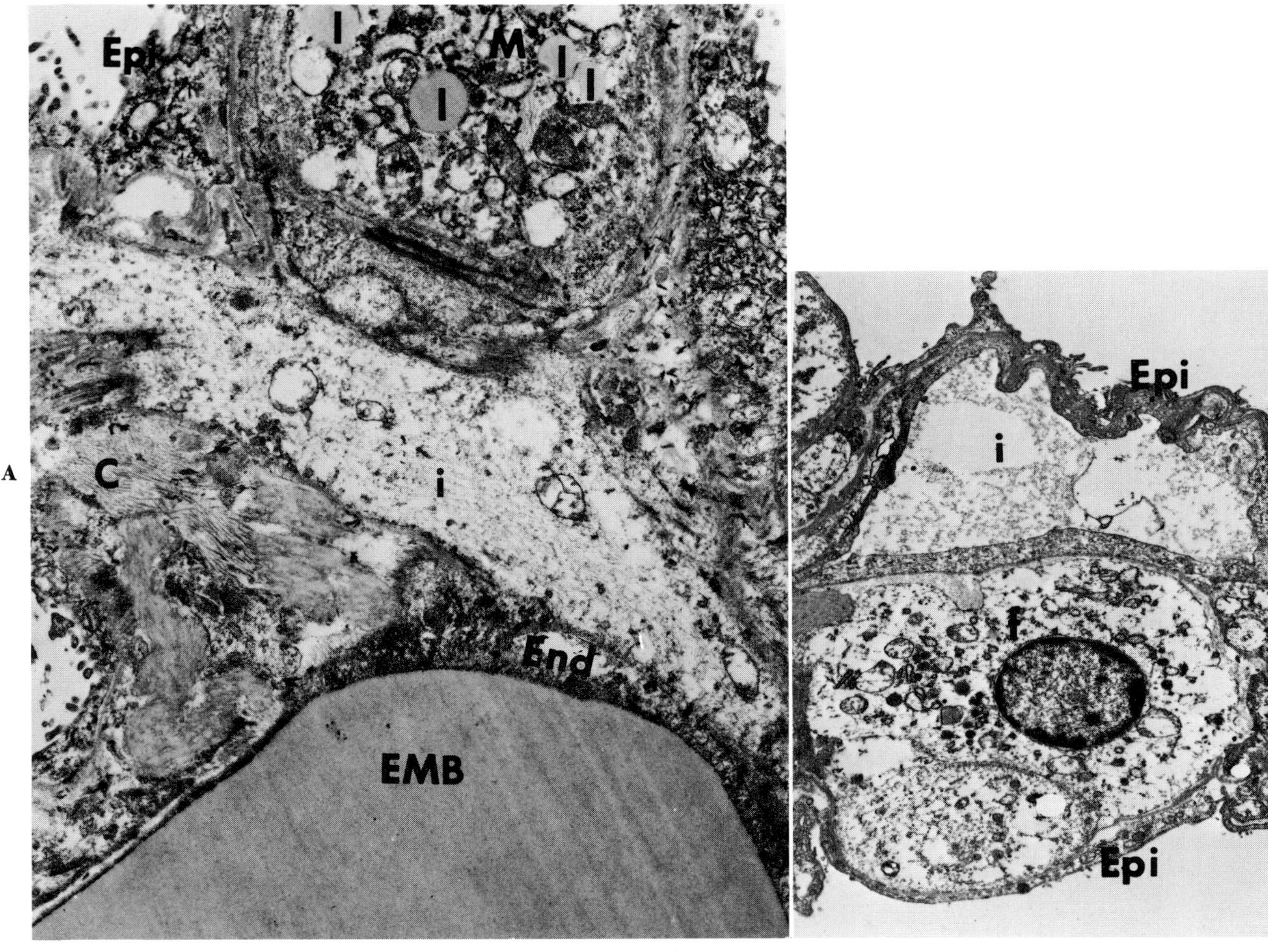

Fig. 2-5. A, Electron micrograph of the lung of a patient dying 4 days after trauma. A capillary embolus, **EMB,** is shown compressing endothelium, **End.** There is dispersion of the interalveolar structures, **i.** An interstitial macrophage, **M,** contains lipid droplets, **I. C,** Collagen. **Epi,** Alveolar epithelium. (×6,600.) **B,** Electron micrograph from same patient as **A.** Marked interstitial edema, **i,** and cellular edema of interstitial cells, **f. Epi,** Alveolar epithelium. (×5,000.)

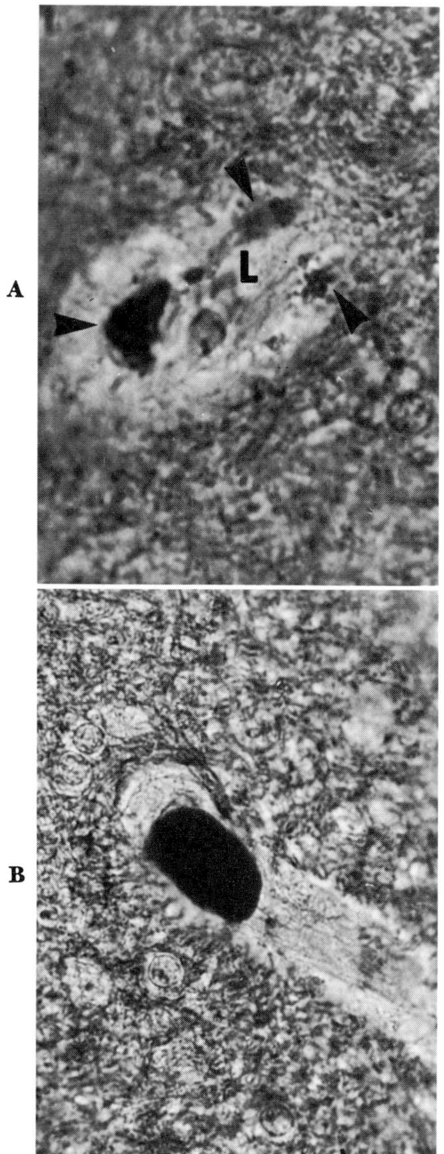

Fig. 2-6. A, Perivascular macrophages, arrows, adjacent to a cerebral arteriole from a patient dying with fat embolism 7 days following trauma. **L,** Lumen of arteriole. (Fat Red 7 B stain; ×1,100.) **B,** Cerebral arteriole impacted with embolic fat. Same patient as in **A.** (Fat Red 7 B stain; ×880.)

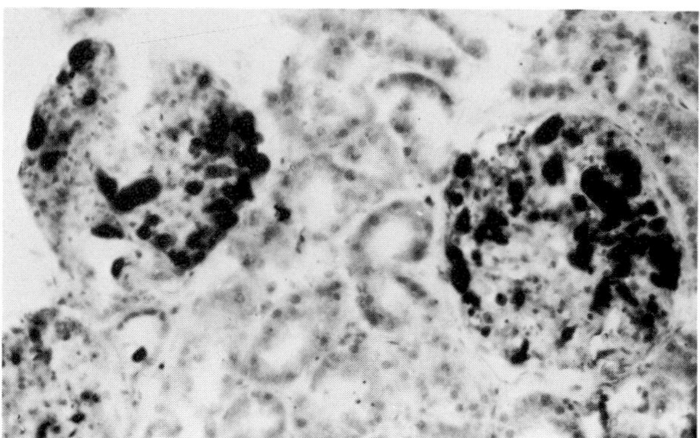

Fig. 2-7. Renal glomeruli impacted with embolic fat from patient dying 8 hours following trauma. (Fat Red 7 B stain; ×200.)

2-7). There may or may not be a tubular swelling and necrosis. One feature in kidney, however, if fat embolism is great, is a finely granular lipid-staining material in the proximal convoluted tubules, especially in the spiral section before entering the loop of Henle. Also, globular lipid may be seen in the lumina of distal segments of collecting tubules. The relationship of these latter findings to embolic fat has not been established, but they may reflect lipid extrusions from anoxic glomerular capillaries with reabsorption by proximal tubular epithelium and elimination of unresorbed lipid in collecting tubules. However, this histologic finding is also seen in animals following an alimentary lipemia and following prolonged starvation.

Other parenchymatous organs such as pancreas, spleen, endocrine glands, as well as muscle, skin, etc., may contain vascular embolic fat. These lesions show no characteristic features other than those already described.

PATHOLOGIC EVALUATION

Pathologists face a dilemma when asked to evaluate fat embolism as a cause of death. This difficulty is due to the frequency of finding embolic fat at necropsy, especially when routine fat stains are employed, and to the lack of a clear-cut series of clinical events with which to correlate pathologic findings. No animal experimental model has been described that allows this correlation, and preceding clinical events cannot be reconstructed precisely, based on morphologic evidence alone. This problem is complicated further by the fact that the cardiovascular system and the lungs are capable of rapid adjustments to embolic events, and the brain, liver, and kidney have great physiologic reserves, as well as rich collateral blood supplies. On the other hand, preexisting disease or associated trauma that might compromise these reserves would set the stage for dire consequences following embolism with what appears histologically as minimal or moderate fat embolism. In addition, the reaction of the lung to shock and nonthoracic trauma with progressive pulmonary insufficiency may be of extreme importance in relating the contribution of fat embolism to the total clinical or pathologic picture.

At the present time, the ranking of fat embolism 1 to 4+, as described by Kent,[52] provides a simple way to evaluate histologic sections of lung. By comparing this ranking with the patient's clinical course, two categories of evidence are emerging: Ranking of 1 to 2+ rarely has had clinical evidence of fat embolism, and those patients with 3 to 4+ ranking frequently have had clinical symptoms compatible with fat embolism. However, there is still a difficult group in the 2 to 3+ ranking in which preexisting disease or clinical complications make the diagnosis of fat embolism as a primary cause of death questionable.

Another impression based on experience, but not on quantitative data, relates to the pulmonary vascular distribution of embolic fat. In patients who have sustained severe trauma, especially to the pelvis or chest, and who die within 24 to 48 hours, embolic fat is more frequently seen in large arterioles with relatively little involvement of capillaries. Fibrin and leukocyte masses enmeshed with embolic fat are seen frequently, and hemorrhage and edema are more pronounced. Patients who develop the so-called classical clinical picture of fat embolism and who survive several days usually have a more marked amount of embolic fat histologically. This is distributed in smaller arterioles, capillaries, and venules.

SOURCES OF FAT

In 1927, Lehman and Moore[53] suggested that sources of fat other than bone marrow fat contributed to the pathogenesis of fat embolism. They suggested that toxic products of tissue necrosis produced an instability of the serum lipids with aggregation and vascular impaction. Subsequently, numerous reports have associated serum lipid instability with the histologic appearance of embolic fat in the lungs of experimental animals; however, the exact mechanism of emulsion instability has not been explained.

It seemed to us that the critical question to be answered to support or deny the concept of serum lipoprotein aggregation as a factor in fat embolism was the precise determination of the lipid composition of embolic fat per se. In order to determine this, histochemical or chemical analysis of embolic fat would have to be achieved, and this presented some difficulty. Ten years ago we reported a histochemical study of fat embolism in nine patients with a pathologic diagnosis of pulmonary fat embolism, and of rabbits subjected to decompression to altitude.[56] The histochemical test used was the Schultz test, which is a modification of the Liebermann-Burchard reaction for cholesterol.[31]

This test is not sensitive to low cholesterol concentration, but if positive, it is quite specific for cholesterol. We reported this test positive in the nine clinical patients, as well as in the animals subjected to decompression. Our results in patients have been questioned recently by Ellis and Watson,[20] who were unable to obtain positive histochemical reactions in twenty-two patients. They did confirm, however, a positive reaction in one patient from our series. We subsequently reviewed our previously reported patients and discovered that their tissues had been stored in 80% alcohol. We now suspect that this may have been a factor in leaching out triglyceride from the embolic fat, resulting in a proportionately higher concentration of cholesterol. Our subsequent experience agrees with Ellis and Watson that fresh tissue only rarely gives positive results.

Ellis and Watson made another point in regard to the birefringent crystals that we described associated with the embolic fat. At the time of our report, birefringent crystals were considered to be microscopic evidence of cholesterol. Since that time, it has been shown that fatty acid crystals are also birefringent, and we agree with Ellis and Watson that the majority of birefringence we described was probably due to fatty acid crystals rather than to cholesterol crystals.

In regard to the lipid composition of embolic fat per se, Holczabek[47] reported that the triglyceride composition of lung extracted by lipid solvents has a much higher concentration of triglyceride in patients in whom histologic evidence of fat embolism is prominent. We feel that this evidence does not define the source of lipid inasmuch as lipid solvent extraction of pulmonary tissue carries with it the inherent error of cell membrane extraction. We have, therefore, attempted to develop a method of retrieval of embolic fat from the lungs of patients at necropsy. This method has been reported[45] and consists of flotation of embolic fat from frozen, unfixed lung, with subsequent chemical assay for total cholesterol[83] and thin-

Table 2-1. Cholesterol content of pulmonary embolic fat in human necropsy material: correlation of recoverable embolic fat with histologic degree of fat embolism

Patient	*Diagnosis*	*Lung embolic fat (mg.)* recovered*	*Cholesterol (mg./100 mg.) lung embolic fat*	*Histologic fat embolism*
V–63–174	Retroperitoneal fibrosis	0	—	Negative
V–68–14	Chronic interstitial nephritis	1.1	Q.N.S.†	Negative
V–63–192	Myocardial infarction	0	—	+
V–63–198	Myocardial infarction	1.0	Q.N.S.	+
M–8–12–64	Gunshot wound	0.6	Q.N.S.	+
V–68–9	Renal failure, infection, hemorrhage	0	—	+
V–68–10	Lymphosarcoma	0	—	+
V–68–11	Muscular dystrophy, pneumonia, hemorrhage	0	—	+
V–68–12	Myocardial infarction	1.3	Q.N.S.	++
V–63–276	Multiple fractures	0.6	Q.N.S.	++
V–68–24	Gunshot wound	0	—	++
V–63–271	Multiple fractures	20.1	11.0	++++
M–7–8–63	Multiple fractures	6.2	7.2	++++
V–66–268	Sickle cell crisis; Gram-negative sepsis	2.3	5.4	++++
V–67–247	Multiple fractures	9.2	7.4	++++
V–68–4	Multiple fractures	5.3	11.0	++++
V–68–104	Multiple fractures	2.3	5.8	++++

*Approximately 10 Gm. wet weight of lung used in each determination.
†Quantity not sufficient for chemical analysis.

layer chromatographic analysis. We have shown that embolic fat can be obtained by this method from patients who have a histologic manifestation of fat embolism that is ranked 3 to 4+ by the method of Kent. Lungs that have minimal fat embolism did not have recoverable fat (Table 2-1).

In five patients, the cholesterol concentration ranged between 5.4% and 11%. Adipose or marrow fat prepared by the identical method routinely contained less than 1% cholesterol. The cholesterol concentration in embolic fat was far in excess of that expected, if the emboli had originated from adipose tissue exclusively. The finding of concentrations of 11% or less also supports the negative histochemical results with the Schultz test as reported by Ellis and Watson.[21] When examined by thin-layer chromatography on silica gel (Fig. 2-8), embolic fat from these same patients showed a greater amount of cholesterol, phospholipid, and cholesterol esters as compared to adipose tissue fat. This evidence has convinced us that sources other than adipose tissue must be considered to play a major role in the pathogenesis of fat embolism and that the most likely source is the serum lipoproteins.

We do not deny that adipose tissue fat contributes to the picture. We, too, have observed bone marrow cellular elements in our cases of fat embolism, and we agree that this is an inevitable source of an as yet undetermined and probably variable amount of embolic fat. However, gross and microscopic examinations of fractured bones do not reveal a massive extravasation of bone marrow fat from around the site of fracture. This would support the evidence that insufficient fat leaves the marrow to produce significant clinical symptoms by the mechanical obstruction of the pulmonary circulation unless the latter is compromised by severe injury or superimposed pulmonary pathology.

The work of Fuschig and associates[28] and Brücke, Blumel, and Gottlob[8] suggested a third mechanism for pulmonary vascular impaction by fat. They reported that in shock, animals manifest an increased lymphatic removal of globular fat from fracture sites or peripheral tissues, with subsequent pulmonary embolization. Szabo, Serenyi, and Kocsar[92] were unable to repeat these results, as were we, using I-131–labeled triolein injected intramuscularly or near the periosteum of long bones in dogs. We did find an equivocal increase in the rate of removal from the site of injection during hypotension. However, this did not manifest itself as an increased localization of radioactivity or as

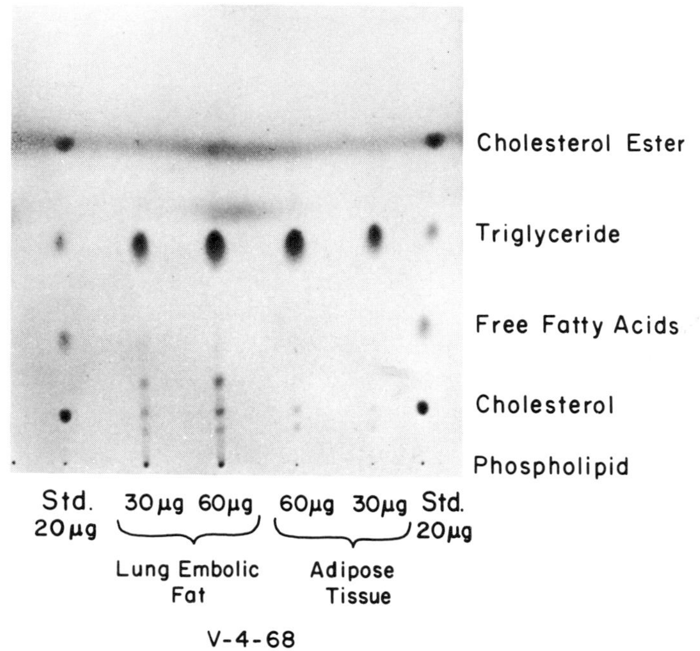

Fig. 2-8. Thin-layer chromatogram comparing pulmonary embolic fat with adipose tissue fat from the same patient. Note the increased concentrations of free cholesterol, cholesterol esters, and phospholipid in the embolic fat. Silica gel-G, 80:20:1 mixture of petroleum ether:ethyl ether:glacial acetic acid. **Std.**, standard.

histologic evidence of embolic fat in the lungs of these animals.[54]

LIPID METABOLISM

Inasmuch as our data support aggregated serum lipoproteins as a major source of embolic fat, we have attempted to direct our studies to lipid transport and its alterations following trauma. Normal pathways of lipid transport are incompletely known at the present time, and many of these are controversial. However, a brief summary of some salient features of these pathways may be helpful as background for subsequent proposals.*

With the ingestion of exogenous fat, emulsification is accomplished in the upper intestinal tract primarily by bile salts. The resultant increase in surface area allows intestinal hydrolytic enzymes to attack triglycerides primarily, breaking them down into fatty acids, diglycerides and monoglycerides, and glycerol. A micelle of fatty acid, bile salt, and monoglyceride is the unit form of absorbable lipid. Upon absorption, fatty acids are esterified to particulate triglyceride again by the intestinal epithelial cells. These are passed through the cell into interstitial tissues, where they subsequently gain entry into intestinal lymphatics and are carried to the bloodstream. In this form, the particulate lipid is known as a chylomicron (2,000 to 4,000 Å in diameter). Chylomicra are thought to be coated by protein that may be derived from gut epithelium, lymph, or possibly from serum. In the form of chylomicrons, the triglyceride-rich fat particle circulates in the bloodstream and is thought to be progressively attacked by a hydrolytic enzyme, lipoprotein lipase. This enzyme (s) is probably derived from or near vascular endothelium, and its concentration in serum can be markedly increased by the injection of heparin. It is now thought that the lipids from chylomicra enter cells of parenchymous tissue primarily in the form of fatty acids rather than as discrete particulate fat, as previously thought, where they are utilized for energy or esterified to triglyceride.

The cholesterol concentration of chylomicra has been shown to be in the range of 10%. This form of fat could contribute to increased concentrations of cholesterol to fat emboli; however, a hyperchylomicronemia, as seen after the absorption of a fatty meal or in metabolic defects such as Type I hyperlipidemia, as described by Frederickson, Levy,

*For recent reviews see references 26, 77, 80, and 81.

and Lees,[26] has not been associated with an increased incidence of fat embolism.

The liver parenchymal cell is of primary importance in fatty acid turnover, and, in a sense, is analogous to the gut epithelial cell, in that it removes free fatty acids from the bloodstream, reesterifies them to triglycerides, and secretes them back into the bloodstream as lipoprotein particles, called very low-density lipoproteins (VLDL). These liver lipoproteins are much smaller than chylomicra, measuring 300 to 800 Å, and they migrate electrophoretically in the prebeta or alpha 2 position. We reported that the Golgi apparatus of the hepatic parenchymal cell participates in the synthesis and secretion of these particles.* Participation of the rough endoplasmic reticulum has also been suggested.[50] We also showed in liver perfusion studies,[35] in the norepinephrine-infused dog,[34] and in the cortisone-treated rabbit[58] that the secretion of these lipoproteins of very low density is markedly increased by increased substrate concentration of free fatty acids. The cholesterol concentration of the lipoproteins of very low density is in the range of 13%, and aggregation of this class of lipoproteins could contribute a significant proportion of cholesterol to embolic fat.

Two other classes of lipoproteins that could contribute high concentration of cholesterol to embolic fat are the beta, or low-density lipoproteins (LDL), and the alpha 1, or high-density lipoproteins (HDL). These lipoproteins contain 45% and 18% cholesterol, respectively. The sites of synthesis of these lipoproteins, as well as their metabolic fate and interrelationships with lipoproteins of very low density, are incompletely known at present.

The pathways for mobilization of adipose tissue fat for metabolic purposes have been under investigation in recent years, and there is good evidence that this is under the hormonal control of norepinephrine.† This hormone presumably has its action through adenyl cyclase in adipose tissue by increasing the concentration of an intracellular lipolytic enzyme, which, in turn, brings about the release of free fatty acids into the circulating blood.[9] Increase in the level of serum-free fatty acids has been well documented following stress and a variety of metabolic alterations that require increased free fatty acids for energy metabolism. Trauma is but one of these conditions.

To complete the cycle, then, free fatty acids derived by hydrolysis of chylomicra or mobilized from adipose tissue increase the substrate concentration to the liver that normally responds by increased synthesis of serum lipoproteins of very low density. It is at this point that the similarity between trauma and other metabolic abnormalities that have been associated with increased incidence of fat embolism comes to a common denominator. Various types of tissue injury, including fractures, burns, diabetes mellitus, steroid hormone injections, and certain drugs and poisons are associated with increased serum-free fatty acid levels and at times with increased serum lipoprotein levels.

The mechanisms by which serum lipoproteins aggregate, coalesce, and contribute to embolic fat are in the realm of conjecture. Such factors as concentration, lowered blood pH, activation of the clotting mechanism, and alteration of lipoprotein surface properties have been suggested. Evidence will be presented in the following section that trauma may induce rapid changes in the lipid composition of particular lipoprotein classes, which may contribute to emulsion instability.

CLINICAL STUDIES

Sixty-seven patients who had sustained major trauma with at least two long bone fractures were selected for these studies. Severe head injuries were not included in order to exclude cerebral contusion as a complicating factor in diagnosing clinical fat embolism. Eight (12%) of the patients developed clinical fat embolism based upon the criteria of rapidly progressing mental confusion with disorientation, decerebrate posturing, and coma following an initial period of lucidity, fever, tachycardia, tachypnea, and shock as prevously described.[13] Blood samples were routinely withdrawn as soon after admission as possible, subsequently at daily intervals for 7 to 10 days, and then weekly until discharge. These serum samples were then analyzed for free fatty acids,[19] lipolytic activity,[55] and electrophoretic mobility.[91] All patients who developed clinical fat embolism received heparin therapy. One patient died (12.5%).

Serum-free fatty acids

Fig. 2-9, *A* presents sequential data of the serum-free fatty acids (FFA) in 47 patients. The normal range in humans is < 0.5 mEq./l. It can be seen that

*See references 34, 35, 58, and 59.

†For recent reviews see references 39, 46, and 90.

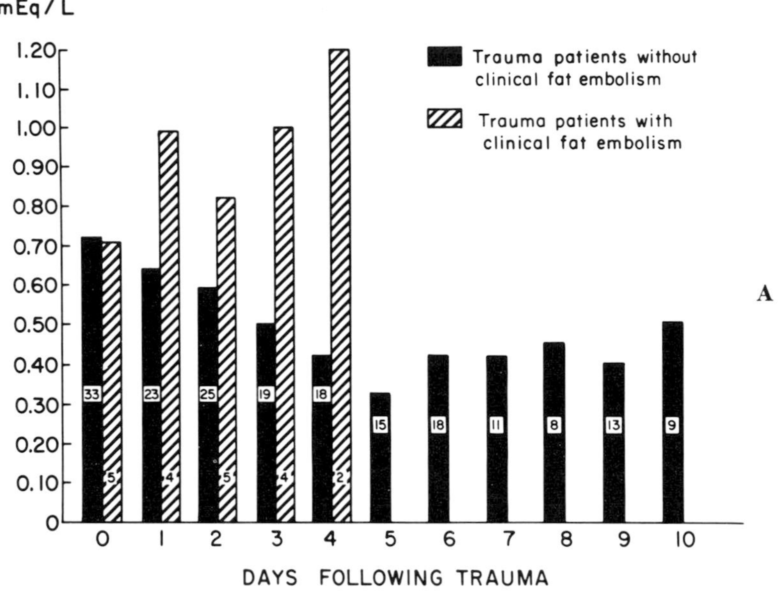

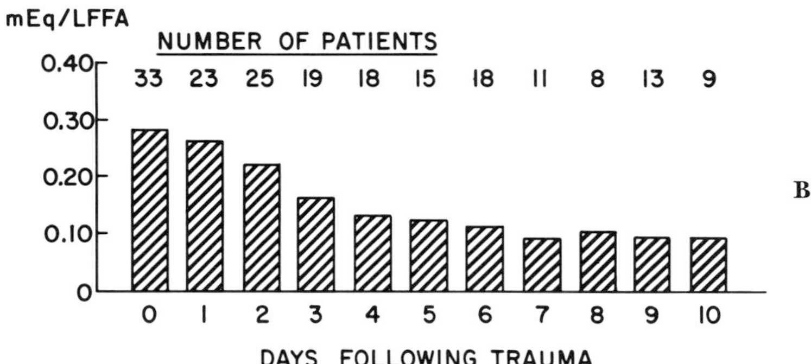

Fig. 2-9. A, Sequential determinations of serum-free fatty acids in forty-seven patients following trauma (solid bars). The initial elevations returned to normal values by the third day posttrauma. Five patients who developed clinical fat embolism (slashed bars) are compared to demonstrate the sustained elevation in free fatty acids before heparin therapy was begun. Numbers in bars represent number of patients studied at each time interval. **B,** Sequential determinations of serum lipoprotein lipase activity in forty-seven patients following trauma. Though there is an apparent decrease in lipase activity over the first 4 days, the level of activity is minimal and within the range of error of the method.

the admission sample, which was routinely obtained within 3 hours after injury, was markedly elevated. By the second and third days of hospitalization, serum FFA levels dropped to normal values and remained in this range. There was considerable individual variation, but this trend in all patients was consistent.

Eight patients of the forty-seven studied developed clinical evidence of fat embolism. Fig. 2-9, *A* also presents serum FFA data on these patients as a group. It can be seen that on admission the serum FFA levels were comparable to those of patients not developing clinical fat embolism, but they were sustained at higher levels for a longer period after trauma.

Serum lipoprotein lipase

Some investigators have placed considerable emphasis on the serum lipase activity of patients following trauma.[74] This interest was based on the assumption that increased levels of serum lipase would increase the rate of embolic fat hydrolysis, with the release locally of "toxic" fatty acids. This, in turn, would produce tissue damage and result in chemical pneumonia, which was suggested as the primary pathologic manifestation of pulmonary fat embolism. Our necropsy studies do not support the concept of a chemical pneumonia with fat embolism. Most observed pathologic findings were compatible with tissue anoxia and congestion from vascular impaction.

Furthermore, assay of serum lipase activity in our series of patients failed to demonstrate any trauma-induced elevation in the level of this enzyme. Our method uses a substrate containing tripalmitin, known to be sensitive to lipoprotein lipase. Fig. 2-9, *B* depicts the daily levels of this lipase in the group of forty-seven patients presented in Fig. 2-9, *A*. It would appear that minimal elevations are present in the first 3 days after trauma; however, these are not significant.

There was no significant elevation of serum lipoprotein lipase in the eight patients who developed clinical fat embolism before they were placed on heparin therapy.

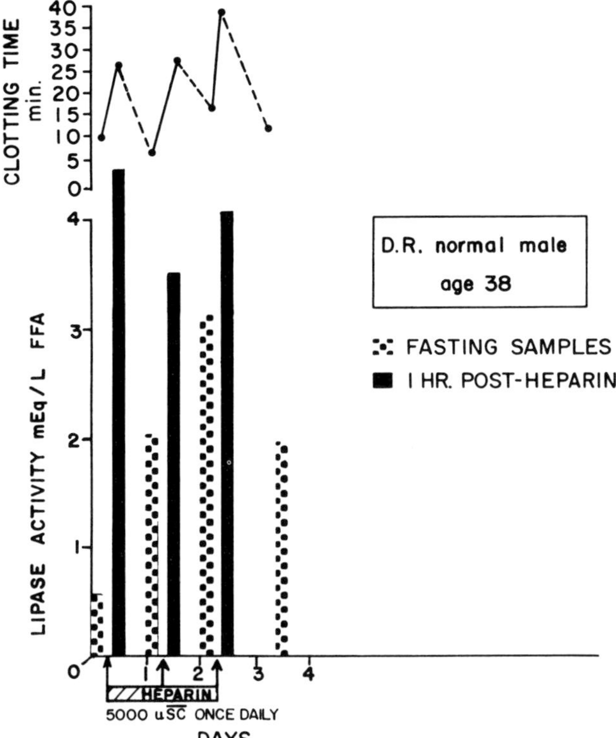

Fig. 2-10. Serum lipoprotein lipase responses to daily injections of sodium heparin subcutaneously (in a normal patient). Maximal activity is seen 1 hour following the first injection and is sustained upon repeated daily injections. Considerable activity persists in fasting samples after the first injection. With this dosage of heparin, the Lee-White clotting time became prolonged to 27 to 40 minutes.

Heparin and serum lipoprotein lipase

Lipoprotein lipase is presumably a tissue lipase localized on or near vascular endothelium. It has been suggested that highly charged macromolecules such as heparin elevate plasma lipoprotein lipase levels by pulling this enzyme off the endothelium and stabilizing its activity.[78] This was one effect of heparin that suggested its use in the treatment of fat embolism. Fig. 2-10 depicts the response of a normal individual to 50 mg. of subcutaneous sodium heparin daily for 5 days. Maximal levels of enzyme activity are present in the plasma by 1 hour after injection. This response is repeatable with the daily injection of heparin, and considerable activity remains 6 hours after heparin. Lee-White clotting times in this individual reached 45 minutes within 1 hour and remained elevated over a 6-hour period.

Fig. 2-11 depicts the plasma lipolytic activity of a patient with clinical fat embolism on heparin therapy (50 mg. q. 6 h.). Samples were withdrawn before and 1 hour after heparin injection. There is a stepwise increase in lipase response to this regimen over a period of 3 days, during which time clinical improvement was apparent. Clotting times of the Lee-White method were 15 to 20 minutes during this same interval and did not become further prolonged during the period of heparin therapy.

Histochemical and chemical evidence of lipase activity in lung

Fig. 2-12 is a photomicrograph of a section of normal human lung prepared by the method of Gomori[31] to demonstrate tissue lipase. It can be seen that the areas of lipase localization consist of bronchial epithelium, macrophages, and vascular endothelium. It is assumed that tissue lipase is a normal constituent of pulmonary tissue, and no quantitative difference was apparent between normal lung and that in which fat embolism was prominent.

Considerable emphasis has been placed on the possible role of pulmonary lipase in the hydrolysis of embolic fat. Increased levels of a serum lipase have been postulated as reflecting increased activity of such a tissue lipase. Tissue lipase activities of lung homogenates were determined from ten random necropsies, two of which had marked fat em-

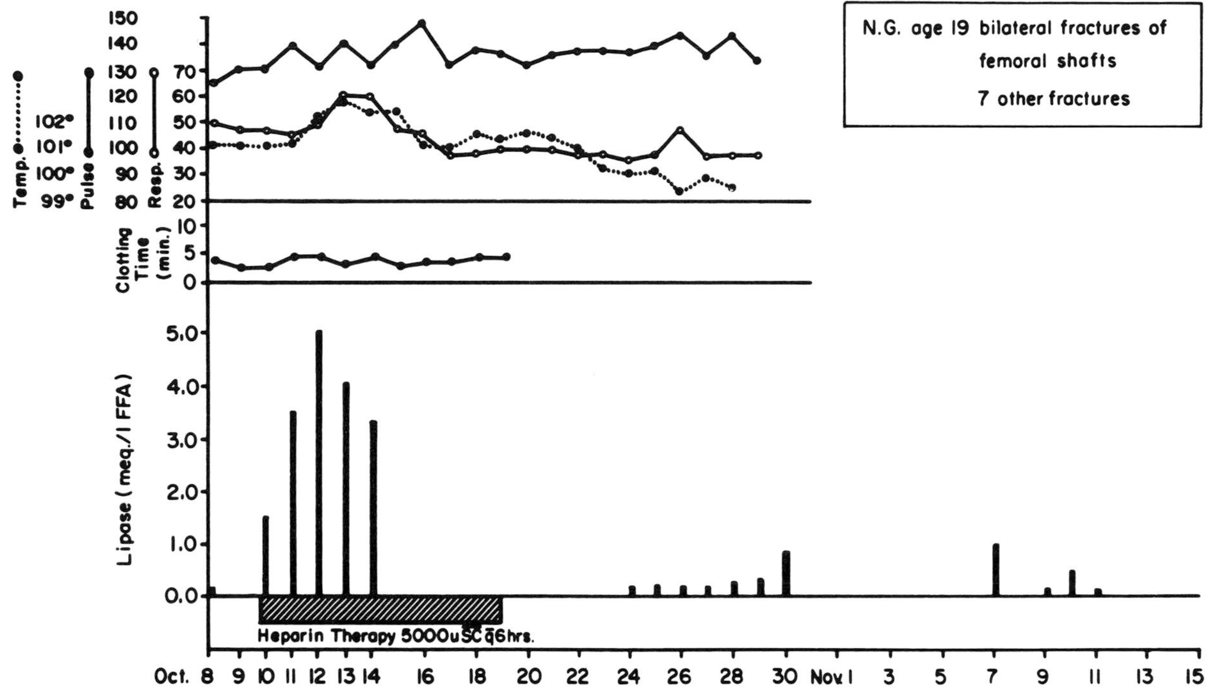

Fig. 2-11. Sequential serum lipoprotein lipase responses 1 hour postheparin in a patient with clinical fat embolism receiving 50 mg. sodium heparin every 6 hours. Insignificant activity was present before heparin, and maximum activity, in comparison to the normal patient depicted in Fig. 2-10, did not appear until the third day postheparin. Clotting times by the Lee-White method were not prolonged during heparin therapy.

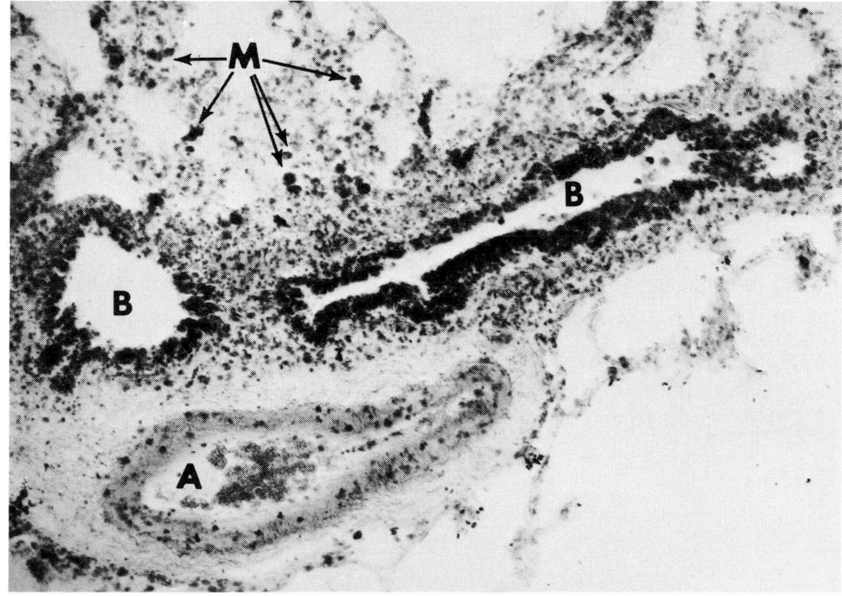

Fig. 2-12. Tissue lipase demonstrated by the histochemical method of Gomori. Granular reactive material is most prominent in the bronchial epithelium, **B,** and in macrophages, **M.** It can also be detected along the vascular endothelium but is not apparent in this illustration. **A,** Arteriole. (×138.)

bolism. The substrate used was Ediol, and incubation was carried out over a 3-hour period at two pH ranges. Considerable lipase activity was present in all homogenates, but there was no correlation of increased activity in the patients with fat embolism.

Serum lipoprotein electrophoresis

Electrophoretic separation[91] of serum lipoproteins was carried out on forty-seven patients presented in Fig. 2-9, *A*. The most striking alteration in the lipoprotein patterns of these patients was an invariable fluctuation in the alpha 2 and beta fractions. This can best be described as a "dropout" or reduced concentration of these fractions. This reduction usually occurred within 24 to 48 hours after injury, with gradual return toward normal over a 10-day period. This occurred in all patients to some degree, but was particularly evident in those patients who developed clinical fat embolism. Fig. 2-13 demonstrates the sequential lipoprotein pattern of one patient (W. C.) typical of this group. The reduction in alpha 2 and beta lipoprotein in this particular patient preceded by a few hours the clinical symptoms of tachycardia, hyperthermia, and disorientation proceeding to coma.

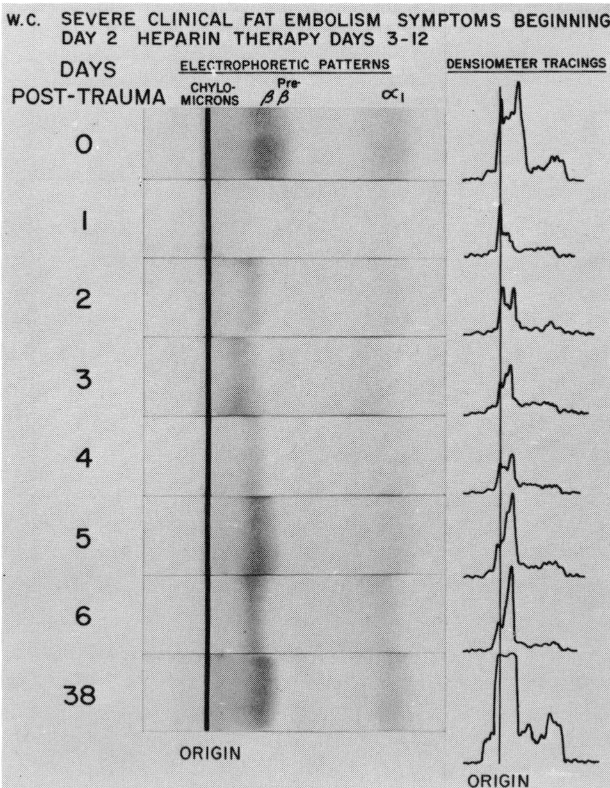

Fig. 2-13. Sequential serum electrophoretic patterns in a patient with clinical fat embolism. Note the marked reduction in the beta and prebeta fractions on day 1 posttrauma. This "dropout" preceded by a few hours the onset of clinical symptoms of fat embolism. On subsequent days these fractions reappeared, fluctuated from day to day, and were apparently normal on the thirty-eighth day posttrauma.

Ultracentrifugal separation of serum lipoproteins

To investigate this phenomenon further, a study was begun on trauma patients, in which the plasma lipoprotein classes were separated by preparative ultracentrifugation,[40] and the lipids in whole serum and serum fractions were analyzed chemically. Serum total cholesterol (TC) and phospholipid were determined on aliquots of a 1:25 extract of serum in acetone: ethanol (1:1). The procedure of determining the total cholesterol was a modification of the method of Searcy and Bergquist[83] in that ferric chloride dissolved in glacial acetic acid, as suggested by Zlatkis, Zak, and Boyle,[99] was used in preference to ferrous sulfate. Phospholipids were calculated on the basis of phosphorus content determined by the colorimetric procedure of Fiske and Subbarow[24] after wet digestion with sulfuric acid.[98]

In the case of serum fractions, it was necessary to adjust the size of the aliquot of any extract so that the amount of the lipid under investigation would fall within optimum range. To date, we have carried out this procedure on six patients, three with no evidence of clinical fat embolism, one in which a diagnosis of fat embolism was equivocal, and two who developed severe clinical fat embolism. The pattern seen in the trauma patients who did not develop fat embolism and the one with a questionable diagnosis was similar. Fig. 2-14 depicts the alterations in cholesterol and phospholipid levels in whole serum and in three different lipoprotein fractions from one trauma patient (F. B.) who recovered without evidence of clinical fat embolism. Since control blood samples were not available on these patients, the normal values indicated in the illustration were borrowed from Furman and associates.[29] The serum cholesterol and phospholipids followed the same trends but did not strictly parallel each other. Both decreased progressively for the first 24 to 48 hours after trauma, remained below normal for 4 to 5 days, then returned rapidly to normal. The cholesterol and phospholipids in the three different lipoprotein classes are also depicted in Fig. 2-14. The most obvious changes were those in the concentrations of cholesterol and phospholipid in the low-density or beta lipoprotein fractions, both of which fell abruptly to approximately 50% of their expected pretrauma levels.

Both LDL cholesterol and phospholipid followed very closely the curves for whole serum and undoubtedly provided the changes accounting for the marked reductions in both these lipid categories. The changes in HDL cholesterol and phospholipid amounted to little more than minor fluctuations that did not appear to be significant. The initial fall in VLDL phospholipid and cholesterol on first glance does not appear to be very dramatic, probably because of the relatively small amount of phospholipid and cholesterol in this fraction. Actually, by the third day posttrauma, there had been a decrease in VLDL cholesterol of about 60% and a decrease in VLDL phospholipid of about 80%. When one remembers that the VLDL is a triglyceride-rich plasma fraction found usually in concentration of approximately 174 mg./100 ml., the fall in VLDL cholesterol and phospholipid indicates a substantial decrease in this fraction that would be more apparent if we had the triglyceride values on this patient. In none of the patients did the HDL show any significant changes. Our results are comparable to those of Birke, Carlson, and Liljedahl[7] in their study of severely burned patients. Their patients, however, did not reestablish their theoretical pretrauma plasma phospholipid and cholesterol levels until 6 to 12 months after being burned.

In the trauma patient developing clinical fat embolism as a complication, the initial response of the serum total cholesterol and phospholipid and the responses of the cholesterol and phospholipid in the individual serum fraction were the same. After the onset of symptoms the plasma levels of these lipid classes continued to fall. However, these patients were put on heparin as soon as a diagnosis of clinical fat embolism was made, so that the significance of serum lipid changes during this time is difficult to interpret.

From these clinical studies, we have concluded that the quantity of circulating lipoprotein is irrelevant as a factor in initiating plasma lipoprotein aggregation. However, evidence is accumulating that changes in the lipid composition of the lipo-

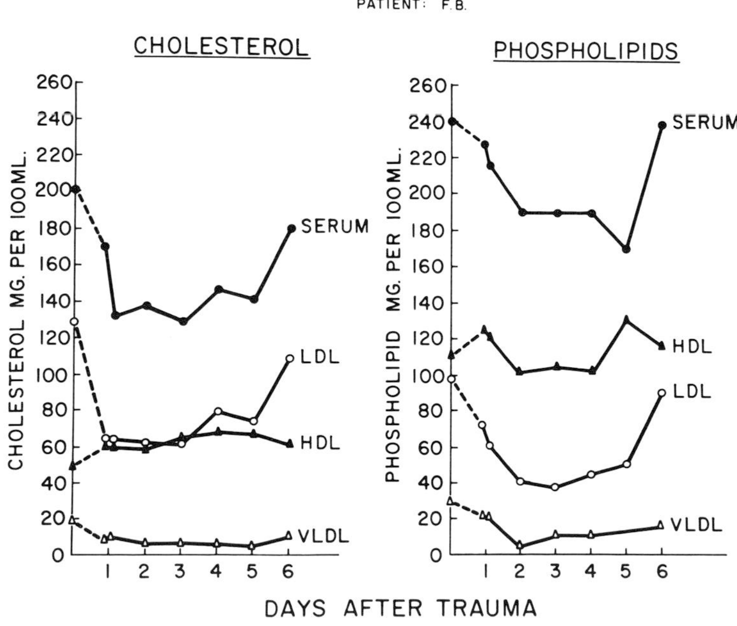

Fig. 2-14. Cholesterol and phospholipid concentrations in serum and in the various lipoprotein classes separated by preparative ultracentrifugation for 6 days posttrauma in a patient who did not develop clinical symptoms of fat embolism. (See text for description.)

protein particles themselves accompany trauma. Table 2-2 is a study of the plasma cholesterol to phospholipid (C/P) ratios in one trauma patient (G. S.) who did not develop clinical fat embolism. The C/P ratio fell in the VLDL fraction and had not recovered by 7 days. This would indicate a proportionately higher phospholipid content. The changes in LDL cholesterol/phospholipid ratio are of less magnitude but in the same direction. In the HDL fraction, the C/P ratio was slightly elevated on admission and remained so for the seven days. Comparable studies on three other patients gave similar results.

Table 2-3 shows a similar study on a patient (E. S.) who had moderate symptoms of fat embolism. In this patient, the admission sample showed a high C/P ratio in the VLDL fraction, indicating a proportionately high level of cholesterol. We have seen this elevation in C/P ratio

Table 2-2. Cholesterol/phospholipid ratio, patient G. S., trauma without fat embolism

	Serum	*VLDL*	*LDL*	*HDL*
Control*	0.84	0.68	1.3	0.45
Days posttrauma				
1	0.86	0.42	1.21	0.52
2	0.82	0.41	1.06	0.58
3	0.80	0.57	0.88	0.71
4	0.77	0.66	0.86	0.55
5	0.54	0.40	0.92	0.49
6	0.68	0.49	0.91	0.37
7	0.85	0.36	1.15	0.55

*Furman, R. H., Howard, R. P., Lakshmi, K., and Norcia, L. N.: Amer. J. Clin. Nutr. **9**:73, 1961.

Table 2-3. Cholesterol/phospholipid ratio, patient E. S., trauma with fat embolism

	Serum	*VLDL*	*LDL*	*HDL*
Control*	0.81	0.69	1.3	0.43
Days posttrauma				
1	0.82	0.94	1.2	0.57
2	0.71	0.68	1.3	0.74
3	0.64	0.70	—	0.84
4	0.70	0.70	1.2	0.91
5	0.55	0.70	1.1	0.50
6				
7	0.84	0.70	0.9	0.64

*Furman, R. H., Howard, R. P., Lakshmi, K., and Norcia, L. M.: Amer. J. Clin. Nutr. **9**:73, 1961.

in the VLDL fraction on admission in another patient (M. C.), who promptly developed severe fat embolism. In this patient, the C/P ratio did not change in the LDL fraction. The C/P ratio in the HDL fraction was slightly elevated on admission and remained so for 7 days.

During the course of these clinical studies, we have made several observations that indicate change in the properties of plasma lipoproteins, particularly in fat embolism patients. These data are fragmentary, but we think they are interesting. Recently, we observed a patient in whom the serum VLDL fraction was totally absent until the eighth day following injury. We began studying this patient on the third day following injury, after she had developed the clinical picture of fat embolism. It was first noted that electrophoretically she had very little lipoprotein in the beta position and none in the prebeta position. On ultracentrifugation, no VLDL fraction floated, so without removing any material the density of the serum was raised to 1.063, it was ultracentrifuged again, and the lipoprotein floating at $d < 1.063$ was removed and negatively stained for electron microscopy.[35] Theoretically this fraction should have contained the VLDL (300-900 Å) and the LDL (200 Å). Fig. 2-15 is an electron micrograph of this fraction, negatively stained with phosphotungstic acid. Note the uniform particles that measured approximately 200 Å in diameter corresponding to the low-density or beta lipoproteins. The VLDL were absent. With clinical recovery, the VLDL reappeared in the serum. In another patient, who developed the clinical picture of fat embolism, a fraction of very low density failed to float at $d < 1.006$, but 300-900 Å particles similar to VLDL were found floating with the LDL at a density between 1.006 and 1.063.

From these observations, it appears that trauma brings about a prompt and, in some cases, sustained elevation in plasma-free fatty acids, together with an equally prompt decrease in the other plasma lipids and indications of a shift in plasma lipoprotein lipid composition. To assign any significance to these changes in the pathogenesis of fat embolism, it is necessary to examine the accompanying changes in both extrahepatic and hepatic morphology.

Moore[64] pointed out that after trauma, oxidation of endogenous fat replaces oxidation of exogenous carbohydrate as an energy source. However, trauma-induced fatty acid mobilization may be in excess of caloric need, a situation that does not

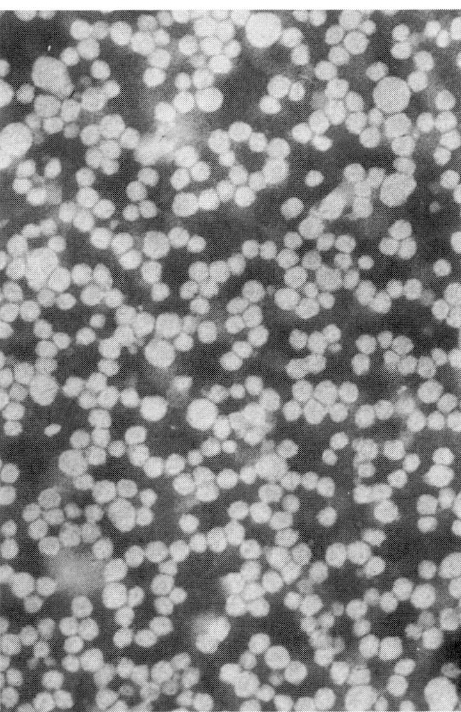

Fig. 2-15. An electron micrograph of negatively stained lipoproteins from a fraction (d<1.063) that should have contained both VLDL (prebeta) and LDL (beta) lipoproteins. The particles are uniform and measure approximately 200 Å in diameter. This is compatible with LDL or beta particles. VLDL or prebeta particles are absent. From a patient with clinical fat embolism on the third day posttrauma. (Phosphotungstic acid stain; ×180,000.)

appear to serve an entirely useful purpose. In extrahepatic tissues, sustained elevation in plasma FFA can lead to accumulation of cytoplasmic lipid droplets that are composed largely of triglycerides.[10,84] Such accumulations are reversible and probably contribute nothing to the pathogenesis of clinical fat embolism, as disappearance of these fat droplets is mediated through intracellular metabolic pathways. On the other hand, trauma-induced hepatic accumulation of triglyceride-rich cytoplasmic lipid droplets may be very significant, since the reversal of this condition involves the release into the circulating blood of a secretory product, the lipoprotein particle of very low density.

Trauma appears to affect the triglyceride secretory mechanism variously, producing at least two different expressions. In some animal experiments, trauma-induced elevations in plasma FFA appear only to increase the rate of VLDL output, with development of some degree of endogenous hyperlipidemia.* In this situation, the fatty liver that develops is characterized by large droplets of triglyceride free in the hepatocyte cytoplasm and is an expression of increased uptake and esterification of FFA, which produces triglycerides faster than they can be secreted as VLDL. In the human trauma patient, there is evidence that fatty liver accompanied by decreased concentrations of plasma lipids is indicative of impaired VLDL secretion,[58] which may involve synthesis of the protein moiety of the lipoprotein, lipid moieties other than triglyceride, or the complexing of these moieties into a particle. The fatty liver that develops experimentally under these conditions is characterized by the presence of numerous liposomes, membrane-enclosed lipid droplets ranging from 1,000 to 4,000 Å in diameter.[4,58]

Resumption of VLDL secretion after a period of impaired release with liposomal accumulation has been shown to result in the appearance of enlarged lipoprotein particles in the plasma VLDL fraction.[58] These could have been liposomes, or newly formed VLDL enlarged by overloading with triglyceride, or both. We are currently of the opinion that severe trauma, which precipitates a period of impaired VLDL secretion may be followed by release into the circulation of triglyceride-heavy VLDL that are unstable and tend to coalesce. An increase in the cholesterol to phospholipid ratio in these particles would also cause a tendency toward instability. The role of fatty liver in the pathogenesis of fat embolism that we have suggested is not to be confused with that suggested by Hartroft and Ridout[38] and Owens and Northington,[72] who proposed the mechanical rupture of fat-laden hepatocytes with release of droplets and subsequent impaction of peripheral blood vessels.

The data presented in these studies support the concept that lipid metabolism is profoundly affected by trauma. Similar alterations in lipid metabolism have been described in diabetes mellitus, steroid therapy, infection, and stress in general, conditions that are also characterized by a high incidence of fat embolism in the absence of mechanical trauma.

DIAGNOSIS

Until recently, fat embolism was usually diagnosed only at autopsy. Histologic embolic fat was

*See references 37, 48, 49, 62, 63, 88, and 89.

and still is a frequent finding in patients dying from any type of trauma. This fact has led to much confusion, both in the appraisal of fat embolism as a distinct clinical entity and indetermining its exact role in causing the death of the patient. Hardaway[36] correctly listed fat embolism as one of several clinical syndromes that may be associated with an episode of diffuse intravascular coagulation. This classification is especially appropriate for the acute aspect of trauma associated with bone fracture and depot fat disruption with the release of thrombogenic embolic fat (together with other products of tissue damage) into the circulation. In this acute phase following trauma, fat embolism as a distinct clinical entity cannot be separated from microembolization by fibrin or reduced vascular flow from whatever cause.

The diagnosis of fat embolism as a distinct clinical entity should be limited to those patients who have recovered from the initial acute effects of severe trauma, who then apparently regress clinically and exhibit a series of characteristic symptoms. This syndrome, which usually follows fractures of long bones by about 24 hours, consists of the rapid development of delirium, stupor, and coma, accompanied by extreme tachycardia, pyrexia, and decerebrate rigidity. Tachypnea, cyanosis, convulsive seizures, and focal neurologic signs are also often present, but they are not of equal diagnostic significance.[13]

Traumatized patients frequently have received head injuries leading to the formation of an epidural or a subdural hematoma. Thus the differential diagnosis of the neurologic signs and symptoms of intracranial hematoma and those of the symptom complex of the fat embolism syndrome becomes of great importance. Coma, following a period of apparent recovery, may occur in both conditions, but the time relationship and accompanying neurologic manifestations are quite different. With hematoma, coma usually appears in less than 12 hours after injury and is accompanied by headache, vomiting, bradycardia, and slowing of respirations. Decerebrate rigidity occurs only with other signs indicative of severe intracranial pressure.

In contrast, the syndrome of fat embolism is usually ushered in by a cloudy sensorium and tachycardia. The patient is apprehensive, talks incoherently, but does not appear to be in pain. Decerebrate posturing often appears well before the onset of coma while the patient is still talking and restless. Most frequently, coma is delayed until about 24 hours or more after injury, but some features of the symptom complex may appear as early as 1 hour or as late as 3 days following trauma. Numerous other neurologic signs and symptoms are seen with less consistent regularity in some patients with fat embolism.

In our own experience, delirium preceded stupor and coma in all patients. Tachycardia of from 140 to 190 per minute was always present. This rapid pulse rate was rather uniquely characteristic, in that it appeared or persisted long after any initial fall in blood pressure immediately following trauma had been corrected, and the blood pressure was normal at the time of onset of symptoms. At times tachypnea was noted, but any more marked respiratory symptoms were rare. Petechiae appearing about 24 hours before the onset of symptoms were seen in about half of our cases. Isolated and intermittent neurologic manifestations, including convulsions, facial paralysis, and pupillary dilatation, were seen in some patients.

There are no laboratory studies that give any specific aid in the diagnosis of fat embolism. Fat droplets have occasionally been noted in the urine,[2,15,65] blood,[5,94] and spinal fluid,[17] but these are merely interesting phenomena that may occur in normal persons.

The changes in the serum lipoproteins as presented in this article may be supportive evidence but do not carry any specificity. Electroencephalograms are also contributory to the diagnosis, but not specific. They are usually abnormal with a diffuse slow wave disturbance.[12]

Sequential chest radiographs may be of help in the diagnosis when the characteristic "snowstorm" appearance develops along with the clinical symptoms.[6,60] However, this pattern is not specific for fat embolism.

TREATMENT

Our experience in the management of the severely traumatized patient, together with the results of our experimental studies, indicates that the syndrome of fat embolism is a reflection (1) of vascular impaction by disrupted adipose and medullary fat and (2) of a profound alteration in lipid metabolism associated with the aggregation of serum lipoproteins. The instability of serum lipoproteins is most likely the result of their altered composition, which occurs rapidly following tissue injury. This is supported by the evidence that fat embolism is encountered in patients who have not sustained trauma, but have similar abnormalities in lipoprotein metabolism. Our treatment of fat embolism, therefore, is directed not only to the well-recognized supportive measures to ensure adequate vascular flow and metabolic support, but also to the more efficient metabolism of lipoproteins in general.

The excellent article by Schumer and Sperling[82] on shock and its effect on the cell points out that the metabolic derangements of shock revolve about exaggerated anaerobic glucose metabolism, which produces increased amounts of lactic acid, amino acids, fatty acids, and phosphoric acids. The resultant local metabolic acidosis is accompanied by a decreased production of the energy component, ATP, and eventually cell death. In order to prevent a resultant vicious cycle, adequate perfusion by oxygenated blood, control of activated coagulative factors, availability of normal cellular substrates in adequate amounts, and elimination of abnormal concentrations of metabolites are of paramount importance.

Careful monitoring of the physiologic and biochemical status of a severely traumatized patient is the best guide to appropriate supportive treatment. Prompt and aggressive measures may not only be lifesaving in the immediate posttrauma period, but it is our strong clinical impression that they also prevent the later development of the syndrome of fat embolism. An excellent outline for the clinical management of shock is given by Hardaway.[36]

The immediate management of traumatic shock requires restoration of circulating blood volume. This may require whole blood transfusion if significant hemorrhage has occurred, or restoration of plasma volume in situations of extensive soft tissue trauma with massive extravasation from the intravascular fluid compartment. Sequestration of large amounts of blood in stagnant vascular beds, such as the mesenteric system, spleen, and liver, may also lower the effective circulating blood volume. Serial hematocrits and, if possible, serial red cell or plasma volume measurements, as well as monitoring of central venous pressure, are helpful guides toward restoration of adequate circulating fluid volumes.

Another immediate concern in shock is the preservation of cellular metabolic integrity. With hypotension, profound peripheral vasoconstriction occurs to preserve an effective circulating blood volume. This leads to inadequate tissue perfusion. Anaerobic glycolysis results, and large amounts of lactic acid accumulate. The blood lactic acid levels rise, lowering the pH as blood returns from peripheral tissues. As metabolic acidosis advances, hyperventilation occurs as partial compensation. Sodium lactate in such circumstances to buffer pH is useless, as the blood lactate is already high and cannot be metabolized fast enough.

If partial respiratory compensation has occurred, arterial pH will be low, P_aCO_2 will also be lowered, but base deficit, a measure of the metabolic component of the acid-base equilibrium, will present an accurate picture of the magnitude of the problem. In situations in which respiration is either impaired, such as in chest injury, or depressed such as in head injury, combined metabolic and respiratory acidosis may exist. The arterial pH will be extremely low, P_aCO_2 high, and base deficit will still reflect the metabolic component of the hydrogen ion accumulation. In very severe cases it is not uncommon to observe a blood pH between 7.10 and 7.0 or lower. This degree of acidosis represents a clinical emergency in which immediate and aggressive measures to raise the pH to a more tolerable range must be instituted if the patient is to survive. When profound acidosis, either metabolic or combined, exists, 0.3 M THAM (tris hydroxymethyl aminomethane) is the buffer of choice. We use it in instances in which arterial pH is below 7.10 or in which P_aCO_2 is above 60 mm. Hg.

Once arterial pH is above 7.15 or 7.20, we prefer sodium bicarbonate unless profound respiratory acidosis exists. THAM[67] is a powerful buffer, capable of combining with both metabolic acids and with carbonic acid—hence its usefulness in combined acidosis. Its disadvantages are that it is very strongly alkaline pH $>$ 10) and capable of causing tissue slough if extravasated. Also, because it is such a good buffer for carbonic acid, as pH approaches physiologic levels, it is capable of suppressing respiratory drive from CO_2. We always monitor arterial pH frequently during THAM administration and have the means of tracheal intubation and assisting or controlling ventilation at hand.

As peripheral blood flow begins to be restored, the pH may again fall to extremely low levels, as lactic acid, which has been pooled in poorly perfused areas, is washed into the central circulation. Repeat buffering may again be necessary.

Once the initial emergency of shock has been treated successfully, attention should be focused on expectant preventative and supportive treatment of the later symptoms of the syndrome of fat embolism that may develop.

Most prophylactic measures are of undetermined value, but it is generally accepted that immobilization of the injury and avoidance of unnecessary manipulation are worthwhile. Since moderate amounts of embolic fat are mobilized from the lungs in about 5 days,[13] it is probably wise in patients with multiple fractures of long bones to delay manipulations or operations for at least this length of time. More radical measures such as ligature of veins and draining fracture sites are of no proved benefit.

Another important prophylactic measure is to provide the patient with a high caloric nonfat supply of food. Glycogen stores are rapidly depleted following trauma, with a resultant demand upon mobilized free fatty acids for energy. The excessive load of free fatty acids upon the liver appears to us to be the key feature in stimulating abnormal lipoprotein synthesis and secretion. Therefore, minimizing the stress and starvation-induced component of posttraumatic lipid metabolism is highly desirable. This may be accomplished by providing adequate oral carbohydrate intake when possible and by intravenous infusion of 10% glucose, when oral nutrition is not feasible. In addition, glucose can be given with hydrolyzed amino acids and vitamins.

Additional supportive measures are of proved value. Additional blood loss should be constantly replaced, and fluid and electrolyte balance should be frequently monitored. Measurement of daily intake and output is essential. Serial determinations of urine specific gravity may also be helpful in assessing the degree of hydration. Cardiac status should be carefully followed, and the patient should be rapidly digitalized if signs of congestive failure appear.

Supportive treatment is especially important in the presence of coma. Sevitt[85] compared this situation with that of a patient in acute renal failure, treated by dialysis until return of renal function.

The significance of respiratory insufficiency and hypoxemia cannot be overemphasized. The administration of oxygen is extremely important and should be based on early and frequent measurement of arterial gases, rather than on clinical evidence of respiratory distress alone. In the face of respiratory depression, no matter the cause, or of profound respiratory insufficiency, where P_aCO_2 approaches 100 mm. Hg., the use of oxygen alone for hypoxemia may exaggerate central respiratory depression and even stop respiration altogether. In such instances the hypoxia itself is the respiratory drive, and once this is alleviated with oxygen administration, assisted ventilation becomes necessary. If arterial oxygen saturation falls below 75% ($PO_2 < 40$ mm. Hg.) in the presence of corrected pH and 100% oxygen by mask, regardless of the P_aCO_2, then the use of positive pressure ventilation with a respirator is indicated. One should not hesitate to employ tracheostomy if necessary.

The use of corticosteroids or ACTH has been advocated by several authors.* The salubrious effect of these steroids is presumably due to their local antiinflammatory action. Evidence is accumulating that steroids may be of value in shock.[36] While use of corticosteroids as antiphlogistic agents may be justified on a short-term basis, extended use is unwise because of the well-established effects of these agents upon lipid metabolism,† which would enhance the metabolic abnormalities induced by trauma. In fact, fat embolism can be the result of corticosteroids in animals[54] and immunosuppressive drugs in humans.[23,51]

Recently clofibrate has been reported to show promise as a prophylactic agent for fat embolism.[71] This agent is reported to block the mobilization of free fatty acids from depot stores, which could remove the increased load upon the liver in the synthesis of lipoprotein. Inasmuch as mobilization of free fatty acid is a normal physiologic process following a variety of stress, and free fatty acids are a primary energy source under these conditions, the use of this drug may not be without harmful side effects. Its role in the treatment of fat-embolism has yet to be established.

The use of ethanol has been recommended in the treatment of fat embolism.‡ The rationale behind this cites its value as a lipase inhibitor, its emulsifying effect in vivo, its vasodilatation of the pulmonary capillaries, and its sedative or analgesic effects. We have found no evidence that ethanol inhibits lipoprotein lipase except in lethal concentrations in vitro.[54] There is contradictory evidence that it has an emulsifying effect in vivo,[11,14] and the fact that it is a sedative should preclude its use when the mental state of the patient must be assessed for diagnostic purposes. Recent studies indicate that in the presence of glucose and insulin, alcohol actually stimulates lipolysis in rat adipose cells and inhibits reesterification of free fatty acids.[76] Metabolically this is the opposite effect that

*See references 3, 61, 93, and 96.

†See references 16, 27, 44, and 58.

‡See references 1, 42, 43, 75, and 97.

one would hope to achieve in correcting the alteration of lipid metabolism following trauma.

Several investigators in experimental studies have been unable to demonstrate that intravenous ethanol had any effect on the mortality of their experimental animals.[43,66,97] Clinical studies likewise have failed to show that ethanol alters the prognosis of patients with fat embolism.[1,3] For these reasons, it is our opinion that the use of alcohol, prophylactically or therapeutically, in cases of fat embolism is unwarranted and, in fact, is contraindicated.

We have long advocated the use of heparin in the treatment of fat embolism.[11-13] This recommendation was intially made on the basis of the ability of heparin to increase the rate of hydrolysis of embolic fat, with earlier removal of embolic fat from the lungs of animals. This effect is due to the release of lipoprotein lipase by heparin from the vascular endothelium. This enzyme hydrolyzes lipoprotein fat[77] and improves metabolic oxidation of fat.[87] In addition, the pharmacologic action of heparin on blood coagulation would indicate that it has additional value in correcting accelerated clotting known to accompany trauma as well as in controlling microembolization by fibrin.[36]

Our experience indicates that the trauma patient is less responsive than a normal person to small doses of heparin. A dose of 50 mg. intravenously, which in a normal person increases the clotting time to 30 to 45 minutes, did not prolong the Lee-White coagulation time significantly in trauma patients. Our routine is to give patients who are suspected of having clinical fat embolism 50 mg. every 4 to 6 hours, with careful monitoring of the clotting time to ensure that it does not exceed 15 to 20 minutes. This therapy is continued for 5 to 7 days following injury, but it may be prolonged beyond this if coma is still present. In our experience no complications have resulted from the use of heparin.

We wish to thank Dr. Ann Minot and Dr. Mildred Stahlman for their assistance in preparing this manuscript, and we also wish to acknowledge the excellent technical work of Mr. John McKissack, Mrs. Joy Adams, and Mr. Jesse Britton.

REFERENCES

1. Adler, F., Lai, S., and Peltier, L. F.: Fat embolism: prophylactic treatment with lipase inhibitors, Surg. Forum **12**:453, 1961.
2. Adler, F., and Peltier, L. F.: The laboratory diagnosis of fat embolism, Clin. Orthop. **21**:226, 1961.
3. Ashbaugh, D. G., and Petty, T. L.: Use of corticosteroids in treatment of respiratory failure associated with massive fat embolism, Surg. Gynec. Obstet. **123**:493, 1966.
4. Baglio, C. M., and Farber, E.: Reversal of adenine of the ethionine-induced lipid accumulation in the endoplasmic reticulum of the rat liver, J. Cell Biol. **27**:591, 1965.
5. Bergentz, S. E.: Studies in genesis of posttraumatic fat embolism, Acta Chir. Scand., supp., **282**:1, 1961.
6. Berrigan, T. J., Jr.: Fat embolism. Roentgenographic pathologic correlation in three cases, Amer. J. Roentgen. **96**:967, 1966.
7. Birke, Gunnar, Carlson, L. A., and Liljedahl, Sten-Otto: Lipid metabolism and trauma. III. Plasma lipids and lipoproteins in burns, Acta Med. Scand. **178**:337, 1965.
8. Brücke, P., Blumel, G., and Gottlob, R.: Ueber die Fettresorption bei Volumenmangel: Ein Experimenteller Beitrag zur Pathogenese der Fettembolie, Arch. Clin. Chir. **313**:1049, 1965.
9. Butcher, R. W.: Role of cyclic AMP in hormone actions, New Eng. J. Med. **279**:1378, 1968.
10. Carlson, L. A., and Liljedahl, Sten-Otto: Lipid metabolism and trauma. I. Plasma and liver lipids during 24 hours after trauma with special reference to the effect of guanethidine, Acta Med. Scand. **173**: 1, 1963.
11. Cobb, C. A., and Hillman, J. W.: Fat embolism, Instr. Course Lect. **18**:122, 1961.
12. Cobb, C. A., Jr., Hillman, J. W., LeQuire, C. B., and LeQuire, V. S.: Treatment of clinical fat embolism with heparin, Southern Med. J. **53**:1459, 1960.
13. Cobb, C. A., Jr., LeQuire, V. S., Gray, M. E., and Hillman, J. W.: Therapy of traumatic fat embolism with intravenous fluids and heparin, Surg. Forum **9**:751, 1959.
14. Corn, D.: The fat embolism syndrome, Med. Clin. N. Amer. **48**:1459, 1964.
15. Cossman, F. P., Adler, F., Kittle, C. F., and Peltier, L. F.: Lipuria and lipasemia after thoracic surgical procedures, J. Thorac. Cardiov. Surg. **40**:430, 1960.
16. Courtice, F. C., and Munoz-Morus, M.: The composition of the plasma lipoprotein in experimental hyperlipaemia induced by triton WR-1339, cortisone, Alloxan, and haemorrhage in rabbits, Quart. J. Exp. Physiol. **49**:430, 1964.
17. Cross, H. E.: Examination of CSF in fat embolism: report of a case, Arch. Intern. Med. **115**:470, 1965.
18. Dodd, C., and Mills, G. L.: Influence of myocardial infarction on plasma lipoprotein concentration, Lancet **2**:1160, 1959.
19. Dole, V. P., and Meinertz, H.: Microdeterminations of long-chain fatty acids in plasma and tissues, J. Biol. Chem. **235**:2595, 1960.
20. Ellis, H. A., and Watson, A. J.: Studies on the genesis of traumatic fat embolism in man, Amer. J. Path. **53**:245, 1968.
21. Ellis, H. A., and Watson, A. J.: An evaluation of subatmospheric decompression as a means of causing pulmonary fat embolism, Amer. J. Path. **55**:203, 1969.
22. Fazekas, I. G.: Fettembolien Bei Experimenteller

Natriumhydroxydund Ammoniumhydroxyd-Vergiftung Frankfurt, Ztschr. f. Path. **51**:524, 1938.

23. Fisher, D. E., Bickel, W. H., and Holley, K. E.: Histologic demonstration of fat emboli in aseptic necrosis associated with hypercortisonism, Mayo Clin. Proc. **44**:252, 1969.
24. Fiske, C. H., and Subbarow, Y.: The colorimetric determination of phosphorus, J. Biol. Chem. **66**: 375, 1925.
25. Frazer, A. C., Elkes, J. J., Sammons, H. G., Govan, A. D. T., and Cook, W. T.: Effects of Clostridium welchii type A toxin on body tissues, and fluids, Lancet **1**:457, 1945.
26. Fredrickson, D. S., Levy, R. I., and Lees, R. S.: Fat transport in lipoproteins. An integrated approach to mechanisms and disorders, New Eng. J. Med. **276**: 34, 94, 148, 215, 273, 1967.
27. Friedman, M., Van Den Bosch, J., Byers, S. O., and St. George, S.: Effects of cortisone on lipid and cholesterol metabolism in the rabbit and rat, Amer. J. Physiol. **208**:94, 1965.
28. Fuchsig, P., Brücke, P., Blumel, G., and Gottlob, R.: A new clinical and experimental concept of fat embolism, New Eng. J. Med. **276**:1192, 1967.
29. Furman, R. H., Howard, R. P., Lakshmi, K., and Norcia, L. N.: The serum lipids and lipoproteins in normal and hyperlipidemic subjects as determined by preparative ultracentrifugation, Amer. J. Clin. Nutr. **9**:73, 1961.
30. Gomori, G.: The microtechnical demonstration of sites of lipase activity, Proc. Soc. Exp. Biol. Med. **58**:362, 1945.
31. Gomori, George: In Microscopic histochemistry, Chicago, 1952, University of Chicago Press, p. 99.
32. Graber, S.: Fat embolization associated with sickle cell crisis, Southern Med. J. **54**:1395, 1961.
33. Groskloss, H. H.: Fat embolism, Yale J. Biol. Med. **8**:297, 1936.
34. Hamilton, R. L., and LeQuire, V. S.: Electron microscopy of very low density lipoprotein (VLDL) secretion and early fatty liver, Fed. Proc. **26**:575, 1967.
35. Hamilton, R. L., Regen, D. M., Gray, M. E., and LeQuire, V. S.: Lipid transport in liver. I. Electron microscopic identification of very low density lipoproteins in perfused rat liver, Lab. Invest. **163**:305, 1967.
36. Hardaway, R. M.: Clinical management of shock, Springfield, Ill., 1968, Charles C Thomas, Publisher.
37. Horiuchi, Y.: Lipemia in acute anemia, J. Biol. Chem. **44**:363, 1924.
38. Hartroft, W. S., and Ridout, J. H.: Pathogenesis of the cirrhosis produced by choline deficiency. Escape of lipid from fatty hepatic cysts into the biliary and vascular systems, Amer. J. Path. **27**:951, 1951.
39. Havel, R. J.: The autonomic nervous system and intermediary carbohydrate and fat metabolism, Anesthesiology **29**:720, 1968.
40. Havel, R. J., Eder, H. A., and Bragdon, J. H.: The distribution and chemical composition of ultracentrifugally separated lipoproteins in human serum, J. Clin. Invest. **34**:1345, 1955.
41. Haymaker, W., and Johnson, A. D.: Pathology and decompression sickness. A comparison of the lesions in airmen with those in caisson workers and divers, Milit. Med. **117**:285, 1955.
42. Hengel, J. L., Smith, J. H., Pories, W. J., and Burget, D. E.: Fat embolism. Diagnostic challenge of a potentially lethal clinical entity, Amer. J. Surg. **113**:525, 1967.
43. Hermann, L. D.: Effect of dextrose-alcohol mixture on pulmonary fat embolism, Proc. Soc. Exp. Biol. Med. **30**:558, 1933.
44. Hill, R. B., Jr., Drake, W. E., and Hays, A. P.: Hepatic lipid metabolism in the cortisone treated rat, Exp. Molec. Path. **4**:320, 1965.
45. Hillman, J. W., and LeQuire, V. S.: Lipid metabolism and fat embolism after trauma: the contribution of serum lipoproteins to embolic fat, Surg. Forum **19**:465, 1968.
46. Himms-Hagen, J.: Sympathetic regulation of metabolism, Pharmacol. Rev. **19**:367, 1967.
47. Holczabek, W.: Dunnschichtchromatographische Untersuchungen von Lipextracten aus der Menschlichen Lunge unter Besonderer Berucksichtigung der Fettembolie, Deutsch Z. Ges. Gerichtl. Med. **55**:242, 1965.
48. Johnson, S. R., and Svanborg, A.: Investigations with regard to the pathogenesis of so-called fat embolism. Serum lipids and tissue esterase activity and the frequency of so-called fat embolism in soft tissue trauma and fractures, Ann. Surg. **144**:145, 1956.
49. Johnson, S. R., and Waldstrom, L. B.: Serum fat in tourniquet shock, Scand. J. Clin. Lab. Invest. **8**: 323, 1956.
50. Jones, A. L., Rudermann, N. B., and Herrera, M. G.: Electron microscopic and biochemical study of lipoprotein synthesis in the isolated perfused fat liver, J. Lipid Res. **8**:429, 1967.
51. Jones, J. P., Engleman, E. P., and Najarian, J. S.: Systemic fat embolism after renal homotransplantation and treatment with corticosteroids, New Eng. J. Med. **273**:1453, 1965.
52. Kent, S. P.: Fat embolism in diabetic patients without physical trauma, Amer. J. Path. **31**:399, 1955.
53. Lehman, E. P., and Moore, R. M.: Fat embolism: including experimental production without trauma, Arch. Surg. **14**:621, 1927.
54. LeQuire, V. S.: Unpublished data.
55. LeQuire, V. S., Hamilton, R. L., Adams, R., and Merrill, J. M.: Lipase activity in blood from the hepatic and peripheral vascular beds following heparin. Proc. Soc. Exp. Biol. Med. **114**:104, 1963.
56. LeQuire, V. S., Shapiro, J. L., LeQuire, C. B., Cobb, C. A., and Fleet, W. F., Jr.: A study of the pathogenesis of fat embolism based on human autopsy material and animal experiments, Amer. J. Path. **35**: 999, 1959.
57. Lynch, M. J., Raphael, S. S., and Dixon, T. P.: Fat embolism in chronic alcoholism; control study on incidence of fat embolism, Arch. Path. **67**:68, 1959.
58. Mahley, R. W., Gray, M. E., Hamilton, R. L., and LeQuire, V. S.: Lipid transport in liver. II. Electron

microscopic and biochemical studies of alterations in lipoprotein transport induced by cortisone in the rabbit, Lab. Invest. **19**:358, 1968.

59. Mahley, R. W., Hamilton, R. L., and LeQuire, V. S.: Characterization of lipoprotein particles isolated from the Golgi apparatus of rat liver, J. Lipid Res. **10**:433, 1969.
60. Marujama, Y., and Little, J. B.: Roentgen manifestations of traumatic pulmonary fat embolism, Radiology **79**:945, 1962.
61. Mieny, C. J.: The treatment of systemic fat embolism, South African Med. J. **36**:219, 1962.
62. Milch, L. J., Redmond, R. F., and Calhoun, W. W.: Plasma lipoprotein changes induced by acute local cold injury, Amer. J. Med. Sci. **225**:416, 1953.
63. Milch, L. J., Redmond, R. F., and Calhoun, W. W.: Blood lipoproteins in traumatic injury, J. Lab. Clin. Med. **43**:603, 1954.
64. Moore, F. D.: In Metabolic care of the surgical patients, Philadelphia, 1959, W. B. Saunders Co.
65. Morton, K. S.: Fat embolism: incidence of urinary fat in trauma, Canad. Med. Ass. J. **74**:441, 1956.
66. Morton, K. S., and Kendall, M. J.: The failure of IV alcohol in treatment of experimental pulmonary fat embolism, Canad. J. Surg. **9**:286, 1966.
67. Nahas, G. G.: Use of an organic carbon dioxide buffer in vivo, Science **129**:782, 1959.
68. Ney, R. L., Shimizu, N., Nicholson, W. E., Island, D. P., and Liddle, G. W.: Correlation of plasma ACTH concentration with adrenocortical response in normal human subjects, surgical patients and patients with Cushing's disease, J. Clin. Invest. **42**:1669, 1963.
69. Nuessle, W. F.: The significance of fat in sputum, Amer. J. Clin. Path. **21**:430, 1951.
70. Ober, W. B., Bruno, M. S., Sinon, R. M., and Weiner, L.: Hemoglobin S-C. disease with fat embolism, Amer. J. Med. **27**:647, 1959.
71. O'Driscoll, M., and Powell, F. J.: Injury, serum lipids, fat embolism and clofibrate, Brit. Med. J. **4**:149, 1967.
72. Owens, G., and Northington, Mary: Liver lipid as a source of post-traumatic embolic fat, J. Surg. Res. **2**:283, 1962.
73. Peltier, L. F.: Fat embolism: the detection of fat emboli in the circulating blood, Surgery **36**:198, 1954.
74. Peltier, L. F., Adler, F., and Lai, S. P.: Fat embolism: the significance of an elevated serum lipase after trauma to bone, Amer. J. Surg. **99**:821, 1960.
75. Pipkin, G.: Transportation of fat embolism, J. Kentucky Med. Ass. **60**:461, 1962.
76. Rasheeduddin, S., Rasheeduddin, Z., Kruger, F. A., and Skillman, T. G.: Effect of ethanol on epinephrine-stimulated lypolysis in rat adiposites, Clin. Res. **16**:443, 1968.
77. Robinson, D. S.: The uptake and release of lipids by the liver. In Meng, H. C., editor: Proceedings of an international symposium on lipid transport, Springfield, Ill., 1964, Charles C Thomas, Publisher, p. 194.
78. Robinson, D. S., and French, J. E.: The heparin clearing reaction and fat transport, Quart. J. Exp. Physiol. **42**:151, 1957.
79. Rywlyn, A. M.: Hemoglobin C and S disease in pregnancy. Report of a case with bone marrow and fat emboli, Amer. J. Obstet. Gynec. **86**:1055, 1963.
80. Scanu, A. M.: Factors affecting lipoprotein metabolism. In advances in lipid research, New York, 1965, Academic Press Inc., vol. 3.
81. Schumaker, V. N., and Adams, G. H.: Circulating lipoproteins, Ann. Rev. Biochem. **38**:113, 1969.
82. Schumer, W., and Sperling, R.: Shock and its effect on the cell, J.A.M.A. **205**:215, 1968.
83. Searcy, R. L., and Bergquist, L. M.: A new color reaction for the quantitation of serum cholesterol, Clin. Chem. Acta **5**:192, 1960.
84. Sevitt, S.: Burns, pathology and therapeutic applications, London, 1957, Butterworth & Co., Ltd.
85. Sevitt, Simon: Fat embolism, London, 1962, Butterworth & Co., Ltd.
86. Shelley, W. M., and Curtis, E. M.: Bone marrow and fat embolism in sickle cell anemia and sickle cell-hemoglobin C disease, Bull. Johns Hopkins Hosp. **103**:8, 1958.
87. Shoulders, H. H., Jr., Meng, H. C., and Tuggle, S.: Effects of heparin in body temperature and plasma lipids following IV administration of fat emulsion in man, J. Lab. Clin. Med. **52**:599, 1958.
88. Spitzer, J. J., and Spitzer, J. A.: Haemorrhagic lipaemia. A derangement of fat metabolism, J. Lab. Clin. Med. **46**:461, 1955.
89. Starup, V.: Einige Untersuchungen uber Die Hamorrhagische lipaemia. Biochem. Z. **270**:74, 1934.
90. Steinberg, Q.: Catecholamine stimulation of fat mobilization and its metabolic consequences, Pharmacol. Rev. **18**:217, 1966.
91. Strauss, Reuben: In Lipids and the steroid hormones in clinical medicine, Philadelphia, 1960, J. B. Lippincott Co., chap. 8.
92. Szabo, G., Serenyi, P., and Kocsar, L.: Fat embolism: fat absorption from the site of injury, Surgery **54**:756, 1963.
93. Taquini, A. C., Roncoroni, A. J., and Aramendia, P.: Fat embolism of the lungs, Amer. Heart J. **51**:468, 1956.
94. Tedeschi, C. G., Castelli, W., Kropp, G., and Tedeschi, L. G.: Fat macroglobulinemia and fat embolism, Surg. Gynec. Obstet. **126**:83, 1968.
95. Vance, B. M.: The significance of fat embolism, Arch. Surg. **23**:426, 1931.
96. Wilson, T. H.: Treatment of fat embolism. Report of two cases, Med. Ann. D.C. **37**:215, 1968.
97. Yale, C. F., and Herrmann, L. G.: Pathology and pulmonary fat embolism, mechanical and chemical alterations with an effective antidote, Surg. Forum **12**:451, 1961.
98. Youngberg, G. E., and Youngberg, M. V.: Phosphorus metabolism. I. A system of blood phosphorus analysis, J. Lab. Clin. Med. **16**:158, 1930.
99. Zlatkis, A., Zak, B., and Boyle, A. J.: A new method for the direct determination of serum cholesterol, J. Lab. Clin. Med. **41**:486. 1953.

Chapter 3

The incidence and prevention of thromboembolic disease

WILLIAM H. HARRIS, M.D.
Boston, Massachusetts

Pulmonary emboli used to be the leading cause of death on the Orthopaedic Service at the Massachusetts General Hospital. Moreover, Fitts and associates[2] found pulmonary emboli to be the leading cause of death following all forms of trauma in a group of patients who survived their trauma by one week. From that study, among a group of 161 patients who died following hip fractures and on whom *autopsies were performed,* this diagnosis was listed as a cause of death in *38%*. In marked contrast with this, the diagnosis of pulmonary emboli was listed as a cause of death in only 2% of the eighty-six similar patients in the same study who did not have an autopsy! The importance of this discrepancy is obvious. Clinically these lesions are not being recognized, and therapeutically the efforts to date have been grossly ineffective.

This problem has been ignored far too long. It is a problem of great seriousness both in terms of *frequency* and in terms of *severity*. The opinion is widely held that the incidence of pulmonary embolism is very low, that the problem arises only sporadically, that its occurrence is unpredictable, and that most patients who have an embolus do well anyway. Such is certainly not the case.

Three *controlled, prospective* studies on the incidence of pulmonary embolism at the Massachusetts General Hospital have recently been completed.[4,7,8] These have brought home very clearly the high incidence of thromboembolic disease. The first study dealt with a consecutive series of 184 patients over the age of 75 who were admitted with fresh fractures of the hip. Of a total of 101 patients who were not treated (the eighty-three control patients and the eighteen patients who had contraindications to treatment), there was a total of twenty-five patients with thromboembolic disease and eight with pulmonary emboli. This is an incidence of 25% thromboembolic disease in this group.

A second group consisting of 135 consecutive patients undergoing 169 mold arthroplasties of the hip was similarly studied. Among the sixty-seven patients in this group who did not receive prophylactic anticoagulation, that is the control group plus the contraindicated group, there were twenty-three patients with phlebitis and four patients who had both thrombophlebitis and pulmonary emboli. Seven patients had proved pulmonary emboli. This is an over-all incidence of 39% of thromboembolic disease, and 10% of the group had pulmonary emboli!

A third study was carried out on a series of 1,223 consecutive patients on the General Surgical Service in which the patients were classified in terms of being "normal"-risk or "high"-risk patients. Prolonged bed rest, obesity, pelvic surgery, visceral malignancy, and prior thromboembolic disease were the factors distinguishing the high-risk group. The incidence of thromboembolic disease in the high-risk group was 10%.

These figures appear excessively high to many physicians. There are several factors behind their documentation that are important to appreciate. In the first place, all three of these studies were *prospective* studies. Experience with the study of thromboembolic disease has clearly shown that retrospective studies of thromboembolic disease are useless, or virtually so. One needs to consider only the frequency with which the patient is not *examined* for thromboembolic disease, the ease with which the dignosis is overlooked, the difficulty that may exist in making a firm diagnosis when suggestive symptoms are present, and the inherent ability of mankind to forget unpleasant disasters, to realize that retrospective studies are of extremely limited value.

In order to offset these disadvantages in present studies, a team of investigators was formed who worked together over a 4-year period of time. Every patient was seen each day by his own physician and specifically examined for the presence of thromboembolic disease. When any question was raised concerning the presence of thromboembolic disease, one or more members of the study group saw the patient "blind," that is to say, without knowing whether or not he was receiving anticoagulation and without prejudice concerning the onus of establishing the diagnosis.

Each suspected episode of thrombophlebitis and pulmonary embolism was classified as "definite," "probable," "possible," or "none." As the course of events evolved, appropriate adjustments were made in classifying that episode into one of these categories. This meant that comparable data from the treated and nontreated groups would be examined, despite the fact that a firm diagnosis could not be made in some cases. In fact, only "probable" and "definite" cases were included in analysis of the data.

Another important factor that has played a major role in these studies is the use of all the current diagnostic tools in the questionable instances. Specifically, this means the use of pulmonary angiography, radioactive iodine scan, and venography, in addition to LDH and SGOT enzyme studies and all of the other established diagnostic methods. This approach enabled us to make definitive diagnosis of pulmonary emboli in a number of instances that had all of the clinical appearance and, in fact, the clinical diagnoses of postoperative pneumonia.

In addition, all patients were reviewed 6 months after surgery. The presence of chronic venous obstruction at that time confirmed the diagnosis in several cases of thrombophlebitis that had been uncertain earlier.

If anything, these figures are too low. They are too low because of the proved experience in autopsy studies, such as that of Fitts and associates[2] and also Sevitt and Gallagher[10] and Hampton and Castleman,[3] which clearly demonstrate the high incidence of both thrombophlebitis and pulmonary emboli that occurs *without* detectable clinical signs or symptoms.

This experience of such high figures for thromboembolism is neither unique nor unprecedented. Tubiana and Duparc[11] reported an incidence of 9.6% of pulmonary emboli in 389 hip operations. Ferguson[1] reported a 5% incidence of emboli in fifty-seven osteotomies of the hip. Neu, Waterfield, and Ash[6] reported a 10% incidence of pulmonary emboli in a series of fractures of the pelvis and lower extremities. Sevitt and Gallagher[9] reported an 18% incidence of pulmonary embolization in the control group of 150 cases in a prospective study of hip fractures in patients over the age of 55. What is more, 10% of this group had *fatal* pulmonary emboli.

Therefore, the first major point is that *the prevalence of thromboembolic disease is far higher than many physicians are willing to acknowledge and is certainly far higher than we should accept.* This applies not only to the mortality of pulmonary embolization, but also to the disability and morbidity of thromboembolic disease.

Secondly, the diagnosis *can* be established with a high degree of accuracy in a large number of cases. This requires basically astute clinical observation, high index of suspicion, daily check of the calf and lower extremities, alertness to pulmonary symptoms and signs, and the clear recognition that it is a common threat. These are the ingredients out of which the diagnosis must come. Moreover the newer techniques, such as pulmonary angiography, must be used in every suspicious situation that cannot otherwise be resolved.

The third major point is the emphasis on the *elimination of the disease*—not treatment, but prevention! I cannot emphasize too strongly that *thromboembolic disease can effectively and safely be prevented.* In the study of the mold arthroplasty patients, among the seventy patients who received crystalline sodium warfarin (Coumadin),* the "treated" group plus a special group that was not

*Endo Laboratories Inc., Garden City, N. Y.

randomized but was treated because of previous thromboembolic disease, there were only five cases of phlebitis and no pulmonary emboli. This is an over-all incidence of 7% of phlebitis and zero emboli, in contrast with the incidence of 39% in the control group that had a 10% incidence of pulmonary emboli and one fatality. These differences are highly significant with P values of < 0.002 for the difference in phlebitis and < 0.02 for the difference in pulmonary emboli. In the study of patients over the age of 75 with hip fractures, none of the eighty-three patients who received treatment sustained a pulmonary embolism during the time they were on treatment. The total incidence of thromboembolic disease in the treated group was seven out of eighty-three, or 8%, compared with 25% in the control group. The difference between the treated and the control group is highly significant, with a P value of less than 0.01.

In the large series of General Surgical patients, the incidence of thromboembolic disease was 10% among the patients in the high-risk group who were not treated, and in a comparable group of high-risk patients treated with prophylactic anticoagulation the incidence was 1.7%.

In the past 4 years, since prophylactic anticoagulation was initiated as a routine for all patients (without a contraindication) undergoing mold arthroplasty, only six pulmonary emboli have been clinically evident in over 1,000 consecutive patients, and none was fatal. In contrast, from the control data of our own series, at least ten deaths and 100 clinically evident pulmonary emboli would have been anticipated. From the figures reported from the Mayo Clinic, over *twenty* deaths from pulmonary emboli would have been anticipated in their experience in elective hip surgery in the adult.[5]

These figures clearly demonstrate that it is possible to reduce markedly the threat of thromboembolic disease by prophylactic anticoagulation. Moreover, all three of these studies showed that the incidence of wound hematoma was only slightly increased in the treated group compared with the control group. In none of these studies was this difference statistically significant. In the study on hip fractures, there were twelve instances of wound bleeding in the control group and sixteen in the treated group. In terms of other bleeding, there were four instances of major bleeding in the control group and six in the treated group. These differences are quite small.

Even more important, the same holds true in terms of sepsis. There was no significant difference in the incidence of wound infection in the mold arthroplasty group. The incidence of major wound sepsis in the control group of the fracture study was three out of eighty-three, and in the treated group it was five out of eighty-three.

A most important point is this. Anticoagulant administration should *not* be delayed until after the signs of phlebitis or pulmonary embolism have occurred. The risk of pulmonary embolus was just as great in those who did not develop clinically recognized phlebitis as it was in those who did! Only two of the seven pulmonary emboli in the control group of mold arthroplasty patients could possibly have been prevented by starting treatment after the development of the signs of phlebitis, because in fact the other five of these emboli occurred *prior* to the signs of phlebitis. This same finding has been reported by Tubiana and Duparc[11] and also by Neu, Waterfield, and Ash.[6] This means that the risk of a pulmonary embolus is just as great in the patient who does *not* develop the *clinically* detectable signs of phlebitis as it is in the patient who does. Many of the patients who throw emboli will subsequently have signs of phlebitis, but *at the time of the embolization* the risk is the same in both groups. Thus it is perfectly clear that if one waits until signs of phlebitis are present, the majority of patients destined to have pulmonary embolus will not be protected! Treatment is too late. Prevention is required.

MECHANICS OF PROPHYLACTIC ANTICOAGULATION

We recommend the use of crystalline sodium warfarin (Coumadin). The control of the daily dose is by the one-stage Quick prothrombin time test, and the desired dose range is between 20% and 30% or 1.5 to 2 times control. Some variation exists in the results of the prothrombin time determination, depending on the type of anticoagulant used in the specimen tube, on the technique of the determination, and on the time interval between drawing the blood and performing the assay. For this reason, it is advisable to discuss the exact level of anticoagulation to be obtained with the director of the laboratory doing the determination. The basic rule is that in the post-surgical or posttrauma patient the desired level of anticoagulation is slightly less than the level used in the treatment of medical conditions. For example, our laboratory currently recommends prothrombin time prolongation to a value between 2 and 2.5 times the control value for management of medical problems. For postoperative patients we now use 1.5 to 2 times control as the desired range. The absolute value of the desirable range may vary slightly depending on the laboratory. A conference with the laboratory director and with the hematologist is necessary before establishing the ideal value for each hospital.

It is true that an even more effective prophylaxis can be obtained by aiming for a longer prothrombin time, but this is done at the risk of a higher incidence of hemorrhage and sepsis. Treatment is contraindicated in all patients who have active peptic ulcer disease, a hemorrhagic diathesis, hemoptysis, melena, or hematuria, previous cerebral hemorrhages and gastrointestinal malignancies, or systolic hypertension above 200 mm. Hg.

In patients who have a history of a duodenal ulcer, if possible, obtain a current upper gastrointestinal series. If this is negative and the patient is asymptomatic, our current practice is to place the patient on a full ulcer regime and administer anticoagulation. Three asymptomatic patients who were denied anticoagulation because of the history of an ulcer have had pulmonary emboli and then required anticoagulant treatment. Because of that experience, we no longer use simply a history of an ulcer in an asymptomatic patient as an absolute contraindication.

In patients who have received trauma with the possibility of internal bleeding, for example, from a ruptured liver or spleen or from retroperitoneal hemorrhage, or who are in danger of intracranial bleeding, anticoagulation is obviously contraindicated until that danger has subsided. Also, patients who have had spinal cord surgery should not be anticoagulated in most instances.

A base line prothrombin time must be obtained prior to beginning therapy. The usual loading dose is 15 mg. for a 60-Kg. adult in good health. However, experience has shown clearly that both the loading dose and the maintenance dose will often need to be *much* lower in the elderly. It is not at all unusual for 7 mg. to be an effective loading dose for an 86-year-old woman weighing under 100 pounds. Her maintenance dose may be 1 mg. per day or even 1 mg. on alternate days.

No sodium warfarin is given the following day, and then the daily dose is calculated based on the prothrombin time. Because the maximum effect of sodium warfarin usually occurs at 36 to 48 hours following administration, it is necessary to take this into account when deciding the effectiveness of a given dose.

The influence of certain drugs, other than sodium warfarin, on the prothrombin time must be kept clearly in mind. Specifically, aspirin and those antibiotics that decrease gastrointestinal bacterial synthesis of vitamin K will produce an augmentation of the sodium warfarin effect.

Phenylbutazone and, in some people, barbituates will also augment the prolongation of the prothrombin time. Any change in the sensitivity of the patient must be watched closely, and the possibility of drug effects such as these must be borne in mind.

Following elective surgery, the loading dose should be given the night of the operation. In patients who are admitted with a hip fracture, the anticoagulation should be started on admission to the hospital, if their general status and their prothrombin time tests are normal. Several reasons exist for this.

First, very often one or several days has already passed since the trauma occurred. In fact, a number of such patients arrive at the emergency ward with thrombophlebitis already well established.

Second, these patients are a very high-risk group, not only because of the swelling and venous compromise that the fracture causes, but also because of their age and the necessity for bed rest.

Third, since it will take on the average 2 to 3 days before the therapeutic range is reached even after sodium warfarin is started, no delay should be permitted.

If the surgery is done within 18 hours of admission, the loading dose will not interfere. If surgery is delayed beyond this, then an additional preoperative prothrombin time is required to be sure that the prothrombin time exceeds 25% or is at 1.5 times control. It is safe to perform any necessary surgery on patients if their prothrombin time is 25% or above or at 1.5 times control. If, however, their prothrombin time is prolonged beyond this level, it should be brought into a safer range by delaying the operation until the prothrombin time recovers spontaneously or by the administration of aqua phytonadione (Mephyton).

If aqua phytonadione (Mephyton) is required, one dose will often hold the prothrombin time above the therapeutic range for 4 or 5 days. For this reason it is much better to avoid its use unless it is really needed.

In situations in which additional surgery is needed while a patient is on anticoagulants, such as the second arthroplasty in a patient with bilateral hip disease, it is preferable to reduce the maintenance dose slightly 72 to 48 hours prior to the second operation to be certain that the prothrombin time will be at this safe range for the surgery. This avoids disrupting the anticoagulation completely for 4 or 5 days, as aqua phytonadione (Mephyton) would do.

It is necessary to check the stool guaiac and hematocrit every Monday, Wednesday, and Friday in order to be sure that any gastrointestinal bleeding that may occur does not pass unrecognized. There have been six major gastrointestinal bleeding episodes, all but one due to unrecognized disease, either ulcer, cancer, or diverticulitis. There have been no cerebral vascular accidents. Urinary bleeding has been a problem only twice.

Anticoagulation is discontinued when the risk has subsided, meaning when the patient is walking five or six times a day, bearing some weight on both legs. If the patient is unable to resume weight bearing, we have arbitrarily set 3 months as the duration for anticoagulation.

The sodium warfarin is stopped abruptly, without tapering the dose. There has been no evidence of a rebound phenomenon or of a hypercoagulable state in the large series of patients so treated.

SUMMARY

The incidence of thromboembolic disease in any patient over the age of 40 who will be in bed for a week or more following surgery or trauma is so high that prophylactic anticoagulation must be used unless a specific contraindication is present. It must be administered well and run safely. If it is so done, the incidence of complication secondary to the anticoagulation is low, acceptable, and more than offset by the reduction in thromboembolic disease.

REFERENCES

1. Ferguson, A. B., Jr.: High intertrochanteric osteotomy for osteoarthritis of the hip. A procedure to streamline the defective joint, J. Bone Joint Surg. **46A:**1159, 1964.
2. Fitts, W. T., Jr., Lehr, H. B., Bitner, R. L., and Spelman, J. W.: An analysis of 950 fatal injuries, Surgery **56:**663, 1964.
3. Hampton, A. O., and Castleman, Benjamin: Correlation of postmortem chest teleroentgenograms with autopsy findings. With special reference to pulmonary embolism and infarction, Amer. J. Roentgen. **43:**305, 1940.
4. Harris, W. H., Salzman, E. W., and DeSanctis, R. W.: The prevention of thromboembolic disease by prophylactic anticoagulation, J. Bone Joint Surg. **49A:**81, 1967.
5. Ivins, J. C., Benson, W. F., Bickel, W. H., and Nelson, J. W.: Arthroplasty of the hip for idiopathic degenerative joint disease, Surg. Gynec. Obstet. **125:**1281, 1967.
6. Neu, L. T., Waterfield, J. R., and Ash, C. J.: Prophylactic anticoagulation in orthopedic patient, Ann. Intern. Med. **62:**463, 1965.
7. Salzman, E. W., Harris, W. H., and DeSanctis, R. W.: Anticoagulation for prevention of thromboembolism following fracture of the hip, New Eng. J. Med. **275:**122, 1966.
8. Salzman, E. W., and Skinner, D.: Anticoagulant prophylaxis in surgical patients, Surg. Gynec. Obstet. **125:**741, 1967.
9. Sevitt, A., and Gallagher, N. G.: Prevention of venous thrombosis and pulmonary embolism in injured patients, Lancet **2:**981, 1959.
10. Sevitt, S., and Gallagher, N. G.: Venous thrombosis and pulmonary embolism: clinico-pathological study in injured and burned patients, Brit. J. Surg. **48:** 475, 1961.
11. Tubiana, R., and Duparc, J.: Prevention of thromboembolic complications in orthopaedic and accident surgery, J. Bone Joint Surg. **43B:**7, 1961.

Chapter 4

Clinical applications of electrodiagnostic studies

WILLIAM F. HEJNA, M.D.
Chicago, Illinois

This course is an introduction to electrodiagnosis and is intended as an aid to the clinician in taking advantage of the various uses that are available. It deals also with the technique of performing the studies under discussion, namely, nerve conduction velocity and electromyography, and with the interpretation of these studies to the extent that reports received may be properly understood. Several categories of problems that confront the orthopedic surgeon will be presented, with case illustrations in each to point out more specifically the type of information that can be gained from these studies.

HISTORICAL NOTE

Electricity and its effect on man has been of interest since about the time of Lyon in 1559, who said, "The marine torpedo (an electrical eel) eases prolonged headache when applied to the top of the head, and relieves all other chronic pains of the body." Galvani discovered "spontaneous electricity" in about 1790. There was, however, no real impetus to this area of study until the 1820-1830's, when the galvanometer and wet cell were better developed. Saladiene proposed the heroic theory of electropuncture in 1825, and in 1833 Duchenne became so interested that he spent much of the remainder of his life devoted to electrical stimulation. In fact, he described the use of faradic current as it is used today. In 1838, Carlo Matteucci proved that electrical currents did originate in muscle. Du Bois-Reymond registered action potentials in 1851. Other studies such as strength duration curves and chronaxy determination were accomplished in the laboratory by Engelmann in 1870 and in the human by Adrian in 1916. With the equipment available, however, these were tedious, and they were all but abandoned until after World War II. Electromyography itself probably originated in 1907 when Lipen recorded voluntary forearm flexion contractions in man. Each world war then brought tremendous interest in the field. By 1950 some clinical examination centers were in use, but by 1960 virtually all centers had such equipment, and clinical diagnosis was launched on a large scale. As in many other areas the technical equipment is production built, it is no longer outrageously expensive, and many standards of interpretation are well defined.

GENERAL USES

Data obtained from the performance of each electromyograph and nerve conduction velocity is applicable only to an abnormality in the lower motor neuron or motor unit, the motor unit consisting of anterior horn cell, its axon, the neuromuscular junction, terminal branches of a single axon, and all of the muscle fibers supplied by a single axon. Perhaps the most important information that the electromyographer can give the clinician is an accurate localization of the disease or abnormality to a portion of a motor unit. Having localized the process to a portion of the motor unit, the electrodiagnostic equipment cannot provide the exact etiologic basis. For example, one can readily define that the abnormality exists in the end organ or muscle fibers, but it is extremely difficult to differentiate whether the patient has muscular dystrophy or myositis. Such localization, however, is extremely valuable since many other diseases have been ruled out, such as Werdnig-Hoffmann disease, poliomyelitis, peripheral neuropathy, etc. By the addition of clinical information such as enzyme studies, one can more accurately make the exact etiologic diagnosis. Table 4-1 lists various diseases and abnormalities that may occur specifically in one or another portion of the motor unit.

A second type of localization that can be provided by the electrodiagnostic equipment and that is of great help at times is pinpointing a root level at which compression of the nerve is occurring. This is done by mapping the myotome involved, and such patterns have been worked out by various authors. In our laboratory the root levels shown in Table 4-2 have been used and are found to correlate fairly well with myelographic findings and surgical findings. Thus, fibrillation or denervation potentials that are occurring in a certain pattern will lead one to suspect a given nerve root or intervertebral space to the exclusion of others.

A third type of localization of disease involves the studying of the muscles supplied by single nerves in proximal distal fashion in an attempt to localize the lesion at a point along a nerve. For example, if one finds abnormal potentials in the opponens muscle but not in the pronator teres, one might assume that the lesion was located between those two points. If, however, one found abnormal potentials in the pectoralis major, the lesion must be proximal to the point at which the nerve to the pectoralis major leaves the brachial plexus. Study of the various muscles about the shoulder girdle and the erector spinae muscles is extremely important, particularly when attempting to define the extent of the brachial plexus lesions. Study of proximal musculature in the shoulder and pelvic girdle and the comparison of these findings with a more peripheral muscle is also some help in determining the distribution in generalized processes such as muscular dystrophy and poliomyelitis.

Apart from localization as described previously, electrodiagnosis is of great importance in several other spheres. One such use is determination of the degree of injury that a peripheral nerve has sustained. This will be described in more detail in the case presentations. It should be noted, however, that several studies formerly in common use are not absolutely necessary in this regard, that is, the chronaxy determination, reaction of degeneration (R.D.), and faradic-galvanic stimulation. Relative to peripheral nerve injury, a further use is prognostication. Using electromyography and nerve conduction velocity, the rate of return can be defined. This appears to be less complicated than the use of strength duration curves, although this is another acceptable method.

Detection of malingerers is accomplished with ease, and such data are admissible in the courts of many states. Information relative to the actual existence of neuromuscular disease is also of increasing importance in workman's compensation arbitration, and in simply providing appropriate care for those patients who are poor historians.

Several other uses for neuromuscular diagnostic studies exist that may, however, be of less importance to the practicing clinician. Determination of neuromuscular excitability, for example, by the use of varying intensity and duration of stimu-

Table 4-1. Localization of pathology in motor unit

Anterior horn cell	*Axon*	*Neuromuscular junction*	*Muscle fiber*
Poliomyelitis	Root level	Myasthenia	Dystrophy
Spinal tumors	Disc	Familial paralysis	Myositis
Trauma	Tumor	Myotonia	
Amyotrophic lateral sclerosis	Spurs		
Cysts	Plexus		
Hemorrhage	Erb's palsy		
	Trauma		
	Wounds		
	Peripheral		
	Stretch injury		
	Compression		
	Laceration		
	Neuropathy		

lation can easily be done. Family members and, in particular, siblings of patients with certain diseases can be studied to determine genetic patterns of transmission, as occasionally electrical abnormalities exist when the problem has not been of such severity to bring the person to a physician. This is true with such afflictions as Charcot-Marie-Tooth disease, muscular dystrophy, and myasthenic syndrome. The entire field of clinical research deserves comment since much has been done to define gait pattern, kinesiology of various joints, etc.

NERVE CONDUCTION VELOCITY

The nerve conduction velocity is simply a test to determine the rate with which a segment of peripheral nerve will conduct an impulse, and this is reported in meters per second. This value is compared to normal standards. Should the conduction time be slower than normal, one can state that abnormality exists in the peripheral nerve or in the axonal portion of the motor unit. By measuring the nerve conduction velocity on different segments of the nerve, one can localize the pathology, as is done in the entrapment syndromes such as carpal tunnel syndrome. The equipment necessary to perform this test includes stimulator and recording electrodes that are connected to an oscilloscope via an amplifier. The stimulator is built into the electromyographic unit and delivers an impulse of variable duration from approximately 0.001 msec. to 0.2 msec. that can be varied in intensity up to approximately 5.0 ma. The recording electrodes are of the skin type, generally being metal discs approximately 0.75 cm. in diameter. The oscilloscope is calibrated in time in milliseconds on the horizontal axis and in potential amplitude in millivolts on the vertical axis.

Table 4-2. Most commonly tested muscles with their root level innervation

	C5	C6	C7	C8
Median				
Pronator teres		xx*	xx	
Flexor carpi radialis		xx	xx	
Opponens			x	xx
Ulnar				
Flexor carpi ulnaris		x	xx	x
Interossei			x	xx
Musculocutaneous				
Biceps; brachialis	x	xx		
Radial				
Triceps		x	xx	
Brachioradialis	xx	x		
Extensor carpi radialis		x	xx	
Extensor carpi ulnaris			x	xx
Abductor pollicis			x	xx
	L3	*L4*	*L5*	*S1*
Adductor longus	xx	x		
Gluteus medius		x	xx	
Gluteus maximus			xx	xx
Internal hamstring		x	xx	x
External hamstring			x	xx
Peroneal				
Tibialis anterior		x	xx	
Extensor hallucis		x	xx	
Peronei			xx	x
Extensor digitorum brevis			xx	
Tibial				
Gastrocnemius				xx
Toe flexors			x	xx

*A double *x* indicates a major contributor; a single *x* indicates a minor contributor.

The nerves most accessible to performing this study are the median and ulnar in the upper extremity, and peroneal and posterior tibial in the lower extremity.

With the patient grounded, the test is performed by first taping the skin electrodes over the motor point and an adjacent area on a muscle such as the opponens, which is supplied by the median nerve. The stimulator is then placed over the nerve at the elbow, where it lies just medial to the antebrachial artery. The shock amplitude is then gradually increased until a response is noted in the form of a biphasic potential on the oscilloscope. The time necessary for the impulse to get from the point of stimulation to the point of recording is easily obtained from the oscilloscope, since the scope is calibrated in time. The distance between these two points is then measured with an ordinary tape measure, and the calculation to determine the velocity is simply made. The velocity thus obtained is the "nerve conduction time," which includes conduction across the neuromuscular junction, along a portion of muscle fiber, and transmission through some adipose tissue and skin. One then makes a similar nerve conduction time determination, stimulating the same nerve 6 cm. proximal to the recording electrode.

One can eliminate the neuromuscular transmission portion simply by subtracting the distalmost nerve conduction time from the total. The shorter conduction is known as the "distal latency," and normal standards have also been determined for the various nerves. Conduction velocity is the meters per second traveled by an impulse on the more proximal segment of nerve, that is, the conduction time minus the distal latency. Thus conduction time determinations can be done on such nerves as the radial, sciatic, and facial, whereas conduction times as well as conduction velocity and distal latencies can be determined for nerves that have two areas accessible for stimulation. Normal values are shown below.

	Distal latency	*Normal conduction velocity*
Ulnar	Up to 4.2 msec.	40-60 m./sec.
Median	Up to 4.5 msec.	40-58 m./sec.
Peroneal	Up to 7.0 msec.	43-57 m./sec.
Posterior tibial	Up to 7.0 msec.	40-55 m./sec.

ELECTROMYOGRAPHY

Electromyography is the study of spontaneous and voluntary electrical wave forms generated in the motor unit and recorded from muscle fibers. The electrical impulse recorded is initiated in the anterior horn cell and is propagated down the axon, exciting the electrical mechanism in all of the muscle fibers supplied by a single axon. This system is called a motor unit, and all such muscle fibers of a motor unit fire synchronously in an "all-or-none" fashion. The oscilloscope wave form or so-called motor unit potential, when voluntarily produced, has a predictable phasicity, amplitude, duration, and frequency of discharge. Some normal variation does occur in motor units; for example, the gastrocnemius muscle has about 2,000 muscle fibers per unit, whereas the platysma has about twenty-five. Hence, the duration and the amplitude vary. Anatomic cross sectional area also varies from muscle to muscle. Spontaneous firing of the muscle fibers which produce motor unit potentials while the muscle is at rest is an abnormal phenomenon.

Equipment necessary for performing electromyography includes a recording electrode, which is generally a coaxial needle electrode of about number 22 gauge. It contains both the probe and distant electrodes for obtaining a potential difference. The potentials picked up with this electrode are passed through an amplifier to the oscilloscope and loudspeaker for recording. Thus, both audible and visual displays are utilized to determine the character of the motor unit potential. In addition, motor unit potentials can be recorded on a tape recorder to replay for later study or teaching purposes.

On actual performance of the test, the scope is observed during insertion of the needle electrode, at rest, on partial voluntary effort, and on maximum effort. On insertion, a short burst of involuntary potentials, called the insertional potentials, occurs. At rest there is normally electrical silence; at full voluntary effort normally the screen is obliterated by vertical deflections in a so-called "interference pattern"; and at partial voluntary effort individual motor unit potentials can be observed. Several samples are studied in each muscle belly by changing the position of the probing electrode. Fig. 4-1 is a schematic representation of pathologic situations that may exist in the motor unit and the effect of such abnormality on the motor unit potential.

Fig. 4-2 is a representation of the more common types of spontaneous and voluntary potentials that can be seen when performing the study. A complete electrical study should include both the nerve con-

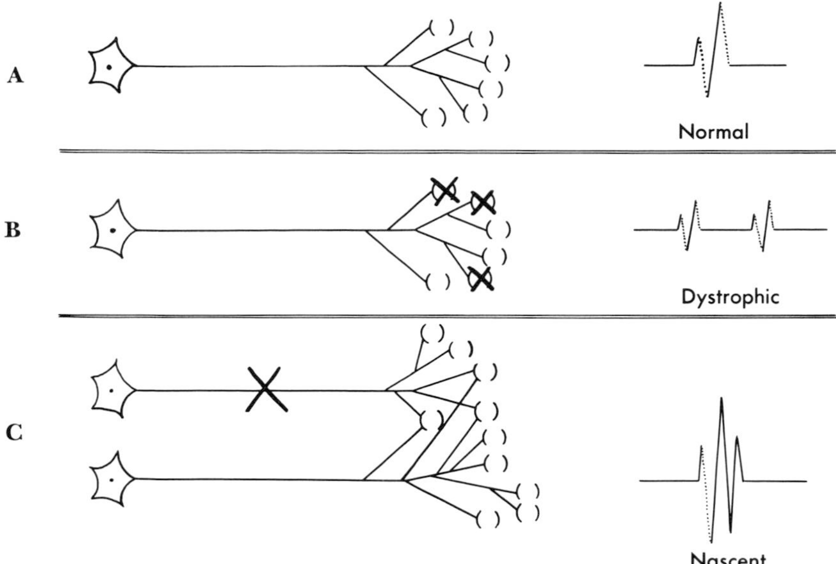

Fig. 4-1. Physiologic basis for some of the commonly seen motor unit potentials (M.U.P.). **A,** Normal motor unit with its M.U.P. demonstrating the "all-or-none" phenomenon. **B,** With several of the muscle fibers destroyed, the resultant "all-or-none" M.U.P. is of decreased amplitude and shorter duration. **C,** Following axon or anterior horn cell destruction neurotization or terminal filament outgrowth and branching from another axon occurs, and the M.U.P. has a greater amplitude and a longer duration.

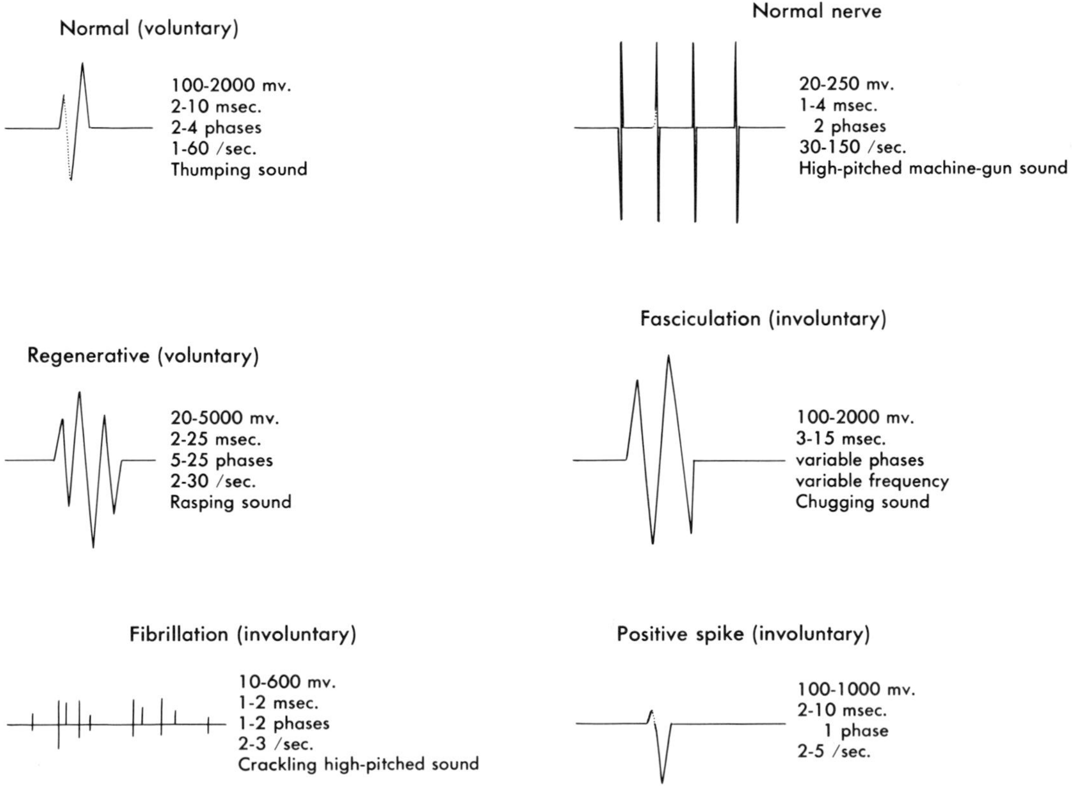

Fig. 4-2. The most commonly encountered M.U.P. patterns with their individual characteristics.

duction velocity and electromyography, since localization of pathology in the motor unit, that is, anterior horn cell, axon, neuromuscular junction, or muscle fiber, can best be done when one has both the nerve conduction velocity and electromyographic interpretation. In addition to the motor unit potentials that are presented, certain other observations can be made referable to the study as a whole. Thus, the insertional potentials usually last only 0.1 second. However, when these are significantly prolonged for several seconds or minutes, upper motor neuron disease or irritated muscle, such as is seen in myositis, may be present. Further, although the classical potential of denervation is the fibrillation, one occasionally may see positive spike potentials 100 to 500 mv. in amplitude and 2 to 10 msec. in duration, which indicates similar pathology. Diseased muscle also occasionally produces spontaneous rhythmic bizarre potentials that have a variable contour, the source of which is poorly understood. When such spontaneous volleys of fading potentials occur with a "dive bomber"-like sound on the loudspeaker, amyotonia congenita is probably the diagnosis.

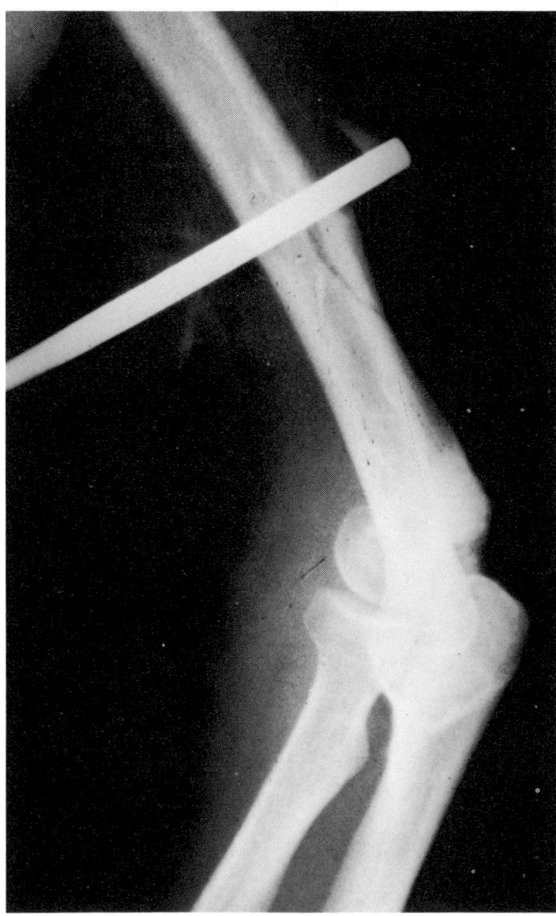

Fig. 4-3. A piston stud that entered the biceps anteriorly, fracturing the humerus, with subsequent radial nerve palsy.

CLINICAL MATERIAL

The case presentations are arbitrarily divided into seven clinical categories. These categories were chosen simply on the basis that they seem to group conveniently the various types of problems that present to the electrodiagnostician, and they in no way represent a formal classification of electrical abnormalities.

Category I. Peripheral nerve injuries

Case 1. A 42-year-old carpenter was working with a stud gun when a faulty piston was ejected backward, penetrating his biceps and humerus and a portion of the triceps, as seen in the radiograph (Fig. 4-3). On initial physical examination there was marked weakness in the brachioradialis and the extensor groups of the forearm. Initial treatment consisted of standard surgical debridement. On the following day the palsy was complete, and in spite of initial observation question arose as to whether the radial nerve was intact or not. The simple maneuver of supramaximal stimulation of the radial nerve proximal to the site of injury produced contraction in the forearm and extensor group. This proved that the lesion was a neurapraxia according to Seddon's* classification, which is presented below.

Seddon's classification of nerve injury:

Neurapraxia	Physiologic loss of conduction
Axonotmesis	Axonal degeneration with sheaths intact
Neurotmesis	Severance of nerve trunk

Discussion. This simple test is based on the fact that wallerian degeneration of the axon is not complete until 4 to 5 days following the injury. After this amount of time, an impulse will not be propagated down the nerve even with morphologically intact structures. Note that at 21 days denervation potentials may be present; however, function in the patient discussed eventually fully recovered. Thus, in a peripheral nerve injury in which there

*Seddon, J. H.: Three types of nerve injury, Brain **66**:237, 1943.

is question as to the actual intactness of the nerve, stimulation prior to wallerian degeneration may prove to be of value.

Case 2. This patient, a 36-year-old man, had alleged radial nerve injury following penicillin injection. He claimed persistent wrist drop and pain in the forearm 2 months following an injection of penicillin into the midportion of the triceps muscle. Nerve conduction velocity studies of the ulnar and medial nerve were normal. On electromyographic examination there were no fibrillation, fasciculation, or nascent potentials. In fact there were no motor unit potentials on voluntary effort.

Discussion. In the face of absence of any spontaneous potentials, presence of normal insertional activity, and absence of voluntary potentials on apparent effort, it was obvious that the patient was simply not trying to move. When informed of this, his motor power recovered completely within the course of the next week. This case is presented to make the point that it is extremely difficult for a malingerer to outwit the apparatus. A significant point is that the electromyographic examination was done 2 months following the alleged injury. This is of some importance, since it takes 14 to 21 days to develop fibrillation or denervation potentials. Such evidence is concurrently admissible in the courts in most of the United States.

Case 3. This patient, a 7-year-old boy (Fig. 4-4), had a combined median-ulnar nerve lesion following injury to his arm in the conveyor belt of a piece of farm machinery. Ten months after repair of the lesion (Fig. 4-4, *A*), the arm and hand appeared as in Fig. 4-4, *B*, and electromyography was carried out. This revealed fibrillation potentials in the muscles supplied by the ulnar nerve, with no voluntary motor unit potentials present. In the muscle supplied by the median nerve, there were fibrilla-

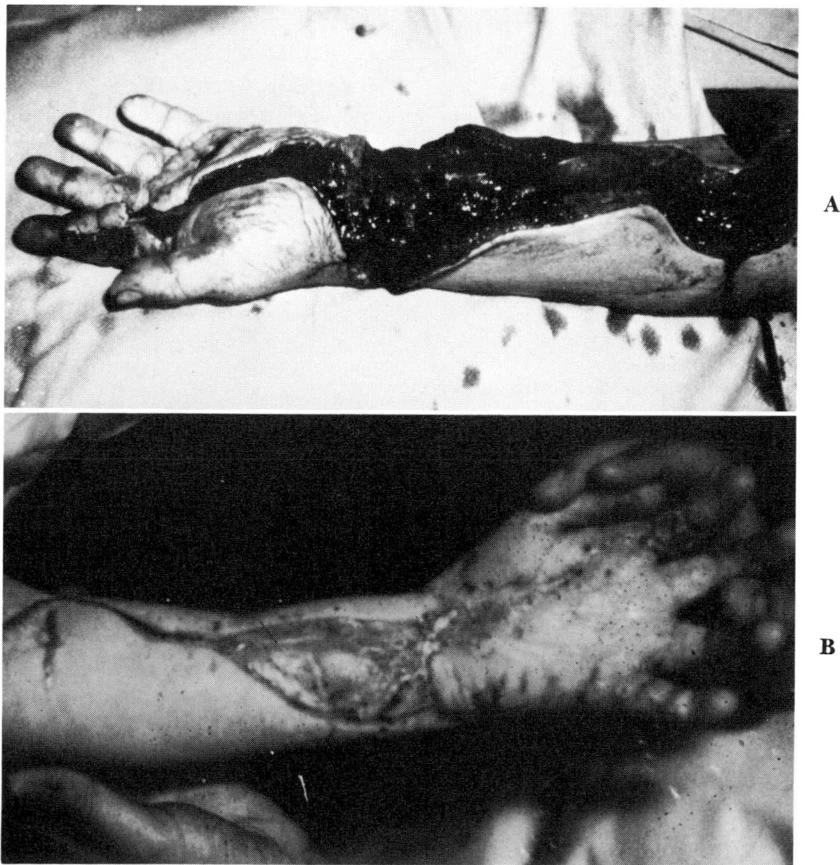

Fig. 4-4. **A,** A child caught his arm in the conveyor belt of a piece of farm machinery. **B,** Photograph of the arm in **A** after initial surgical care had been performed.

tion potentials with a few voluntary motor unit potentials firing on effort. These were of increased amplitude and firing at a rapid rate.

Discussion. One can define a degree or grade of injury to peripheral nerves based on electrical findings such as the availability of motor unit potentials, the number of fibrillation potentials present, and the conductivity of the nerve. A more formal classification of injury based on electrical findings is that of Sunderland, as seen below.

Sunderland's* classification of nerve injury:

Grade	Findings
Grade 1A—Mild	Rest—Silence Effort—Normal or slight decrease in number of potentials Chronaxy less than 1 msec. No R.D.
1B—Moderate	Rest—Very few fibrillations Effort—Few M.U.P. Chronaxy 1 to 10 msec. No R.D.
1C—Severe	Rest—Few fibrillations Effort—No M.U.P. Chronaxy 10 to 20 msec. after 7 days No R.D.
2A—Partial	Rest—Fibrillations in many samples Effort—Few M.U.P. Occasional polyphasics Chronaxy over 20 msec.
2B—Complete	Rest—Fibrillations in all samples Effort—No M.U.P. after 5 days R.D. after 5 days Conduction lost after 4 to 5 days Chronaxy over 30 msec. after 5 to 7 days
3—Severance	Rest—Abundant continuous fibrillations Effort—No M.U.P. R.D. from injury on Chronaxy 30 to 60 msec.

It is apparent from the electromyograph that the ulnar nerve lesion is complete, and attempt at surgical correction should be via direct attack with graft or tendon transfer surgery. Further delay would be a waste of time, as additional return will not occur.

The preceding three examples of peripheral nerve injuries are, of course, but a few types of trauma in which the electrodiagnostic information is of some help. Penetrating wounds, dislocated hip, and obstetrical palsy are a few additional examples. One should have in mind when ordering the study just what information is desired; for example, it may simply be establishing the existence of injury, determining the level of injury, or following the progress of regeneration.

Category II. Weakness in the child

The differential diagnosis of weakness in the child is a problem that frequently confronts the orthopaedist. Information sought from the electrodiagnostic study may be the diagnosis or the distribution of a known lesion or simply the rate of progress after a diagnosis has been made. One example of such a problem is meningomyelocele. In these cases the diagnosis is apparent. Since it is a lower motor neuron lesion, one is aware that fibrillatory activity would be the characteristic pattern. The electromyograph can be of some help, however, in determining the exact level of involvement, the status of the anal sphincter, and whether changes are taking place. Thus, long-range programming of the child's care can be aided.

Charcot-Marie-Tooth disease is another disease in which the diagnosis can be made clinically when the weakness is present in a particular distribution, at a relatively advanced stage, with good clinical correlation. However, in the early case or in those in which ataxia may be a differential diagnosis, the presence of a delayed conduction velocity may make the diagnosis. Fibrillation and fasciculation potentials may also be present at times in this disease.

Residual polio is also occasionally diagnostically unclear. More usually the electrical studies are done to document the distribution of involvement prior to performing reconstructive surgery. The electromyograph will characteristically show fasciculation potentials, as well as fibrillations, and a decreased number of voluntary potentials, placing the lesion at the anterior horn cell level. It should be remembered that the electromyograph does not provide a quantitative estimate of power and therefore should not be used exclusively to plan muscle transplant surgery.

Included in the differential diagnosis of generalized weakness in the child are muscular dystrophy, cerebral palsy, floppy baby syndrome, and Werdnig-Hoffmann disease. When muscular dystrophy is present, the electromyographic pattern

*From Licht, S.: Electrodiagnosis and electromyography, New Haven, Conn., 1956, Elizabeth Licht, Publisher, p. 317.

will be that of low-voltage, short-duration potentials occurring at a normal frequency and normal rate, whereas Werdnig-Hoffmann disease would produce fasciculation potentials characteristic of anterior horn cell pathology. Cerebral palsy is, of course, an upper motor neuron lesion, and findings in the electromyograph are not diagnostic. One will, however, note persistent insertional potentials, particularly when spasticity or hypertonicity is present.

Category III. Lumbar nerve root compression

Case 1. A 47-year-old man had the sudden onset of low back pain that radiated into the leg following lifting a heavy object at work. He had signs typical of S1 nerve root compression on the right side, and conservative management failed to relieve his symptoms. Myelography was done, and it revealed the defect seen in Fig. 4-5. Electromyography was done, revealing fibrillation potentials in the gastrocnemius and posterior tibial muscles, which are supplied by the S1 root. The history, physical findings, myelogram, and electromyograph are thus classical for herniated lumbar disc; this was corroborated by surgical exploration. In our laboratory the accuracy of diagnosis for myelography and electromyography is approximately 80% when either study is done alone. When both studies are done in consecutive cases, the accuracy is 85% to 90%. One source of difference is found when the dural sac is normally several millimeters from the posterior aspect of the vertebral body at the S1 level. In these instances a bulging or herniated disc may be present but not impinging on the dural sac. Electromyography for pathology at this level appears to be more productive than myelography. On the other hand, the search for fibrillations on the electromyography must be diligent and thorough, or the abnormal potentials may not be found.

Case 2. This patient was a 72-year-old man who had low backache with sciatica for 2 to 3 months. It was progressive in nature. Neurologic examination was equivocal, and the radiographs of the lumbar spine revealed moderately advanced osteoarthritis. Electromyography was then done, which produced fibrillation potentials in muscle groups of both lower extremities. In view of the electrical findings, myelography was carried out and revealed the complete blockage at the L4-L5 level seen in Fig. 4-6. At surgery a transdural approach was necessary to remove a chordoma that was impinging on the dural sac centrally.

Discussion. When bilateral denervation potentials are found, one must be suspicious of a large central disc herniation, tumor, or a more general-

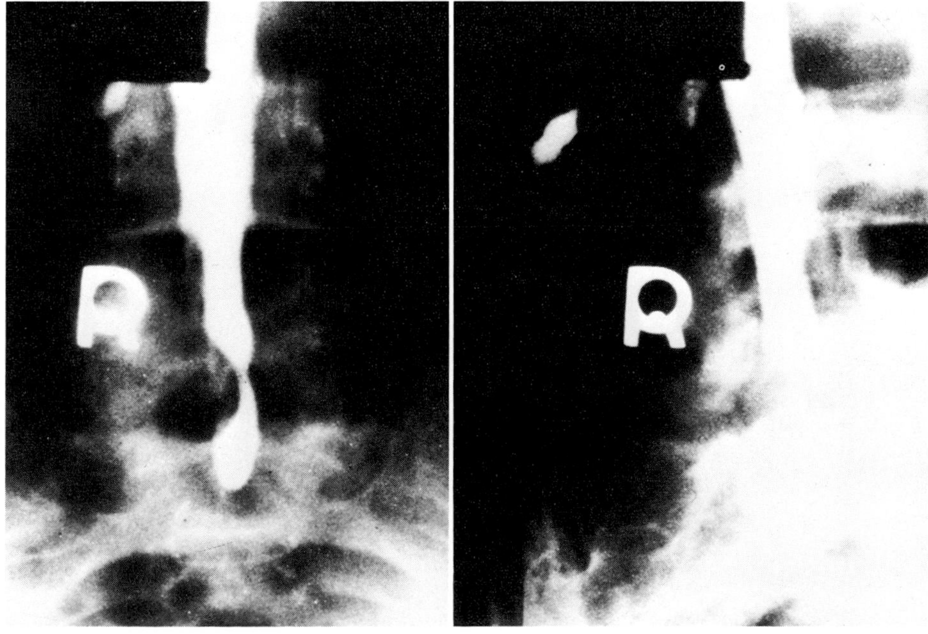

Fig. 4-5. Myelogram demonstrating a defect at the L5-S1 level on the right. This correlated with the electromyographic findings.

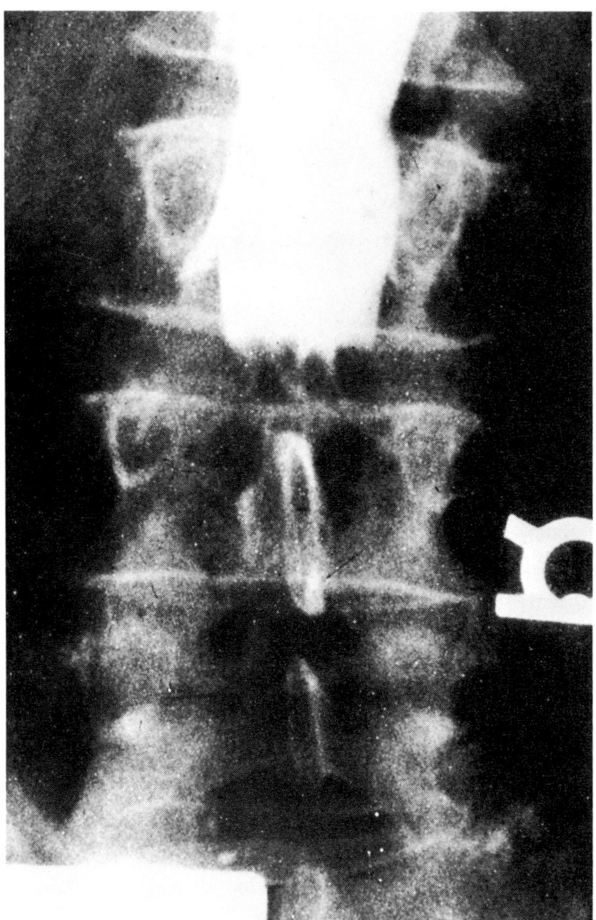

Fig. 4-6. Complete blockage of the dye column from a chordoma. Myelography performed after electromyography demonstrated denervation potentials bilaterally.

ized problem such as poly neuropathy. The latter diagnosis is ruled out by nerve conduction velocity studies. The patient under discussion was doing well 18 months after surgery.

Case 3. A 21-year-old primipara delivered a normal baby under spinal anesthesia. Following delivery she had severe low back pain and paralysis that was flaccid in the right lower limb. Electromyographic examination was done; it revealed fibrillation potentials in the right gastrocnemius and plantar intrinsic muscles. More detailed history revealed that backache with mild sciatica had been present the last half of her pregnancy. Myelography was done revealing an L5-S1 defect.

Discussion. In instances of sudden palsy, electromyography should be done early and again 21 days later, since fibrillation potentials appear at 14 to 21 days. If present in the early study, the lesion must have been present prior to the alleged onset, in this case at the time of the administration of the spinal anesthetic. If the palsy persists but no fibrillation appears, one may be able to prove malingering.

Category IV. Lower limb weakness in adult

This represents a group of patients who come to electrodiagnostic testing with a complaint of weakness in the lower extremities rather than severe pain. These have been separated from the lumbar compression group since the differential diagnosis more appropriately is neuropathy versus amyotrophic lateral sclerosis, versus spine tumor, versus simple senile debility. Characteristically these patients have noted weakness in the lower limbs bilaterally with progressive difficulty in walking or stair climbing and frequently with intermittent mild to moderate backache. Physical examination may show varying degrees of muscle atrophy and weakness in specific muscle groups, for example, those of the anterior compartment or quadriceps. In addition, the deep tendon reflexes may be diminished.

Case 1. H. F. was a 70-year-old woman. She presented a clinical picture of an active woman in whom the nerve conduction velocity was normal. The electromyographic examination, however, showed diffuse bilateral fibrillation potentials in the distal muscle groups. Myelography was carried out and was as seen in Fig. 4-7. The multiple indentations were due to hypertrophic osteoarthritis, and the patient underwent multiple foraminotomies. Eight months following surgery some motor return was occurring.

Case 2. G. J. was a 62-year-old woman with a similar clinical problem with the exception that the weakness in her legs was of relatively shorter duration, and the glutei were not involved. The electromyogram was normal, however, the nerve conduction study showed significant delay in both peroneal nerves. Further work-up produced an abnormal radioactive iodine uptake and B.M.R. with a subsequent diagnosis of myxedema neuropathy. More commonly, of course, the neuropathies of diabetes mellitus, nutritional deficiency, and pernicious anemia are seen.

Case 3. A. B. was a 67-year-old man with a similar clinical problem. He had normal nerve conduction velocities, but his electromyogram showed diffuse fasciculation and fibrillation potentials. In addition, there was a decreased number of volun-

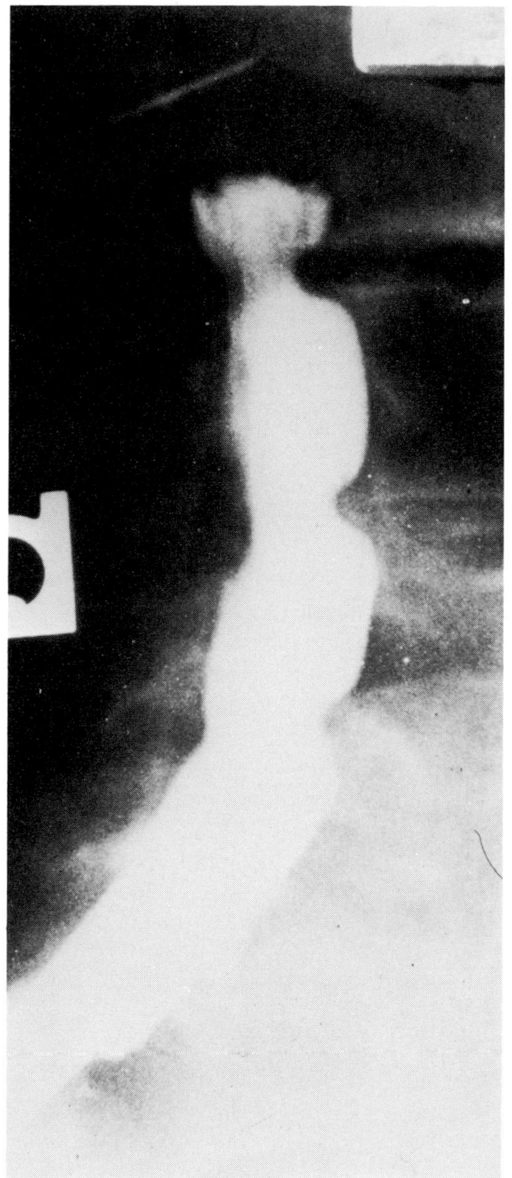

Fig. 4-7. Multiple defects produced by osteophytes.

tary potentials that were firing at a very rapid rate. The diagnosis of amyotrophic lateral sclerosis was made.

Category V. Shoulder hand syndrome

Pain that originates in the neck or shoulder region and radiates to the hand has frequently vexed the clinician. One is hard pressed at times to place the origin of the lesion, since it may arise at the spine or root level, the brachial plexus, the peripheral nerve, or, in fact, be referred from a distant point such as the cardiac diaphragm. Electromyography is of value in these cases when the neurologic system is involved.

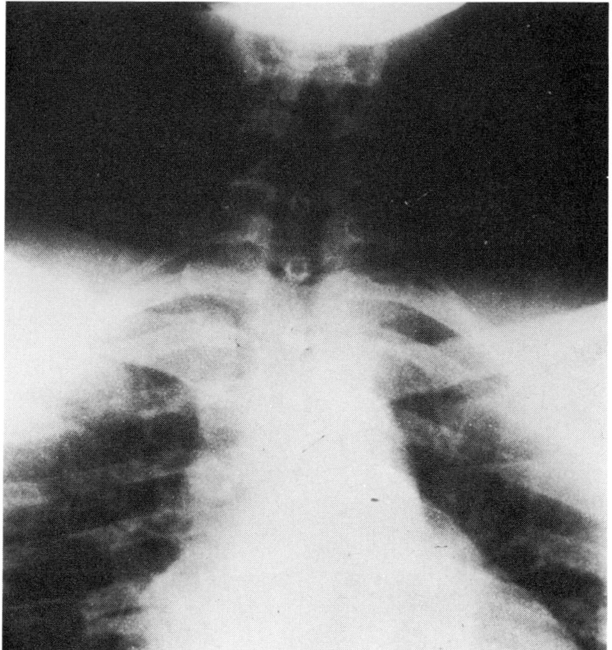

Fig. 4-8. Bilateral cervical ribs as a cause of shoulder hand pain.

Case 1. E. B. had increasing pain in the base of the neck that radiated to the forearm and caused tingling in the fingers. On physical examination all joints had a full range of motion, and the neurologic examination was said to be normal. There were fibrillation potentials in the ulnar nerve distribution, and on further study the radiograph seen in Fig. 4-8 demonstrated cervical ribs. Surgical decompression was carried out, and the symptoms remitted.

Case 2. In this patient (W. F.), persistent pain from the shoulder to the wrist was present. There was a questionably decreased biceps jerk on one side, and the electromyograph produced fibrillation potentials in both the first interosseous muscle and the pronator teres, that is, muscles of the ulnar and median nerves. This suggested nerve root level involvement, and myelography was carried out. The defect seen in Fig. 4-9 was noted, and surgical decompression of the nerve root successfully eliminated his symptoms after several weeks of conservative management failed.

Discussion. As mentioned, pain in the described distribution may be secondary to many types of lesions, from mechanical ones such as osteophytosis

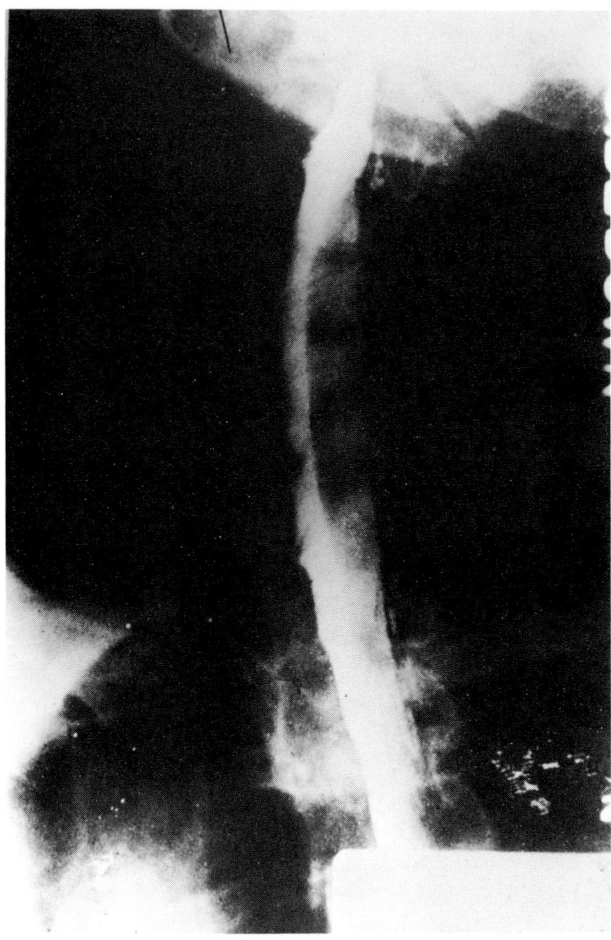

Fig. 4-9. Myelographic defect demonstrated after electromyography suggested nerve root compression.

to vascular ones such as cardiac insufficiency or sympathetic dystrophy. In these instances electrical studies may be helpful in ruling out brachial plexus traction injuries, polyneuropathies, etc. In addition, electrical studies have become popular in our center as a source of obtaining objective data in so-called flexion acceleration injuries or whiplash.

Category VI. Entrapment syndrome

Case 1. H. L. was a 38-year-old woman who complained of pain in the hand at night. Some relief was obtained if she arose and shook the hand, and she was concerned regarding the "circulation." On further questioning, there was slight numbness in the long and index fingers and increasing difficulty with fine movements, for example, buttons and sewing. Physical examination was unproductive except for an equivocal Tinel's sign over the median nerve at the wrist. Conduction velocities in both the ulnar and median nerves were normal, and the distal latency was normal in the ulnar nerve. The distal latency, however, in the median nerve was prolonged, thus placing the pathology in the median nerve at the wrist. When the clinical picture is complete, that is, with thenar wasting, specific hypesthesia, and reproduction of symptoms by digital compression at the wrist, the diagnosis, of course, is clear. However, such is not generally the picture, and there is good argument for early diagnosis and treatment, since rarely does atrophy of the thenar eminence revert following surgery.

Discussion. Entrapment syndromes can also be diagnosed in this manner in the median nerve at the pronator teres, in the peroneal nerve at the neck of the fibula, and in the ulnar nerve. For example, injuries at the upper end of the fibula may produce a delay in conduction over this portion of the nerve, whereas the ulnar nerve most frequently is involved in the groove at the medial aspect of the elbow. The diagnosis in these cases is based on the presence of normal conduction time in one portion of the nerve and delayed conduction time in another portion of the same nerve. When the compression exists for an adequate period of time under enough tension, fibrillation potentials will develop, although these are not necessary to make the diagnosis.

Category VII. Myasthenia

Stimulation and recording apparatus can also be used to aid in documentation of disease at the neuromuscular junction, that is, myasthenic syndrome and myasthenia gravis. Recording electrodes are placed into a muscle, and the muscle is exercised for a 3-minute period. The nerve to this muscle is then stimulated repetitively for 1 minute. One can observe directly from the oscilloscope the decreasing amplitude in motor unit potential as the chemicals at the neuromuscular junction are used up. This phenomenon is the myasthenic syndrome. When the process can be immediately reversed by administration of edrophonium chloride (Tensilon), the diagnosis is a myasthenia gravis.

In addition to the preceding categories of abnormality, the electrodiagnostic equipment is frequently used in the field of clinical research. A bibliography is appended that demonstrates the use of these tools in the study of regional kinesiology as well as as an adjunct in the study of neuromuscular physiology, and in the definition of some biomechanical neuromuscular properties. In our own laboratory clinical studies at the present time include a determination of accuracy of diagnosis correlating electromyography, lumbar myelography, and surgical findings, in consecutive cases. In a second program, simultaneous recordings are being made on a multichannel recorder from the forearm musculature of rheumatoid arthritis patients and normals. It appears that an imbalance exists between the extensor carpi radialis and extensor carpi ulnaris in those patients in whom radial drift of the carpus is present with subsequent ulnar drift of the phalanges.

REFERENCES

Texts

1. Aids to the investigation of peripheral nerve injuries, Medical Research Council War Memorandum No. 7, London, Her Majesty's Stationery office.
2. Cohen, Hyman, and Brumlik, Joel: A manual of electroneuromyography, New York, 1968, Hoeber Medical Division, Harper & Row, Publishers.
3. Haymaker, L., and Woodhall, B.: Peripheral nerve injuries, ed. 2, Philadelphia, W. B. Saunders Co.
4. Licht, Sidney, editor: Electrodiagnosis and electromyography, New Haven, Conn., 1956, Elizabeth Licht, Publisher.
5. Marinacci, A. A.: Clinical electromyography, Los Angeles, 1955, San Lucas Press.
6. Mayo Clinic and Mayo Foundation: Clinical examinations in neurology, Philadelphia, 1957, W. B. Saunders Co.
7. On amyotrophic lateral sclerosis, Mayo Clin. Proc. **32**:425, 1957.

Periodicals

1. Archibald, K. D., and Goldsmith, E. I.: Sphincteric electromyography, Arch. Phys. Med. **48**:387, 1967.
2. Basmajain, J. V., and Travill, A.: Electromyography of the pronator muscles in the forearm, Anat. Rec. **139**:45, 1961.
3. Bonner, F. J., and Schmidt, W. H.: EMG in disc dislocation, Arch. Phys. Med. **38**:689, 1957.
4. Buchtal, F.: EMG in acute polio, Acta Med. Scand. **116**:148, 1944.
5. Buchtal, F.: EMG in polymyositis, Neurology **3**:424, 1953.
6. Buchtal, F.: EMG in muscular atrophy of neurogenic origin, Neurology **3**:591, 1953.
7. Buentnal, F.: EMG is paralyses of the facial nerve, Otolaryngology **81**:963, 1965.
8. Byers, R. K., and Banker, B. Q.: Infantile muscular atrophy, Arch. Neurol. **5**:140, 1961.
9. Cone: Clinical EMG, J. Bone Joint Surg. **39A**:492, 1957.
10. Dedo, H. H., and Ogura, J. H.: Vocal cord electromyography in the dog, Laryngoscope **75**:201, 1965.
11. Denny-Brown, D.: Fibrillation and fasciculation, Brain **61**:311, 1938.
12. Doyle, B. J.: Clinical application of EMG, Arch. Phys. Med. **37**:748, 1956.
13. Eaton, L. M.: Symposium-ALS, Mayo Clin. Proc. **32**:425, 1957.
14. Erlanger, J., and Schoeple, G. M.: A study of nerve degeneration and regeneration, Amer. J. Physiol. **147**:550, 1946.
15. Funey: EMG in neck and shoulder disorders, J. Med. Soc. New Jersey **54**:74, 1957.
16. Gaugen: EMG in cerebral palsy, Amer. J. Ment. Defic. **56**:145, 1951.
17. Gough, J. G., and Koepke, G. H.: EMG determination of motor root levels in erector spinae muscles, Arch. Phys. Med. **47**:9, 1966.
18. Harvey, A. M.: The EMG in myasthenia gravis, Bull. Johns Hopkins Hosp. **69**:1, 1941.
19. Haskell, B., and Rouner, H.: Electromyography in the management of the incompetent anal sphincter, Dis. Colon Rectum **10**:81, 1967.
20. Hoefer, P. F. A.: Localization of spinal cord tumors, J. Neurosurg. **7**:3, 1950.
21. Huddleslon, O. L., and Golseth, J. G.: EMG in polio, Arch. Phys. Med. **29**:92, 1948.
22. Huxley, H. D.: The contraction of muscle, Sci. Amer., November, 1958.
23. Ingbert, H. O., and Johnson, E. W.: EMG evaluation of infants with lumbar meningomyelocele, Arch. Phys. Med. **44**:87, 1963.
24. Inman, V.: Function of shoulder joint, J. Bone Joint Surg. **26**:1, 1947.
25. Jones, R. V., and Lane, R. E.: Tight filum terminale, Arch. Surg. **73**:556, 1956.
26. Katz, R. L., and Gissen, A. J.: Neuromuscular and electromyographic effects of halothane and its interaction with C-tobocurarine in man, Anesthesiology **28**:564, 1967.
27. Kugelberg, E.: "Insertion activity," J. Neurol. Neurosurg. Psychiat. **12**:268, 1949.
28. Kugelberg, E.: Hereditary familial juvenile muscular atrophy simulating muscular dystrophy, Arch. Neurol. Psychiat. **75**:500, 1956.
29. Long, C., Brown, M., and Weiss, G.: Electromyography kinesiology of the hand. Part II. Third dorsal interosseous and extensor digitorum of the long finger, Arch. Phys. Med. **42**:559, 1961.
30. Lundervalt: Technical errors in EMG, Acta Psychiat. Scand. **29**:151, 1954.
31. Marinacci, A. A.: EMG and differential diagnosis neurosurgery versus neuronitis, Bull. Los Angeles Neurol. Soc. **21**:37, 1956.
32. Marinacci, A. A.: EMG in evaluation of neurological complications of spinal anesthesia, J.A.M.A. **168**:1337, 1958.
33. Marinacci, A. A., and Bull, L. A.: The medicolegal application of electromyography in peripheral nerve injuries, Neurol. Soc. **27**:147, 1963.
34. Moek: Postoperative disc EMG, J. Neurosurg. **8**: 469, 1952.
35. Pererson, C. R., and Wise, C. S.: Electromyographic method for objective measurement of muscle relaxant drugs, Arch. Phys. Med. **42**:566, 1961.
36. Reynolds, G. G., Pavot, A. P., and Kenrick, M. M.: Electromyographic evaluation of patients with post-

traumatic cervical pain, Arch. Phys. Med. **49**:170, 1968.

37. Schwab, R. S., and Stafford-Clark: Fasciculations in disorders other than progressive muscular atrophy, American Neurology Association, p. 169, 1950.
38. Shea, P. A.: EMG in diagnosis of nerve root compression syndrome, Arch. Neurol. Psychiat. **64**:93, 1950.
39. Thompson, W., and Kopell, H.: Peripheral entrapment neuropathies of the upper extremity, New Eng. J. Med. **260**:1261, 1959.
40. Thompson, W., and Kopell, H.: Peripheral entrapment neuropathies of the lower extremity, New Eng. J. Med. **262**:56, 1960.
41. Wagman, I. H., and Lesse, H.: Maximum conduction velocity of ulnar nerve, J. Neurophysiol. **15**:235, 1952.
42. Worster Drought, C.: Muscular fasciculation and reactive myotonia in polyneuritis, Brain **75**:595, 1952.
43. Watkins: The EMG in orthopedics, J. Bone Joint Surg. **31B**:823, 1949.
44. Weddell, G., Pattel, R. E., and Feinstein, B.: Electrical activity of voluntary muscle in man under normal and pathological conditions, Brain **67**:178, 1944.
45. Marble, H. C., Hamlin, E., Jr., and Watkins, A. L.: Regeneration of ulnar, median, and radial nerve. Amer. J. Surg. **55**:274, 1942.

Chapter 5

Bracing for patients with acquired spasticity

JACQUELIN PERRY, M.D.
Downey, California

Disabilities requiring orthopaedic attention generally are handled by directly correcting the cause or effect of the lesion. This is rarely possible for the patient with acquired spasticity. The cause of his malfunction lies within the spinal cord or brain, beyond the reaches of direct manipulation. As a result, the orthopaedic surgeon treats only the peripheral manifestations without approaching the primary site of dysfunction.[2]

Several clinical entities create this situation: the most common etiology is a stroke, which causes hemiplegia; brain damage from direct trauma is being seen with increasing frequency; an incomplete cervical or thoracic spinal cord injury results in a similar clinical picture. Multiple sclerosis generally causes less interference with the sensory modalities. Lacking the direct approach, the therapeutic program is focused on the peripheral structures to modify the influences on the central lesion as well as its effects. Bracing, for example, is used to rebalance inadequate motor responses and to modify the sensory input.

The overt dysfunctions are paralysis and spasticity. Paralysis is the inability to perform a desired moton. Spasticity is the exaggerated or prolonged muscle response that occurs. Both of these difficulties represent impairments in the motor–control and sensory–interpretation functions of the central nervous system. The peripheral motor system is intact. The muscles, except for a little disuse atrophy, are normal, as are the peripheral nerves, which provide the final stimulus for action and the immediate reception of sensory information. Generally, the loss of selective motor control is followed by the emergence of primitive patterns of motion. Clinical manifestations, therefore, are a mixture of paralysis, spasticity, and primitive pattern motion. Patients who fail to develop patterns as a substitute for weakened or lost selective control in their lower extremity have less capacity to walk, even though they do have less spasticity.

Selective motor control is the normal ability to move any joint independently, to combine motions as desired, and to vary the strength or duration of the muscle action at will. It is a cortical function. Primitive patterns, in contrast, are stereotyped combinations of flexion or extension generated from more ancient motor centers within the brain stem.

The motions constituting the flexion-extension patterns are the same as those in the withdrawal and thrust reflexes, only their mode of initiation is different. A reflex is a motor response to a sensory stimulus, whereas primitive patterns are initiated by the patient. When the patient has a severe lesion, he has to be in the posture that automatically makes use of the pattern before he can initiate any action. For an example, when lying in bed he may have no control of the lower extremity, but on standing he will be able alternately to stimulate his flexor and extensor patterns, thereby enabling himself to walk.

The strength and completeness of the muscular response in the involved extremities is determined by the nature of the lesion and cannot be varied by the patient. In contrast, the person with poliomyelitis or a peripheral nerve lesion has precise selective control of the remaining active musculature in the extremity and precise sensory perception, so that he can alter his usual mode of function to substitute for the impairment. This type of substitution is not available to the person who has lost selective control and is dependent on primitive patterns.

The spastic patient presents the tantalizing picture of a person who can initiate extremity motions, yet cannot alter them to voluntarily improve his situation. The extent to which this occurs depends upon the degree of impairment in motor control and sensory awareness. Differences between individuals range from slight hesitancy in selective control to complete dependence on patterns. Sensation is intact in some, others have disabling dullness of proprioception, and still a third group may evidence complete anesthesia. Until the clinician accepts and understands the presence of these semiautomatic primitive patterns and the significance of sensation as an influence on motor function, the performance and management of the adult spastic patient is very confusing.

In the lower extremity patterned motions are very useful. Walking is a repetitious act, and considerable variation from normal still permits the patient to move himself about effectively. Customary upper extremity function, however, is highly selective. The daily routines of eating, dressing, and personal care require reaching in numerous directions and working at different speeds. Many tasks are performed beyond the range of vision. Vocational and recreational activities further complicate the demands. Highly varied motions and good awareness of touch, pressure, and position are necessary to perform even simple tasks.

These different performance requirements markedly influence the effectiveness and use of bracing. One may generalize and state that the basic indications for bracing are to prevent deformity and assist function, but beyond this the use of braces in the upper and lower extremities differs so markedly that the management of each must be discussed separately.

Primitive patterns are quite discrete in the lower extremity. The flexion pattern consists of simultaneous hip flexion, knee flexion, and ankle dorsiflexion. Extension of the hip and knee with ankle plantar flexion comprises the extensor pattern. The flexor synergy provides a means of taking a step, and the extensor gives stance stability. Control of the foot is seldom balanced, however. The patterned response may be either excessive or insufficient. Braces cannot provide the basic motions necessary for normal walking, but they are very useful in modifying the patterns to make the gait safe and effective.

ANKLE-FOOT DISTURBANCES

Equinovarus resulting from tightness of the calf musculature is the most common ankle-foot disability. There may also be associated involvement of the posterior tibialis and toe flexor muscles. The tightness may result from contracture, spasticity, or an extremely strong pattern response. Equinus is generally the basic mechanism, with weight bearing twisting the foot into varus as the heel seeks the ground (Fig. 5-1). This occurs because the soleus muscle, inserting on the medial aspect of the os calcis, is commonly the most spastic or contracted muscle.

The customary method of controlling equinovarus due to other types of lesions is to apply a brace with rigid lateral supports, a down-stop at the ankle joint, and a dorsiflexing spring. These components constitute the familiar Klenzak brace.

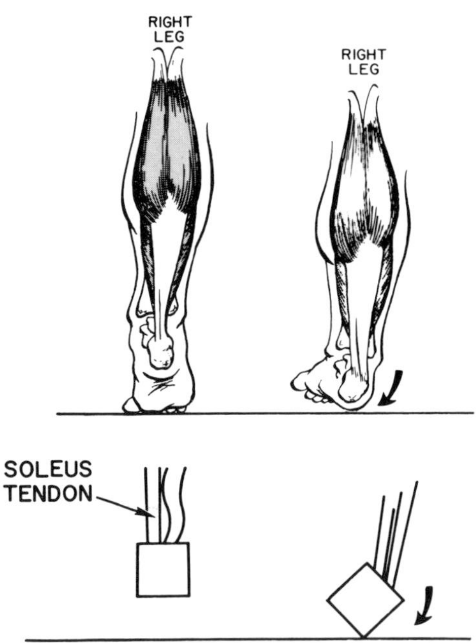

Fig. 5-1. Varus from soleus spasticity. Varus is a common sequel to attempting weight bearing in the face of a tight heel cord. The medial insertion of the soleus muscle on the os calcis creates a deforming lever to cause rotation as body weight tends to stretch the foot toward dorsiflexion.

Such a brace is appropriate if there is only a mild to moderate contracture. If, however, either spasticity or a strong pattern response is present, the Klenzak brace, in our experience, is inadequate. Better control is obtained if no action is permitted at the ankle joint, rather than just limiting movement. Springs are avoided, and the ankle joint is selectively locked in the best position for an individual patient. The improvement in the patient's gait readily demonstrates that the mechanical restraints of a locked ankle are not as disadvantageous as uncontrolled spasticity. A bichannel adjustable ankle locking brace (Bi-CAAL) (Fig. 5-2, *A*) is preferred to precut flanges because the ankle position best for the individual patient cannot be predicted.[4]

A locked ankle joint is a compromise between the range of motion normally used in walking and the need to restrict joint motion to control spasticity or pattern response. Normally, an individual uses about 15° of plantar flexion and 10° of dorsiflexion, as he swings from heel strike through midstance to the push-off position. When the ankle is locked at neutral, heel strike still tends to thrust the foot into plantar flexion. The locked brace transmits this force to the tibia, thereby creating a more vigorous knee flexion force. A little equinus would be desirable at this time. But during midstance, the ankle normally moves into about 10° of dorsiflexion to allow the trunk to pass forward over the flat foot, so that the other leg can reach for a step. Restriction of this range makes it more difficult to balance on the supporting foot and correspondingly shortens the step of the opposite foot. The compromise position is approximately 90°, but there are individual variations that depend on such factors as the hyperextension range within the knee, the height of the shoe heel, and the amount the foot slides within the shoe. To attain the very best position for the patient, walking trials and individual adjustments are necessary. This is readily accomplished with a bichannel (Bi-CAAL) brace. The depth of steel rods in each channel, fixed by setscrews, determines the ankle position (Fig. 5-2, *B*).

If the tightness of the calf structures is excessive, or if the associated involvement of the toe flexors or posterior tibialis is marked, varus often exceeds the stabilizing effect of the brace's lateral uprights, and the foot will twist in the shoe. Customarily, a T strap is applied as an additional stabilizing force. Ocasionally this is effective in the spastic patient, but more commonly the T strap merely serves to mask the disability, the foot still twists, and the patient's gait remains unstable. In this situation the potential of bracing has been exceeded, and more vigorous treatment with corrective casts or surgical release is necessary to attain a stable foot posture.

Occasionally the foot twists into valgus rather than varus. Experience has demonstrated that a large, hard rubber longitudinal arch support is more effective in controlling this deformity than a medial T strap.

Infrequently found is the patient with a passive drop foot, free from spasticity or contracture of the calf muscles, and having no tendency to go into varus. In these isolated instances, a wire coil spring brace is of value. Otherwise, the support this device offers is insufficient, and the stretch induced by the spring is an aggravation rather than a helpful influence. A posterior plastic "shoe horn" support (Fig. 5-3) is able to control mild spasticity, as well as the flaccid drop foot. It is more cosmetic and is a useful training aid for

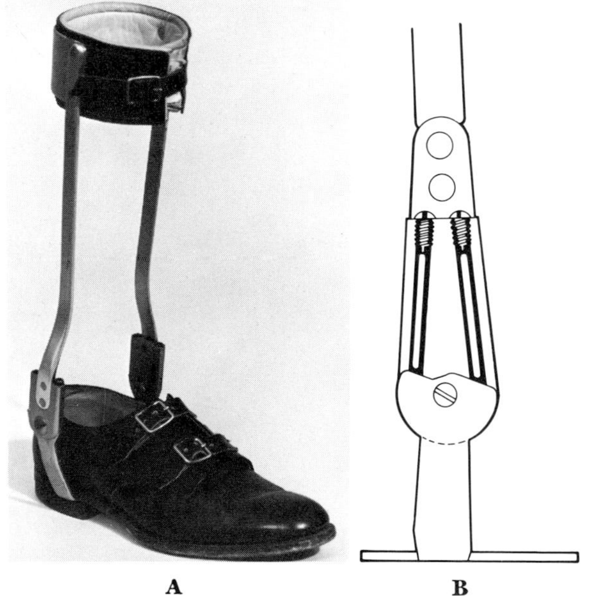

Fig. 5-2. A, Bi-CAAL brace. The basic brace for patients with acquired spasticity. It provides both ankle and knee stability in patients with adequate extensor patterns. **B,** Double channel adjustable ankle lock. Posterior and anterior ankle motion is determined by the depth of the channel rod fixed by the setscrew. This permits locking the joint in any desired position (or selection of a particular range of limited motion, in special circumstances). Adjustments are made merely by turning the setscrews. (From Perry, J.: Clin. Orthop., vol. 63, 1969.)

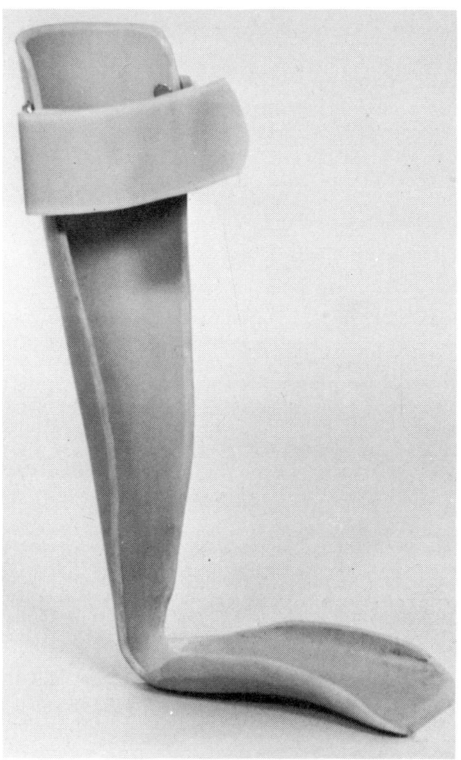

Fig. 5-3. Cosmetic brace. This brace, often called a plastic "shoe horn," provides a moderate degree of rigidity against plantar flexion and is useful in the patient with mild or no spasticity who needs to be supported out of equinus.

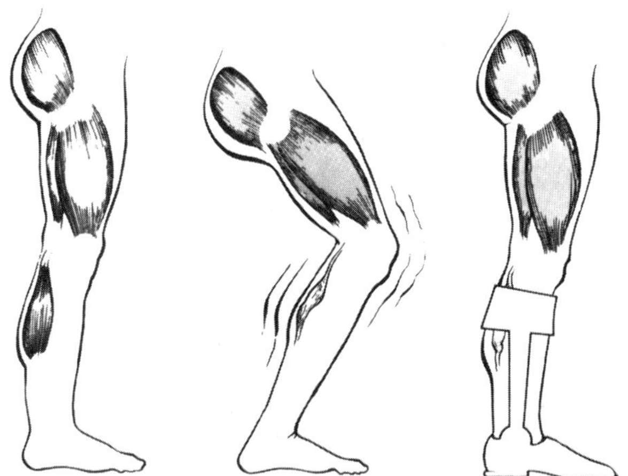

Fig. 5-4. Knee-ankle control relationships. The normal person or the patient with a good pattern response of the hip extensors, quadriceps, and calf muscles maintains adequate knee stability. When the calf muscles fail to participate in the pattern, the knee will flex because the ankle will yield to the dorsiflexion. Insufficiency of the calf muscles can be replaced with a short leg brace, thereby attaining knee stability whenever the extensor pattern is otherwise adequate.

the patient who can be expected to become brace-free.

KNEE

Knee dysfunction is generally one of two types: collapse into flexion or excessive hyperextension. Flexion collapse may result from an inadequate extensor pattern at the hip and knee, failure of the calf muscles to participate in an otherwise good extensor pattern, impaired proprioception, or a flexion contracture. In other types of disability the unstable knee customarily is controlled with a long leg brace, but this is inappropriate for the patient with spasticity. Locking the patient's knee prevents his taking a step unless he can circumduct.

When a patient has sufficient control of the hip and trunk muscles to advance a braced extremity by circumduction, he has good patterns and some degree of selective control. This person's knee instability is the result of inadequate ankle control by the calf muscles or of distal proprioception impairment. Both can be managed with a short leg brace (Fig. 5-4), the mechanism of control being as follows:

As the foot strikes the ground there is an abrupt interruption of its rapid forward travel during swing. Momentum continues to carry the tibia forward, tending both to dorsiflex the ankle and to flex the knee, the latter because body weight is behind the foot. A short leg brace that restricts this ankle dorsiflexion will stabilize the tibia,[3] thereby eliminating the flexion force at the knee. With a stable tibia, extensor pattern action at the hip and knee becomes more effective in stabilizing the thigh so that far less strength is required. In addition, the momentum that is carrying the body forward is made available to help extend the knee rather than add to the collapse.

If the patient's extensor pattern is not adequate to support the hip and knee, despite the aid of an adequate short leg brace, he will also be unable to take advantage of a long leg brace. The hip muscles are usually considered only in relation to their influence on the lower extremity. However, they also have a second function, that of stabilizing the pelvis (and hence the trunk) over the weight bearing extremity. A long leg brace supports only the knee and foot, not the trunk. When the extensor pattern is inadequate, the trunk falls away from the braced extremity toward the other side, preventing the patient from taking a step with the other foot. The reason for this is twofold. First, the trunk muscles on the involved side respond just as poorly as the hip extensors. Second, the patient lacks both the selective control and the sensory proprioception to substitute effectively by other maneuvers.

The patterned response presents a singular advantage over other forms of impaired muscle functions. Consistently, our staff has found that the strength of the quadriceps in the extensor pattern equals or exceeds that of the hip extensors. Thus, whenever the patient demonstrates sufficient hip extensor and trunk muscle response to balance the trunk over a long leg brace (or an extended knee cage), there will also be sufficient quadriceps strength to support the knee if the ankle is stabilized adequately with a short leg brace. As a means of providing anterior ankle stability (dorsiflexion restraint), in addition to controlling the other associated foot impairments, the Bi-CAAL brace is the support of choice.

Patients with poor extensor patterns require knee stabilization during their standing practice periods. Rather than prescribe a long leg brace (which infers that this will be a walking aid), an extended knee cage (Fig. 5-5) is used as a supplement to the short leg brace. The knee cage is not considered a brace because it is part of the therapist's armamentarium rather than a personally prescribed item. This policy is followed because if the patient does develop an adequate extensor pattern, he will need only a short leg brace. If not, he will not be able to walk, even with a long leg brace, because of hip instability.

Recurvatum of the knee is also best managed with a Bi-CAAL brace because of the strength of the deforming force. The deformity occurs in midstance as the patient attempts to bring his body weight forward over the supporting foot, in order to take a step with the other leg. Whether it is

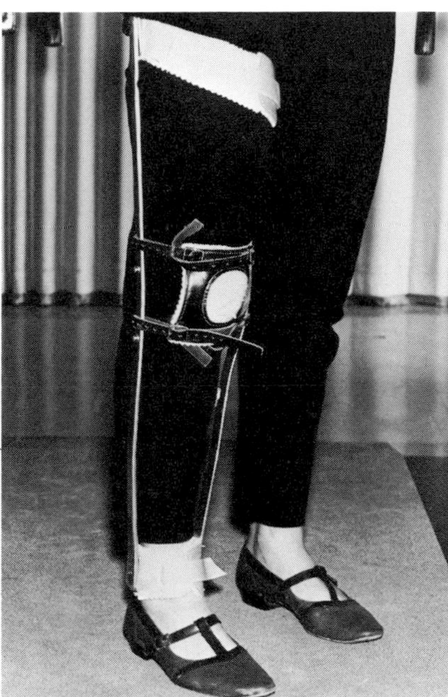

Fig. 5-5. Extended knee cage. The knee cage reaches from groin to ankles, with posterior cuffs at the ends and a knee control pad anteriorly. This length encourages the extremity to fall passively into extension. The usual knee cage with its ends close to the knee actually causes the knee to flex.

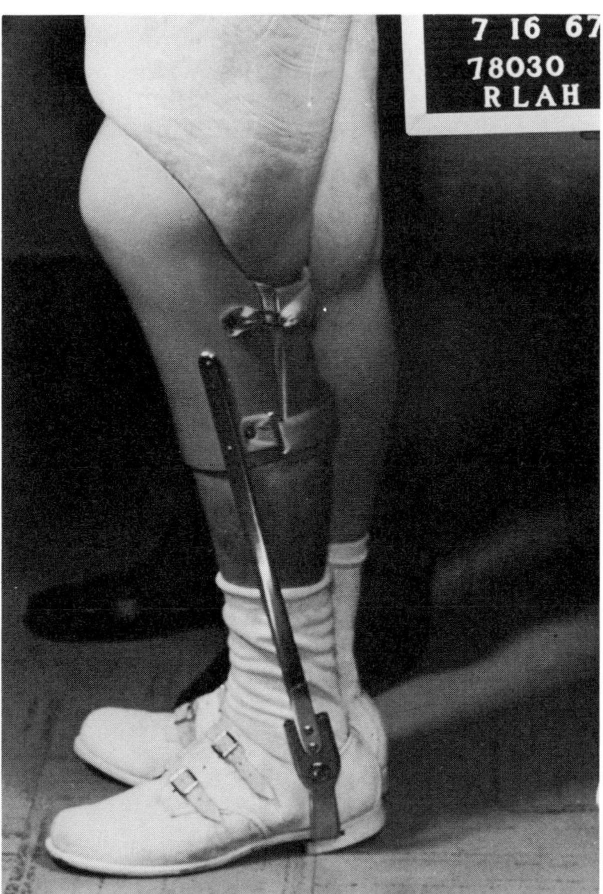

Fig. 5-6. Supracondylar brace. Pretibial shell with the supracondylar extension restricts knee hyperextension by creating pressure against the distal thigh. It is a useful training device but too uncomfortable for long-term use.

due to excessive plantar flexion at the ankle or to hypermobility at the knee, the tibia is angulated posteriorly at the ankle. Utilizing a brace to lock the ankle joint in slight dorsiflexion prevents the patient from assuming this position. It also creates a flexion thrust at the knee to further overcome the tendency to hyperextend. By having locked the ankle, rather than just applying a down-stop, knee stability also is assured when the hyperextension is a substitution maneuver for a weak quadriceps or impaired proprioception. If an overly strong quadriceps response is the cause, the deformity will occur a little earlier in the walking cycle, but the management is the same. Occasionally, a patient with a marked hyperextension range and impaired proprioception at the knee will rock back on his heel, even with the ankle locked. This can be restrained without restricting knee flexion by creating a force against the lower thigh. A pretibial shell with a supracondylar extension (Fig. 5-6) is substituted for the usual calf band on the short leg brace. This is a useful training device, but the pressure against the thigh is too uncomfortable for long-term wear.

UPPER EXTREMITY

In the lower extremity, improvement of a patterned response provided a useful function. This is not true in the upper extremity because simple, patterned action does not meet even the minimum daily needs of arm and hand function. As a result, the value of bracing is far more limited.

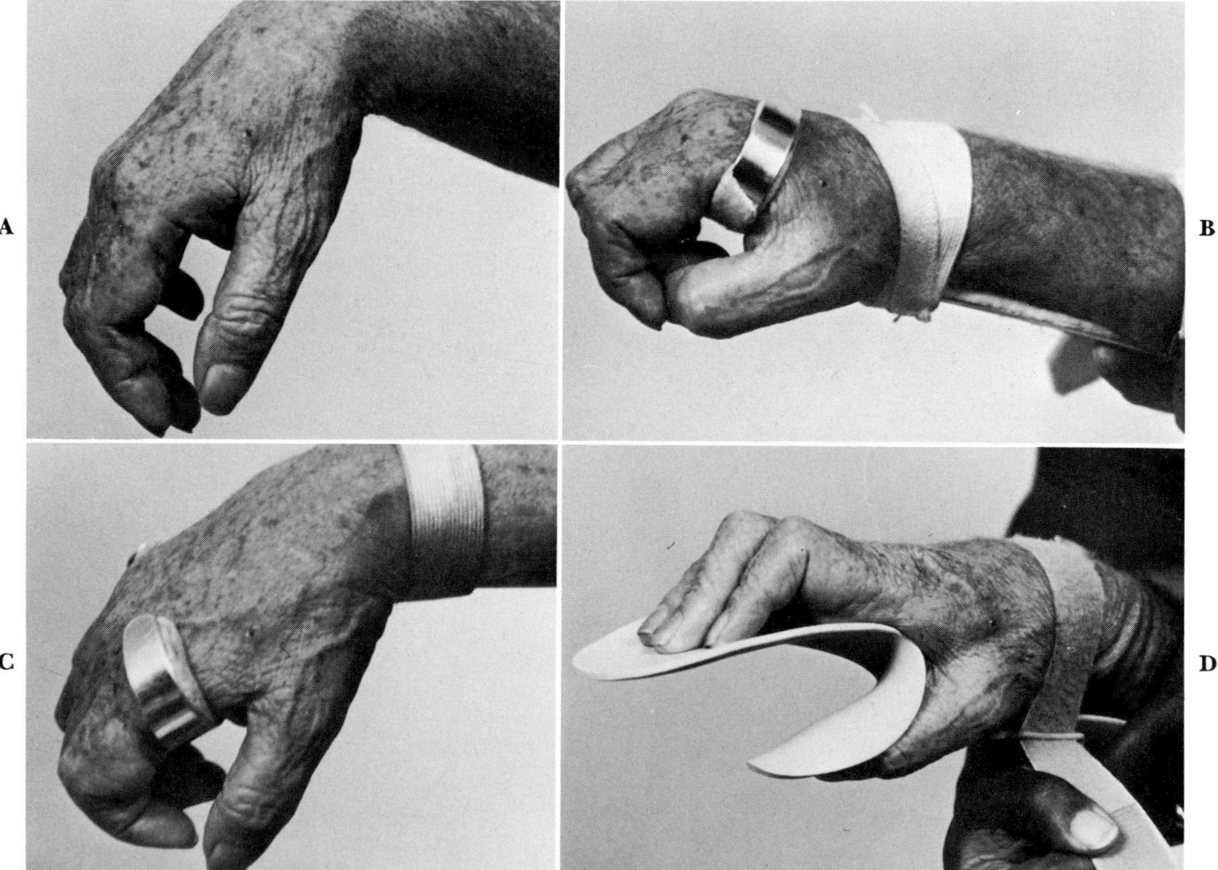

Fig. 5-7. Volar wrist splint. **A,** The degree of tightness (spasticity or contracture) is not apparent in the dangling wrist. **B,** When a volar splint is applied, tension of the fingers must be observed as the wrist is extended. **C,** The volar splint has been partially flexed so as not to cause undue tension on the fingers. **D,** The digital platform will not overcome the tightness. It merely concentrates the pressures in another area, contributing to brace intolerance. It is not indicated for the spastic hand.

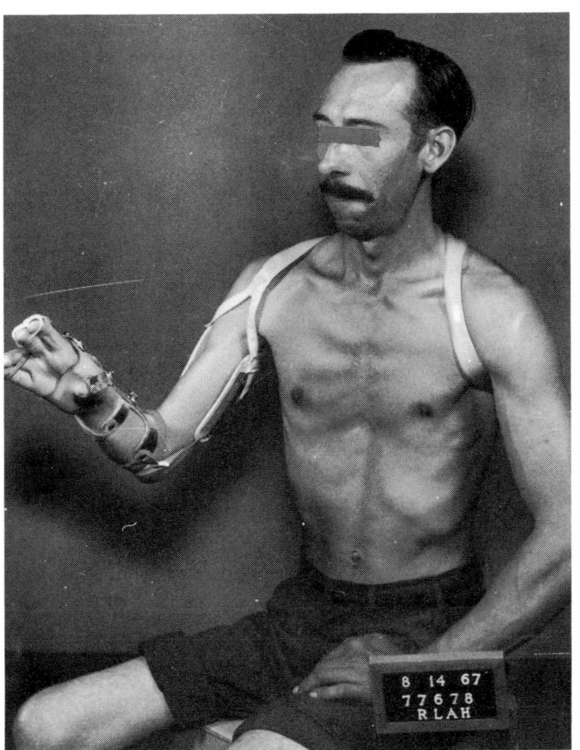

Fig. 5-8. Remote control finger assistance. The flexor hinge hand splint places the fingers in a position of functional pinch. The contralateral shoulder loop provides active opening. Closure is active by a picture of selective control. (From Braun, R. M.: Clin. Orthop., vol. 63, 1969.)

Fig. 5-9. A, Sling. This customary form of arm support is indicated only if it is accompanied with an active range of motion program to avoid aggravating the adduction internal rotation deformities that the spastic patient tends to develop. **B,** Axillary roll. Better positioning of the subluxated shoulder with associated relief of pain is accomplished with the axillary roll. In addition, it avoids maintaining the arm in a deforming posture. Hand edema has not been a complication of this device.

A

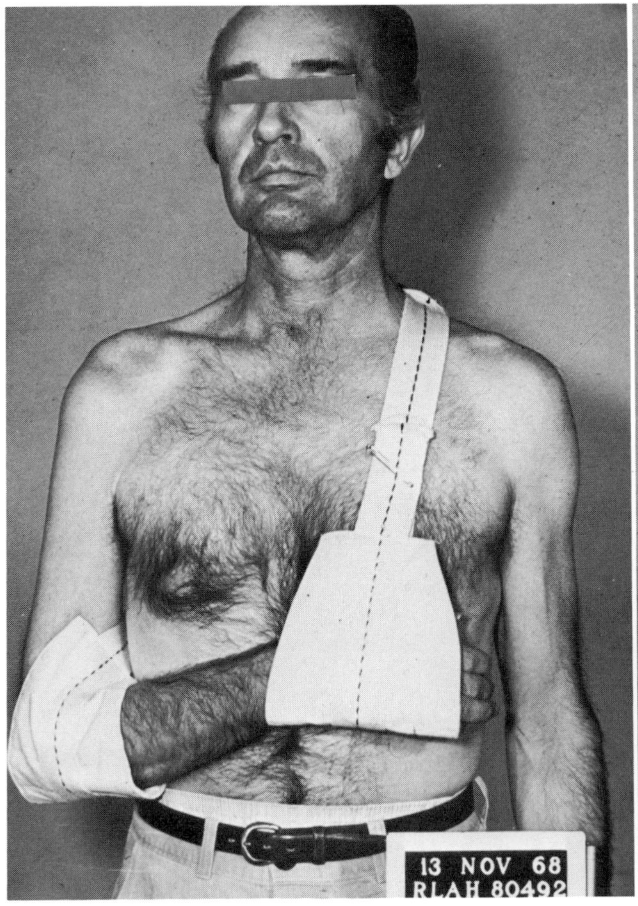

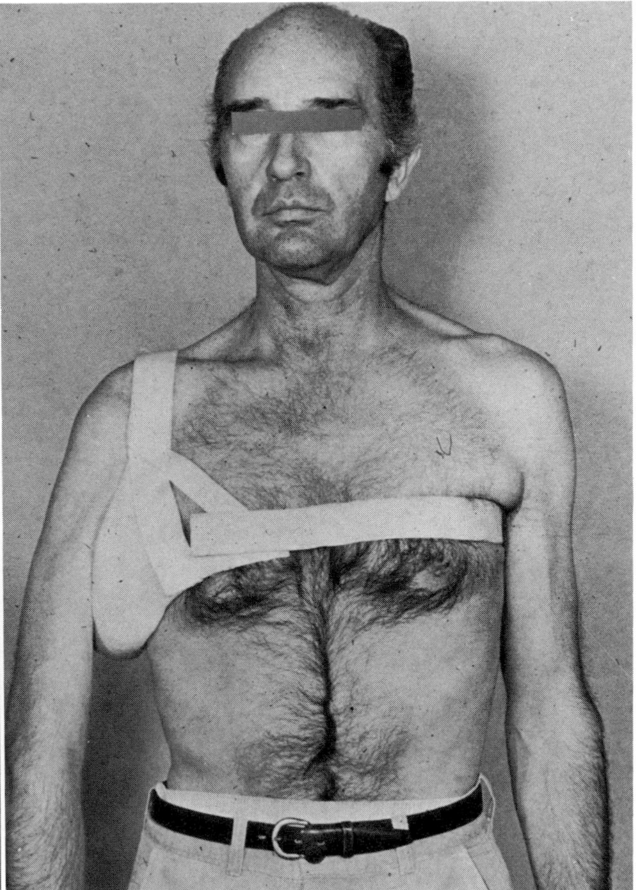

B

The most common indication is avoidance of progressive deformity with a simple volar splint to support a flexed wrist (Fig. 5-7, *A*). When applied early, contractures within the wrist and finger muscles generally can be controlled so that the hand can rest in a functional position. If a patient is seen late or if considerable spasticity develops, then the brace will have to be flexed to accommodate to the degree of deformity and subsequently modified as the patient's condition improves (Fig. 5-7, *B*). When there is either spasticity or contracture, the finger flexors are tightened as the wrist is extended. Attempts to force the wrist onto a preset splint merely cause greater spasticity and an intolerance of the brace. The skin is an intermediate structure between the rigidity of the spastic muscles and that of the brace itself. This is true even with the addition of a volar platform for the fingers (Fig. 5-7, *C*). If physical therapy techniques are unable to decrease the contractures of the muscle, a brace may not be tolerated until surgical release has been accomplished (Fig. 5-7, *D*).

Bracing as a means of assisting function is indicated only when the patient has adequate sensation, some finger extension, and sufficient cognition to operate a remote control unit (Fig. 5-8). The brace provides a more rapid and more complete opening and closing of the hand. Long-term acceptance of such a unit is limited to the patient with a particular vocational requirement. However, dynamic finger assistance is an effective training aid for the patient with brain trauma.

Bracing of the painful shoulder has been difficult. The sling is the most convenient aid (Fig. 5-9, *A*), but this is safe only if it is combined with a daily range of motion to avoid further encouraging the adducted, internally rotated posture. If the patient is dependent upon a wheelchair, a wide armrest and dowel handpiece provide good positioning of the symptomatic arm. Corrective support for the ambulatory patient is more complex. A forearm trough arising from a gun holster base gives good positioning, but this interferes with the ease of dressing and thus is only a part-time aid. The flaccid or mildly spastic shoulder responds to an axillary roll[1] (Fig. 5-9, *B*). All the devices must be combined with a good range of motion program, and, if the condition persists, surgical release of the subscapularis should be considered.

SUMMARY

Lower extremity bracing is an effective means of providing a safe and more efficient method of walking if the patient has an extensor pattern for hip stability and sufficient flexion pattern to take a step. At the same time, bracing of the upper extremity is almost completely restricted to the prevention of deformity, and assisting in its correction. Thus, bracing is used in the adult patient with spasticity to help correct the gait and hand function disturbances resulting from loss of selective control, effects of spasticity and contracture, imbalance, inadequacy of patterned motion, and impaired proprioception.

In either extremity, bracing is restricted to the mild and moderate deformities. When the disability is severe, surgical release or other intensive efforts are required before a brace can be tolerated.

REFERENCES

1. Bobath, Karl, and Bobath, Berta: Personal communication.
2. Mooney, Vert: Personal communication.
3. Sutherland, D. H.: An electromyographic study of the plantar flexors of the ankle in normal walking on the level, J. Bone Joint Surg. **48A**:66, 1966.
4. Young, John: Personal communication.

Chapter 6

Diagnosis and management of internal derangements of the knee joint

ARTHUR J. HELFET, B.Sc. (Capetown), M.D., M.Ch. Orth. (Liverpool)
New York, New York

The successful management of internal derangements of the knee joint is based upon:

1. Exact diagnosis
2. Meticulous gentle surgery
3. Adequate postoperative reablement

MECHANICS OF THE KNEE JOINT

Correct diagnosis depends upon an understanding of the mechanics of the knee joint, the pattern of its movements, and the manner in which these are controlled by the muscles of the thigh and guided by the cruciate ligaments and menisci.

The knee joint is not a hinge joint. In flexion and extension, the tibia navigates a helical course on the lower end of the femur, rotating outward on extension and inward on flexion. When the thigh muscles are relaxed, the tibia may be freely rotated on the femur, but when the muscles are contracted and especially in weight bearing, there is synchronous rotation of the tibia on the femur, that is, the tibia always rotates outward when the knee joint extends, and inward when it flexes.

Examination of the normal knee (Fig. 6-1, *A*) in extension shows that the tibial tubercle is opposite the outer half of the patella with the medial femoral and tibial condyles an exact fit, due to the rotational alignment of the one on the other. If the hand is run along the medial side of the knee joint, the two condyles present a smooth, curved surface.

When the knee is flexed (Fig. 6-1, *B*), the tibia rotates inward, and the tibial tubercle is seen to be opposite the medial half of the patella. Thus, differences in the rotation of one knee, when compared with the other, becomes immediately obvious.

The lower end of the femur is bicondylar in shape. The medial condyle is longer and curved, while the lateral condyle is rounded (Fig. 6-2). It acts as a ball-and-socket joint for the lateral condyle of the tibia. Thus, as the knee straightens, the medial condyle of the tibia rotates outward on the axis of the lateral, taking a longer course on the medial femoral condyle (Fig. 6-3).

The model (Fig. 6-4, *A*) of the knee joint has a ball-and-socket joint representing the lateral condyle and a long, curved facet that represents the medial condyle of the femur. The fibular side of the leg is colored red, the tibial side white.

The model, as also the knee itself, illustrates the synchronous rotation of the tibia and the resultant helical movement. In full flexion the tibial tubercle is well medial, and the fibular part of the model presents.

As the knee joint straightens (Fig. 6-4, *B*), the tibial tubercle moves laterally in relation to the pa-

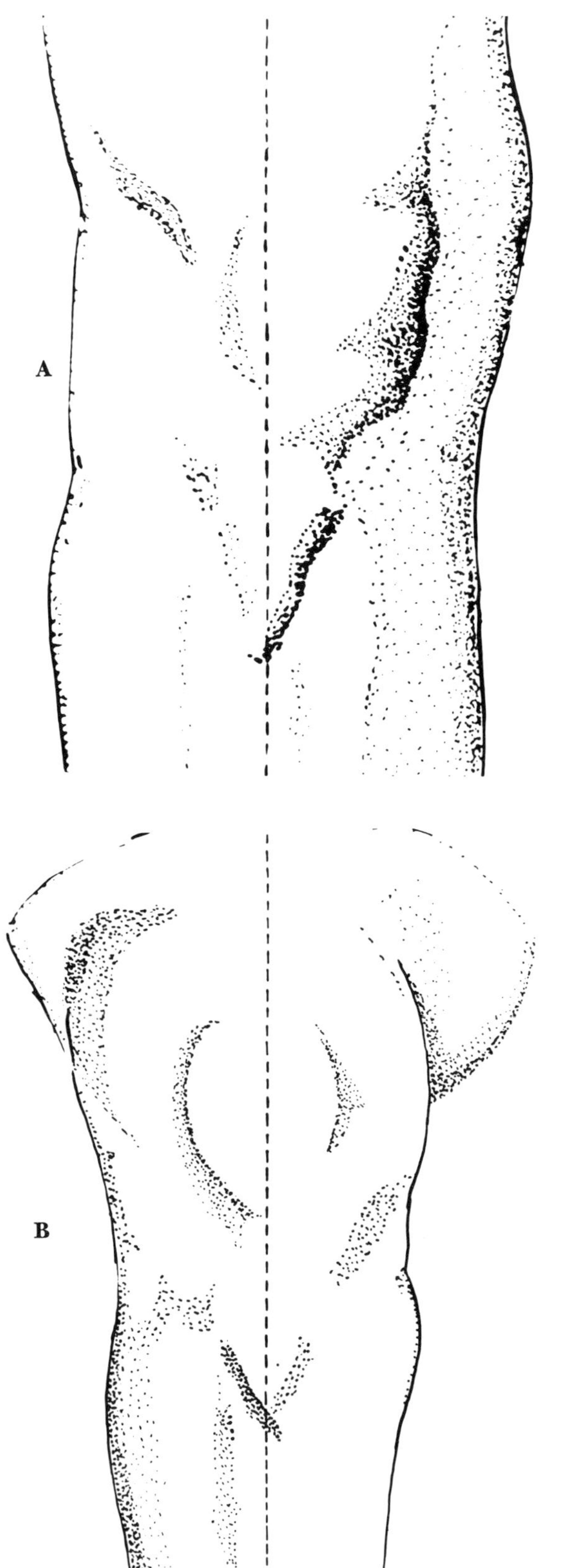

Fig. 6-1. A, Diagram of extended knee. **B,** Diagram of flexed knee.

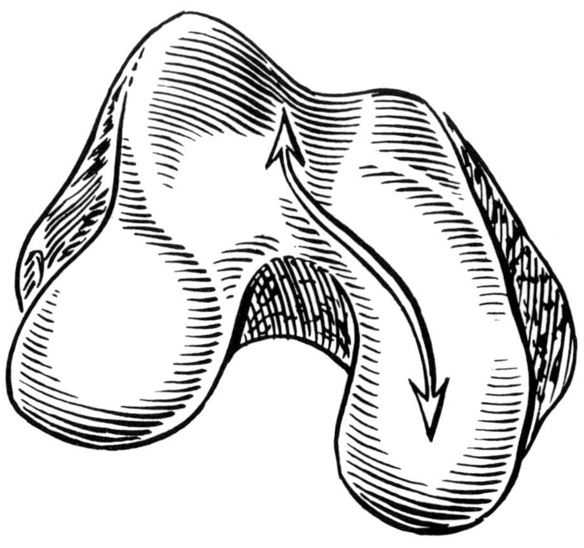

Fig. 6-2. Drawing showing diverse curves of bicondyloid lower end of femur necessitating helicoid movement. (From Helfet, A. J.: The management of internal derangement of the knee, Philadelphia, 1963, J. B. Lippincott Co.)

tella, and the tibial side of the model becomes more obvious (Fig. 6-4, *C*), until finally, in full extension (Fig. 6-4, *D*), the tibial tubercle aligns with the lateral part of the patella, and the tibial half of the model has reached full external rotation.

The medial tibial condyle must obviously take a sinuous course due to the shape of the lower end of the femur (Fig. 6-5). At the same time, the patella has to follow a similar sinuous excursion. In flexion, the medial part of the patella is in contact with the lateral surface of the medial condyle. As the knee straightens, the patella follows a sinus path, to reach, in full extension, its comfortable bed in the trochlear groove. If external rotation is prevented, the contracting quadriceps muscle forces the medial side of the patella to impinge against the medial condyle.

Examination of the opened knee reveals that the anterior cruciate ligament would also impinge on the medial femoral condyle if the tibia is prevented from rotating laterally during extension (Fig. 6-6).

CONTROL AND GUIDE MECHANISMS OF THE KNEE JOINT

The synchrony of rotation with flexion and extension of the knee joint with movement is *controlled* by the muscles of the thigh.

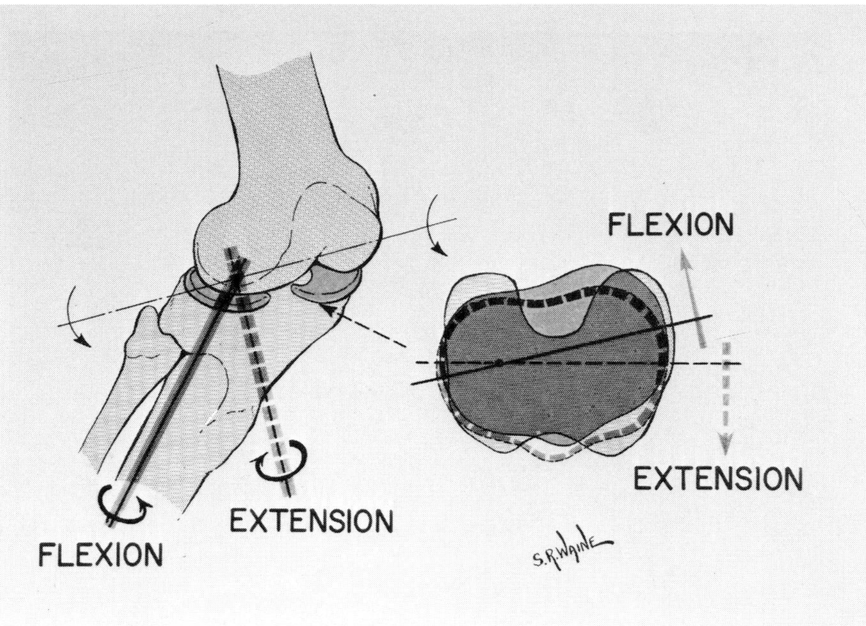

Fig. 6-3. Illustration of tibial rotation.

The extensor muscles run from without inward (Fig. 6-7, *A*), to insert into the patella and by means of the quadriceps expansion and strong medial capsule and ligaments attach to the medial border of the tibia. Extension is necessarily accompanied by external rotation of the tibia.

Those hamstring muscles inserting into the tibia are attached to its medial side, and active flexion must cause a synchronous internal rotation of the tibia. The popliteus muscle is one of the stabilizing muscles. In weight bearing it holds the outer side of the femur while the tibia rotates on the medial condyle. It also has attachments to the posterior end of the lateral meniscus to stabilize this side of the joint in extension and flexion (Fig. 6-7, *B*).

The biceps femoris and tensor fascia lata (Fig. 6-7, *C*) are independent of the knee joint. Running directly to the fibular head, they stabilize the leg when it bears weight, especially when the knee is bent. In this position the tibia must rotate on the femur. This would produce instability if the biceps femoris muscle did not stabilize the leg. The integrity of the superior tibiofibular joint is also essential. Should the joint become unstable, the leg will buckle while flexion is taking place.

The movements of the knee joint are *guided* by a system of menisci and cruciate ligaments that, with the capsular ligaments, keep the tibia in its tracks on the femoral condyles and so maintain the normal stable pattern of movement. This guide mechanism, in the form of a figure-of-eight, with intimate connections between the menisci and the cruciate ligaments, acts rather in the manner suggested in Fig. 6-8. The menisci are morphologically tendinous.

The view that the cruciates exist as "check-straps" to prevent anterior and posterior glide is false. Abnormal glide never occurs after injury unless the capsule of the knee joint has also been disrupted. The menisci have a degree of elasticity and of mobility in their anterior halves, to compensate for the distortion of sudden asynchronous movement (Fig. 6-8).

MANNER OF DERANGEMENT OF MENISCI

Most internal derangements of the knee joint are due to nothing more than the forced interruption of this synchrony. The footballer catches his toe while falling, thus flexing his knee without internally rotating the tibia (Fig. 6-9, *A*). When the natural elasticity of the meniscus or guide rope has been overcome, it splits along the line of its fibers. Similarly, the tibia may be forced to rotate without synchronous extension, or the knee may straighten with rotation prevented. This is illus-

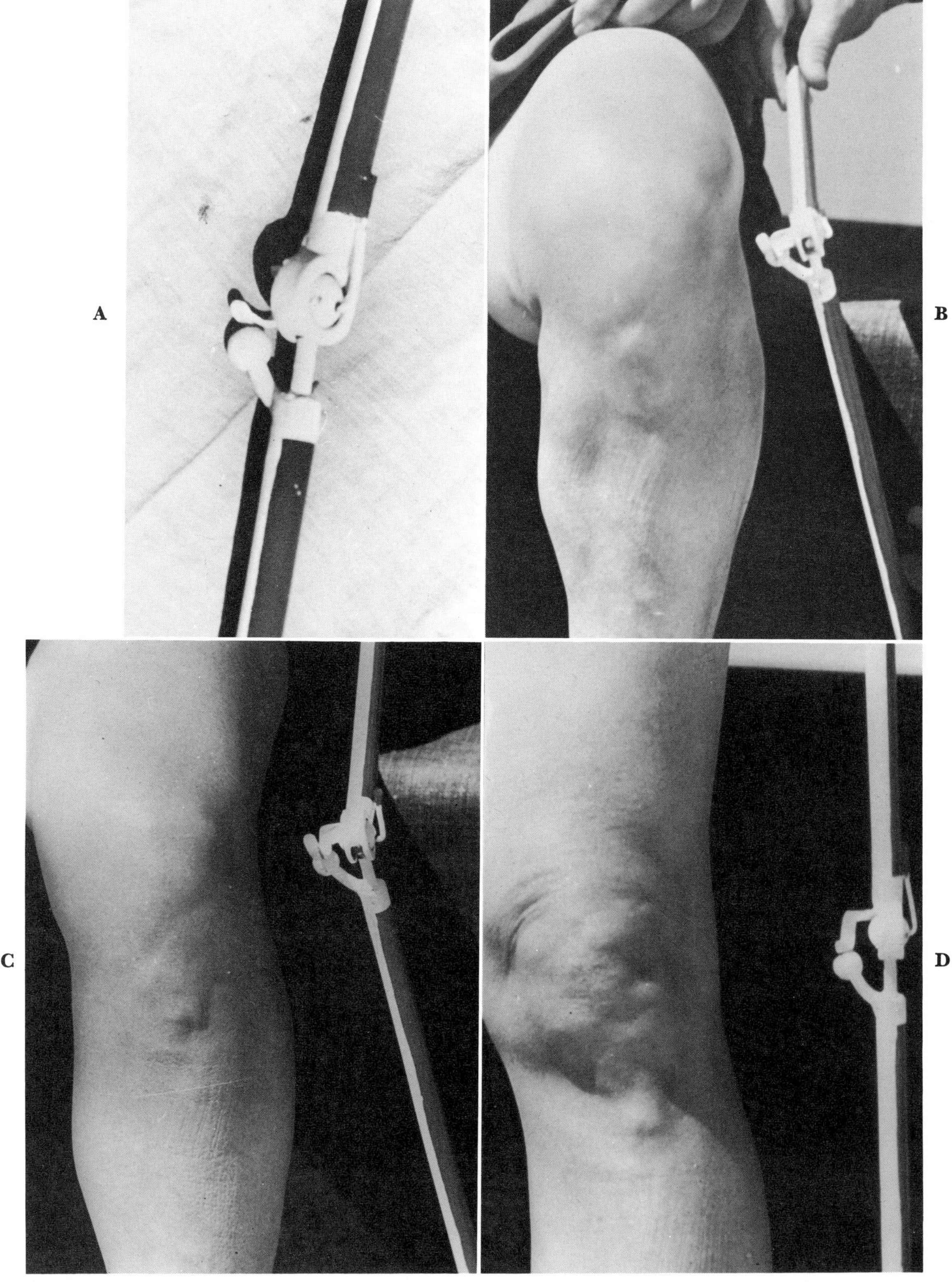

Fig. 6-4. A, The model. **B,** Model flexed. **C,** Model extending. **D,** Model fully extended. (Note movement of tuberosity of tibia in relation to the patella.) (From Helfet, A. J.: The management of internal derangement of the knee, Philadelphia, 1963, J. B. Lippincott Co.)

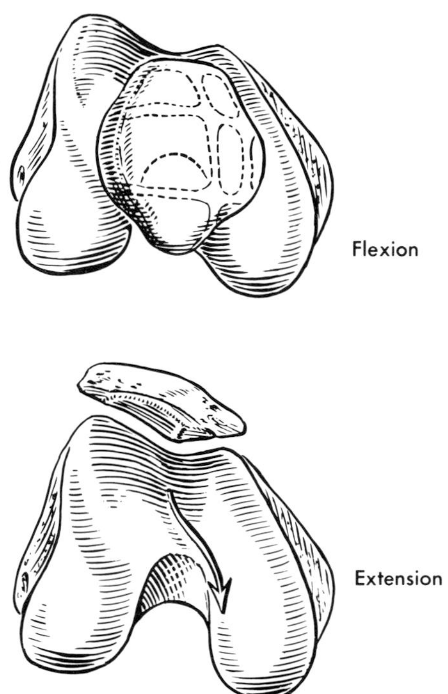

Fig. 6-5. Diagram showing associated sinuous or helicoid excursion of patella. (From Helfet, A. J.: The management of internal derangement of the knee, Philadelphia, 1963, J. B. Lippincott Co.)

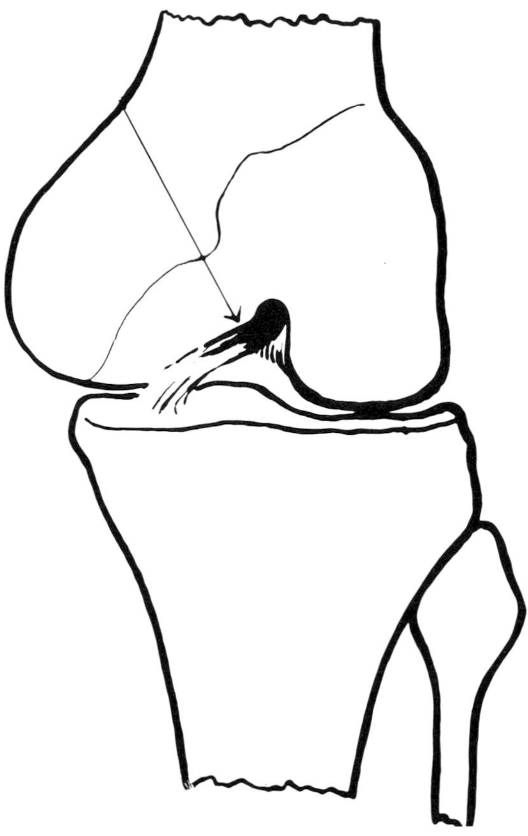

Fig. 6-6. Diagram showing anterior cruciate ligament impinging on medial femoral condyle, when tibia is prevented from rotating laterally during extension. (From Helfet, A. J.: The management of internal derangement of the knee, Philadelphia, 1963, J. B. Lippincott Co.)

trated by the case of a carpenter who crouched before a chest of drawers (Fig. 6-9, *B*), attempting to dislodge one of its drawers. The drawer gave suddenly; the carpenter twisted his weight onto one acutely flexed knee. He developed an intense pain on the medial side of that knee, and to relieve it he threw himself onto the other knee, with similar results. In both instances, rotation took place without extension. Operation confirmed, bilateral medial meniscal tears.

In older people the mechanism is altered by changes in the meniscus and articular cartilage due to the aging process.

What happens when excessive traction is applied to the normal meniscus? It lengthens by either splitting across its shortest border, producing a parrot beak tear, or it splits longitudinally through its substance, so that it may *bowstring* and take a shorter route across the joint (Fig. 6-10, *I*). On the other hand, it may detach from one or the other end, leaving the necessary gap to accommodate the lack of rotation—the *retracted* meniscus (Fig. 6-10, *II*).

The term bowstring meniscus is used to describe what most writers call a bucket handle tear of the meniscus (Fig. 6-11, *A*). A shearing strain has been applied to the meniscus, and it splits longitudinally along the line of its fibers. The injuring force has prevented synchronous rotation, and the split is usually vertical but may be horizontal.

The length of the split is usually of equal extent, namely, about half the width of the patella. The free border of the meniscus *bowstrings* into the intercondylar notch. The knee becomes "locked." A better term would be "blocked." In most cases there is some loss of extension, but careful observation will always reveal an almost total block to synchronous external rotation. Occasionally the patient or the surgeon may reduce the bowstring portion. Often under anesthesia, or even often without it, manipulation results in a sudden freeing of this block, and we think we have reduced it. What really happens is that the bowstring snaps and coils up, usually at the anterior end. The

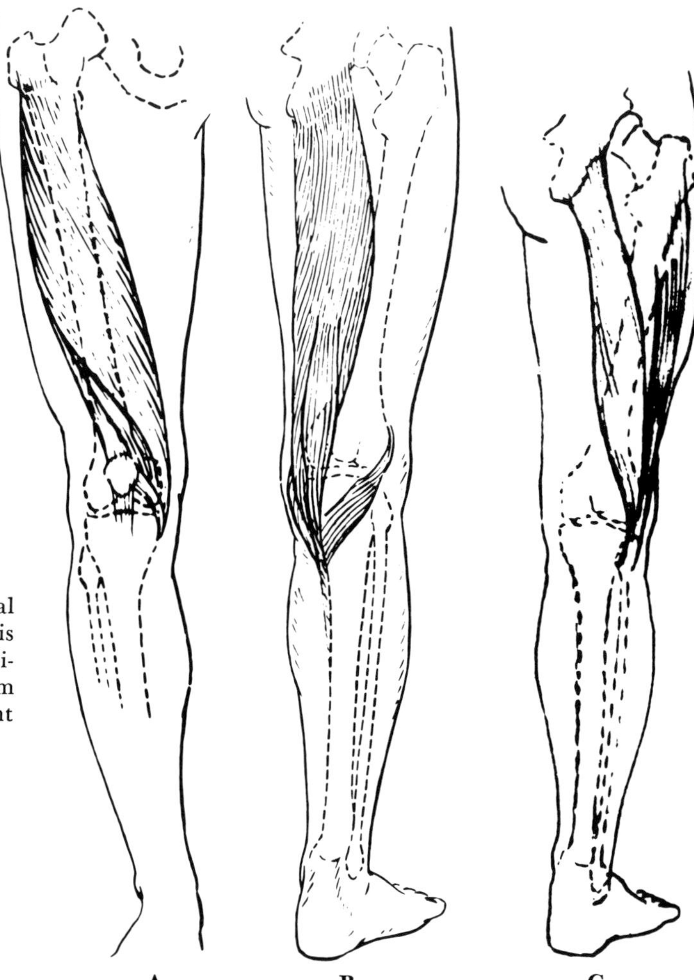

Fig. 6-7. A, Muscular control—extension and external rotation by the quadriceps femoris with vastus medialis prominent. **B,** Muscular control—hamstrings and popliteus. **C,** Biceps femoris and tensor fascia lata. (From Helfet, A. J.: The management of internal derangement of the knee, Philadelphia, 1963, J. B. Lippincott Co.)

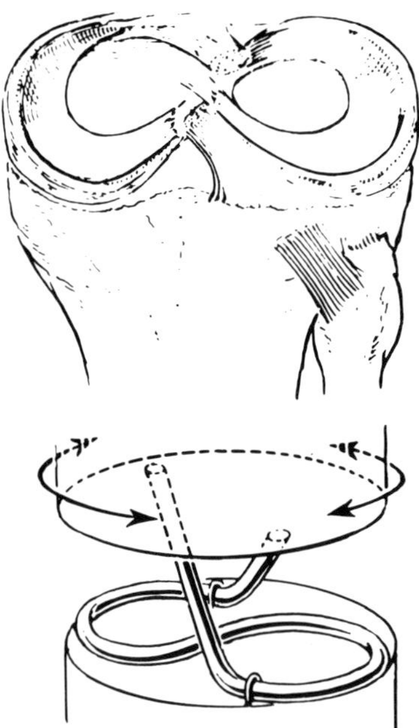

Fig. 6-8. Action of guide mechanism. (From Helfet, A. J.: The management of internal derangement of the knee, Philadelphia, 1963, J. B. Lippincott Co.)

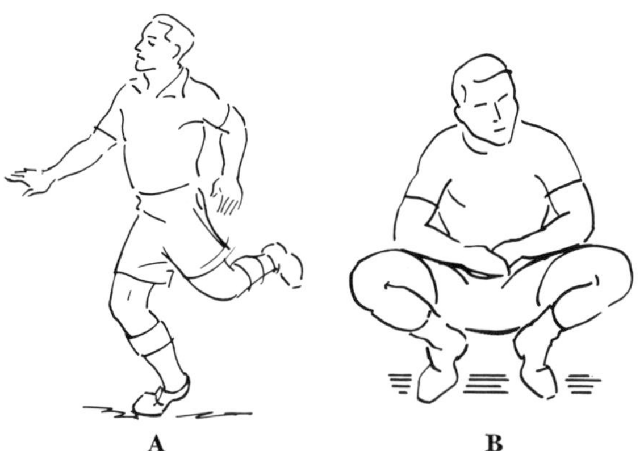

Fig. 6-9. A, Football player. Internal rotation of tibia during flexion is forcibly prevented. **B,** Carpenter squatting. A sudden asynchronous movement would injure the meniscus.

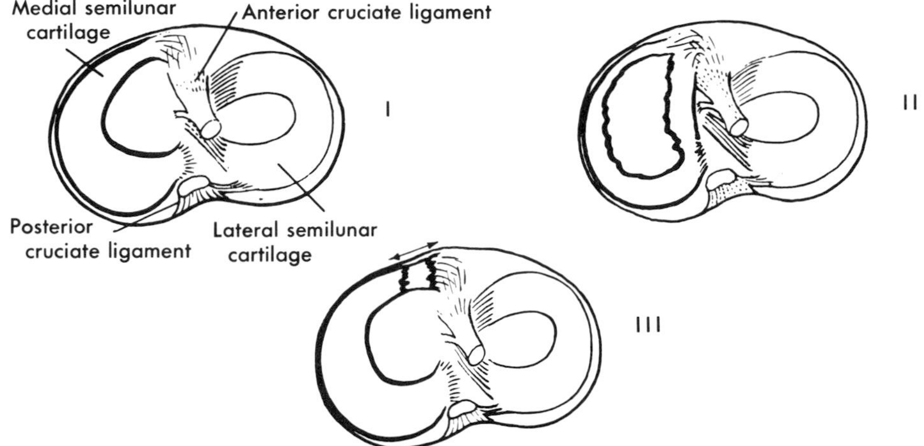

Fig. 6-10. I, Normal figure-of-eight anatomy of menisci and cruciate ligaments. **II,** Bowstring meniscus. **III,** Retracted meniscus.

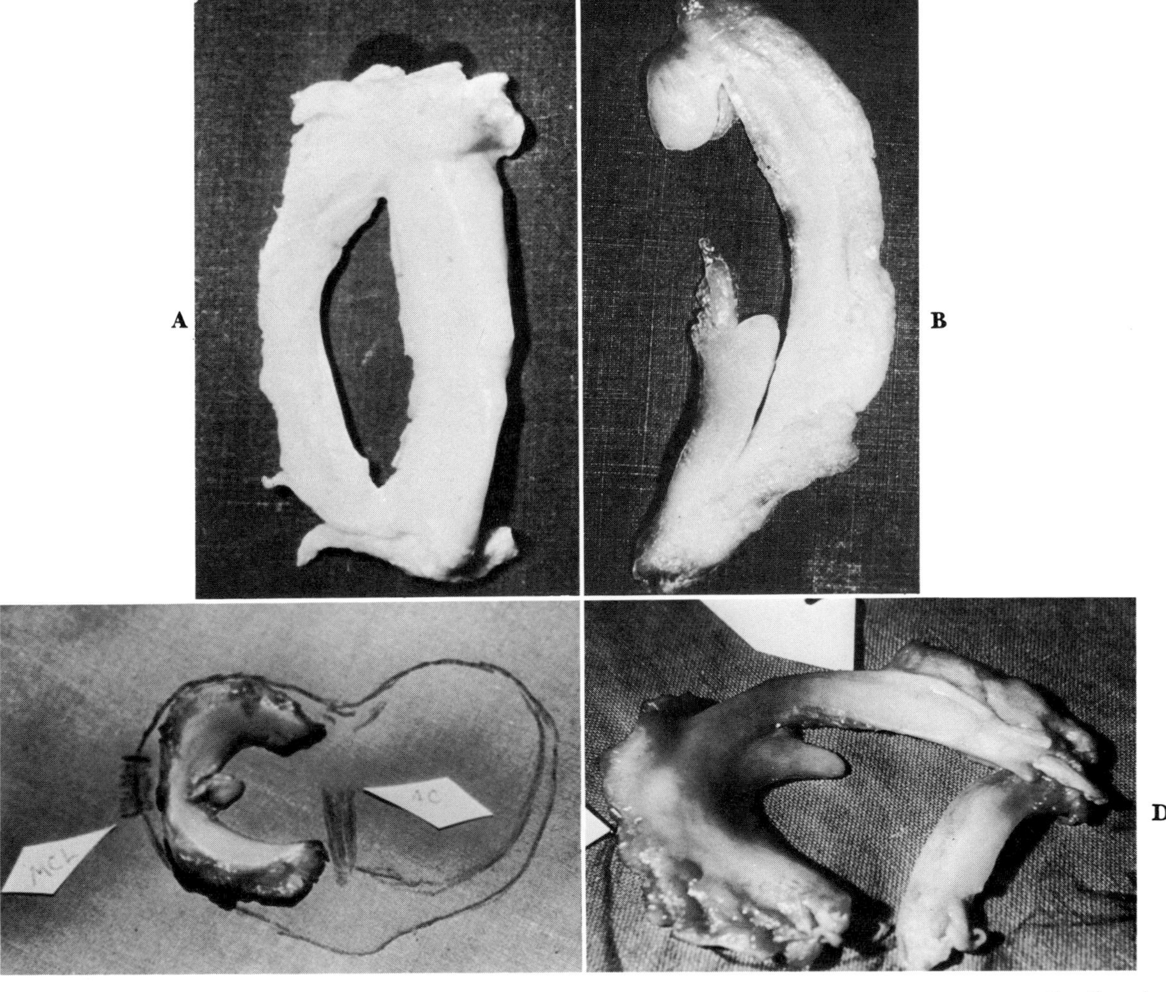

Continued

Fig. 6-11. A, Bowstring meniscus. **B,** Retracted meniscus. **C,** Parrot beak tear. **D,** Detached bowstring and parrot beak.

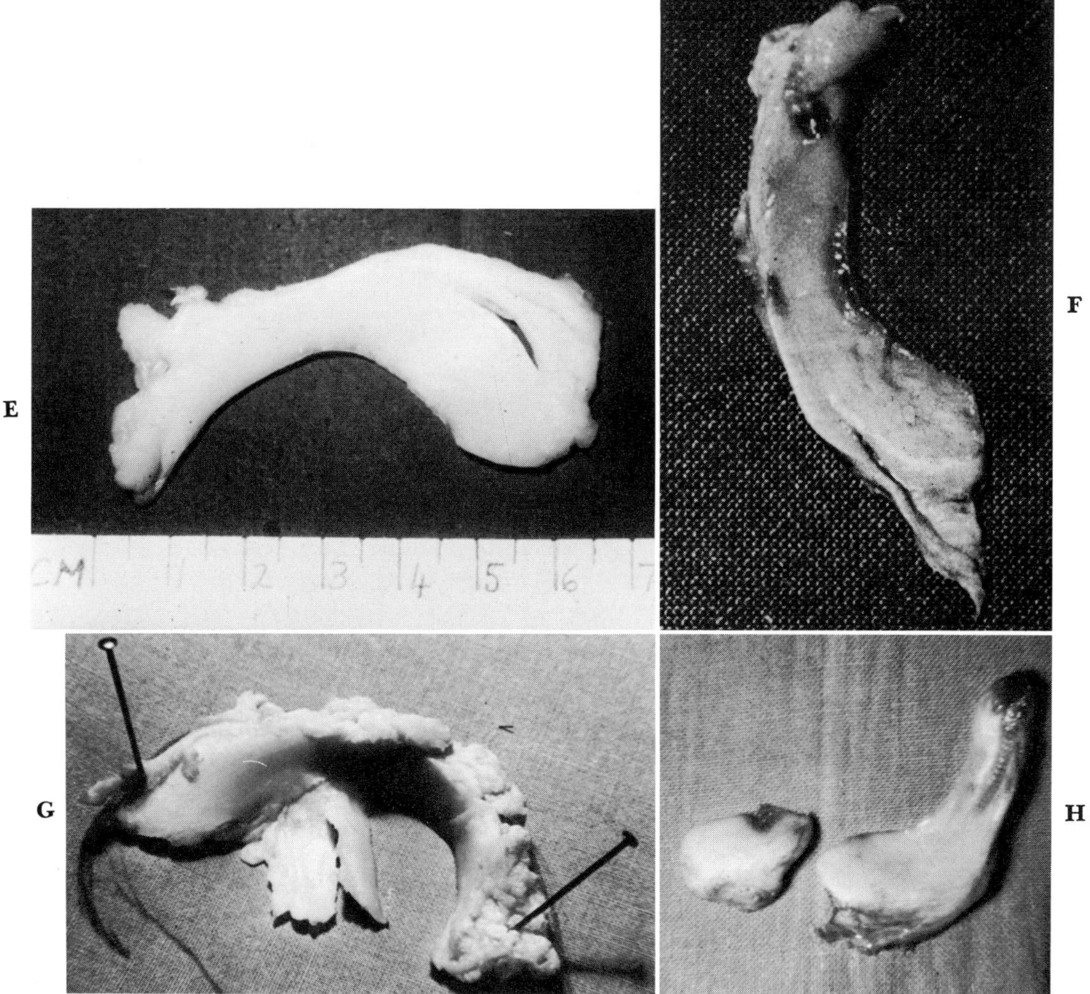

Fig. 6-11, cont'd. E, Ruptured posterior horn. **F,** Retracted meniscus in older patient. **G,** Fishtail meniscus. **H,** Fractured meniscus.

coiled portion constitutes a lump, which may produce the same symptoms and signs as the anterior end of the retracted meniscus (Fig. 6-11, *B*).

The whole meniscus may shear from its capsular attachment, the detached meniscus then being bowstrung. The difference between this and a torn meniscus is that in the latter the fibrocartilage is avascular; therefore, natural repair is impossible, whereas there are blood vessels in the capsular attachment to the meniscus. The process of fibrous tissue repair is possible, and healing may occur. This injury was described by Bristow[2] as a "sprain of the meniscus" because natural recovery was possible.

Fibrosis usually occurs with loss of elasticity. In treating such patients, one first attempts manipulation. All that is required is a freeing of adhesions. This can be obtained by rotational manipulation. Once rotation is recovered, flexion and extension are full. If manipulation fails, meniscectomy should be performed.

One can imagine an elastic meniscus with its shorter free border and longer capsular border being forcibly straightened. The free border is stretched beyond its point of endurance, and a *parrot beak* tear results (Fig. 6-11, *C*). The fibers are first torn across, but the line of tear then runs longitudinally. The free segment resembles a parrot beak. The extent of the longitudinal tear is variable (Fig. 6-11, *D*).

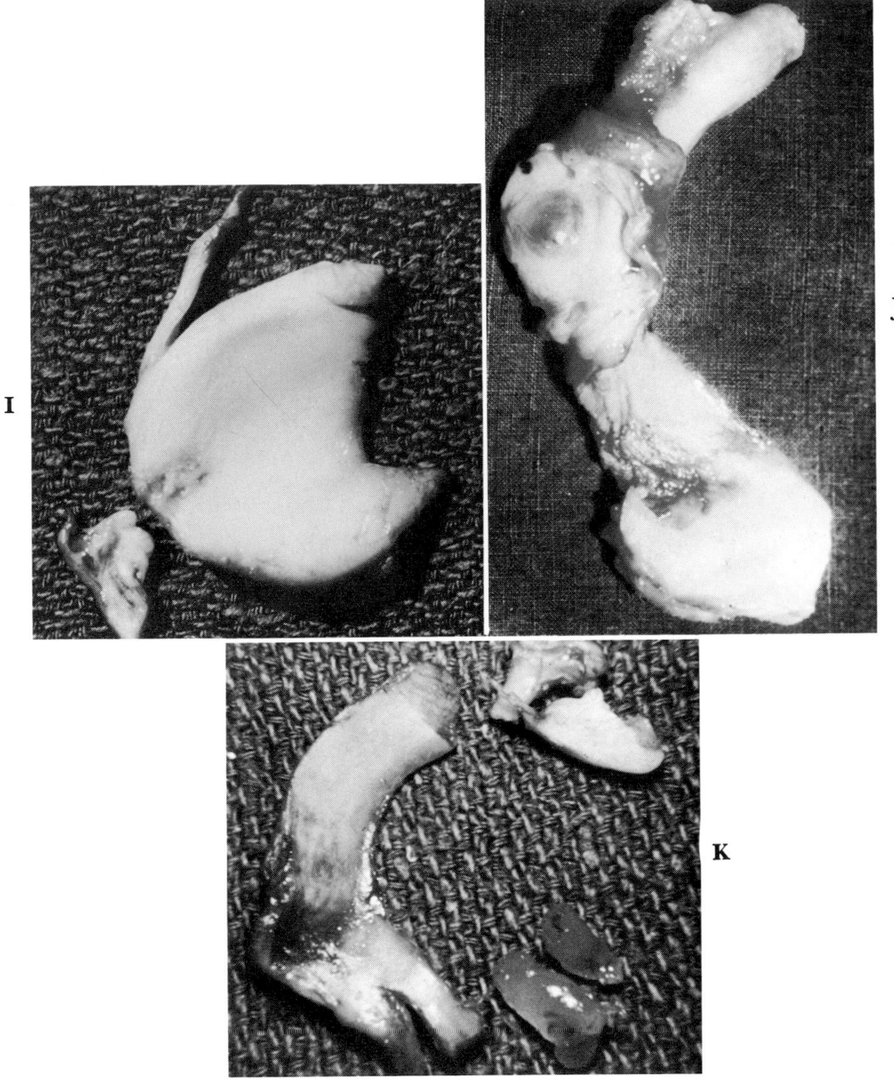

Fig. 6-11, cont'd. I, Discoid meniscus. **J,** Cystic meniscus. **K,** Cysts found between the anterior horn and the cruciate ligament. (From Helfet, A. J.: The management of internal derangement of the knee, Philadelphia, 1963, J. B. Lippincott Co.)

In other instances, prevention of synchronous movement may, instead of splitting the meniscus, disrupt the anterior or posterior horn from its tibial attachment (Fig. 6-11, *E*). Detachment of the anterior horn from the anterior tibial spine results in a loose meniscus. The retracted anterior horn may bunch up considerably (Fig. 6-11, *F*). The posterior horn, however, is more intimately attached to the capsule of the joint and tends to rupture obliquely rather than retract.

In the older patient, after retraction of the anterior horn, the anterior two-thirds contracts slowly. The posterior horn is abraded, squashed, and shredded until the typical fishtail appears (Fig. 6-11, *G*).

Finally, and only in these older menisci, does the meniscus fracture between the retracted anterior two-thirds and the fixed posterior one-third, and this fracture is transverse (Fig. 11, *H*). In this instance the two fragments were completely separated.

The discoid meniscus (Fig. 6-11, *I*), a congenital abnormality, is singularly liable to injury, presumably because of its inefficiency in the guide mechanism. The usual central tear is really a bow-string effect, sometimes the whole meniscus being affected. More than one split may occur, and there may be detachments of a horn. There may even be cyst formation (Fig. 6-11, *J*).

I believe cysts of the meniscus to be traumatic in origin, as I have never seen a cyst in association with an undamaged meniscus. The cyst always occurs in the vascular attachment between the meniscus and the capsule, or at the junction of the meniscus and the anterior or posterior cruciate ligaments. It never occurs along the free border. The cysts (Fig. 6-11, *K*) were found in the ligamentous attachments, between the anterior horn and the cruciate ligament.

The cyst is usually obvious on clinical examination, especially when the knee is fully extended—but not as frequently when the knee is flexed.

If the surgeon's knife or a tear transgresses the vascular attachments of the meniscus, bleeding occurs, and the resulting hematoma may be invaded by blood vessels and fibroblasts. The meniscus may regenerate. It now does not consist of true fibrocartilage, but of a vascular fibrous tissue. It is usually irregular, often tender, and peculiarly liable to recurrent injury.

Following hemarthrosis, with organization of clot, adhesions may form between any of the structures depicted (Fig. 6-12). In the normal meniscus, the anterior two-thirds has long coronary ligaments, which allows movement during rotational alignment. Adhesions of the meniscus result in loss of this elasticity and in a block to rotation, that is, they cause mechanical derangement of the knee joint. The physical signs resulting are the same as those from any meniscal block.

A syndrome of increasing importance is *adhesion of the fat pad* (Fig. 6-13). This results from a direct blow to the flexed knee with injury to the fat pad. Typically it is due to dashboard impact. The infrapatellar pad of fat is a mobile structure. It contains a high proportion of adipose elastic tissue and is enveloped by synovium so disposed as to constitute ligaments that maneuver the lobes of fat, which then act as a cushion and fill the changing space produced in the front of the knee joint during flexion and extension.

Adhesions of the fat pad to the front of the tibia and along the edge of the meniscus often involve the anterior meniscal horn. The fibrous tissue causes a greater block to rotation than that caused by meniscal tears.

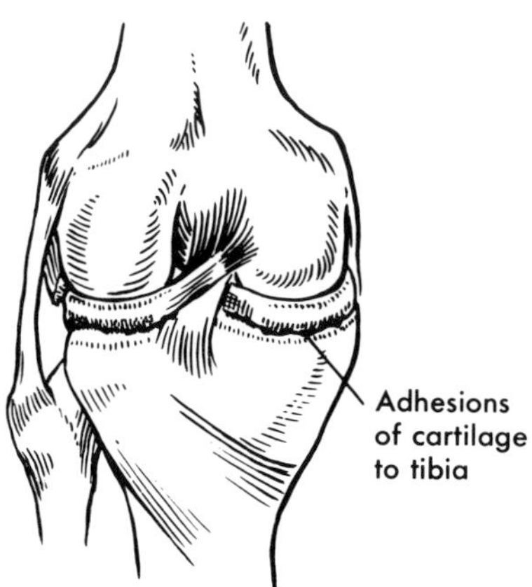

Fig. 6-12. Diagram of meniscal adhesions. (From Helfet, A. J.: The management of internal derangement of the knee, Philadelphia, 1963, J. B. Lippincott Co.)

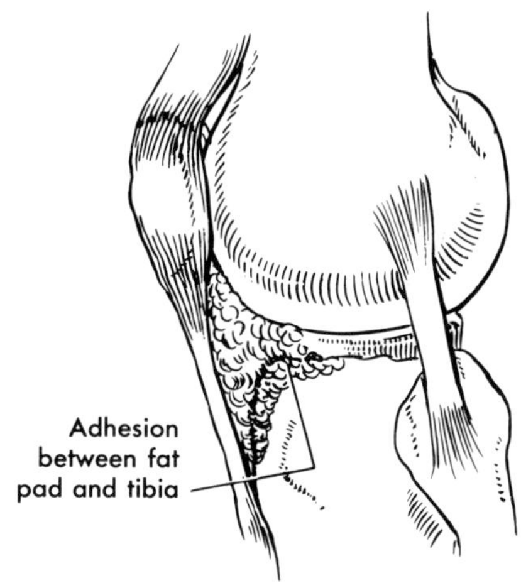

Fig. 6-13. Diagram of adherent infrapatellar fat pad. (From Helfet, A. J.: The management of internal derangement of the knee, Philadelphia, 1963, J. B. Lippincott Co.)

There are two ways of dealing with this problem. One may, under general anesthesia, be able to free the adhesions by manipulation, until the synchronous movement suddenly becomes free. If this is impossible, one should operate to divide the adhesions meticulously. The fat pad is enveloped in white scar tissue. As the adhesions are gently divided, the fat lobules are seen to pout until the fat pad regains its normal structure. The fat pad should not be excised. It performs an important function, and excision results in a creaking, stiffish joint.

Popliteus tendinitis is a rare but disabling condition (Fig. 6-14). The patient develops pain on

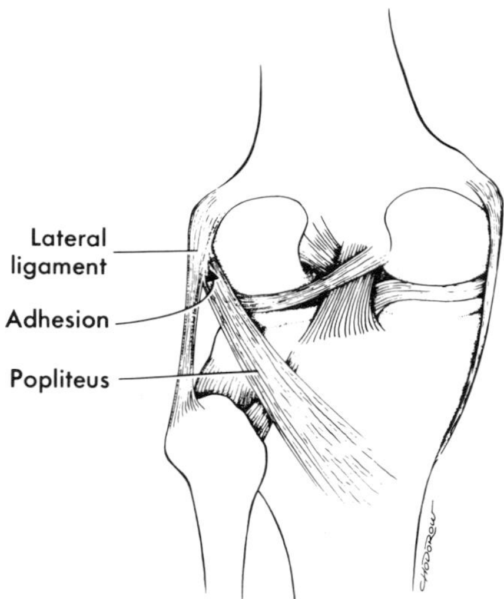

Fig. 6-14. Diagram of popliteal tendinitis.

flexion, especially at its extremes, for example, sitting on his heels. The more he flexes, the more pain he has. There is usually no trouble when the knee is extended. The patient also has pain when he attempts to rotate the tibia externally against resistance. Local tenderness is present. Injection of a local anesthetic into the popliteus sheath gives an exact diagnosis and also relieves the patient of his symptoms.

Instability or arthritis of the superior tibiofibular joint is an uncommon syndrome and is often missed. It simulates derangement of the lateral meniscus, and many patients have this meniscus removed unnecessarily.

Attention has already been drawn to the importance of the superior tibiofibular joint in bearing body weight while the knee is flexed. If the patient is asked to flex the knee while bearing weight solely on the affected leg, he or she will not do so without stabilizing the leg with the opposite foot (Fig. 6-15).

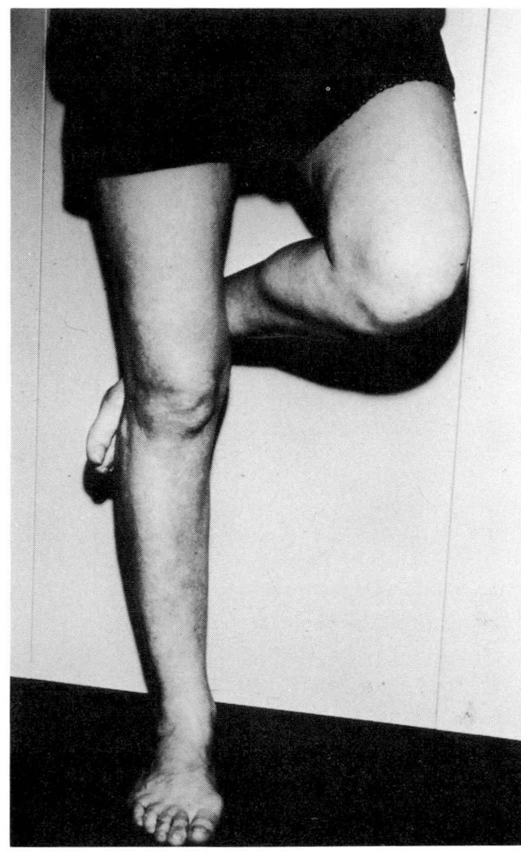

Fig. 6-15. Test for instability of the superior tibiofibular joint.

DIAGNOSIS OF INTERNAL DERANGEMENTS

In diagnosis of internal derangements, the mechanics of the knee joint must again be considered.

If the knee were a hinge joint, a wedge of specific bulk would cause a specific block to movement (either flexion or extension). The thicker the wedge the greater would be the limitation of movement. It is not, however, a hinge joint, but a helix. Any change in the volume of the spiral results in a similar block to rotation.

Thus any obstruction to the synchronous movement of the knee, while causing a greater or lesser degree of loss to extension or flexion, converts movement from a spiral to a hinge type. Whether the obstructing mechanism is a bowstrung meniscus or adhesions to the coronary ligament following hemarthrosis, with consequent inelasticity, a block to rotation is present. This block leads to the appearance of a number of clinical signs.

The diagnostic feature is local or even finger point pain and tenderness (Fig. 6-16). In this instance, forcing extension and external rotation of the tibia on the femur would produce finger point pain and tenderness if the lesion were in the anterior compartment of the joint.

When one attempts to extend or flex the knee, the patient develops finger point pain and tenderness at the site of the block. The localization, either anteriorly or posteriorly along the joint line, is exact and easily differentiates the meniscal injury from collateral ligament injury where the tender

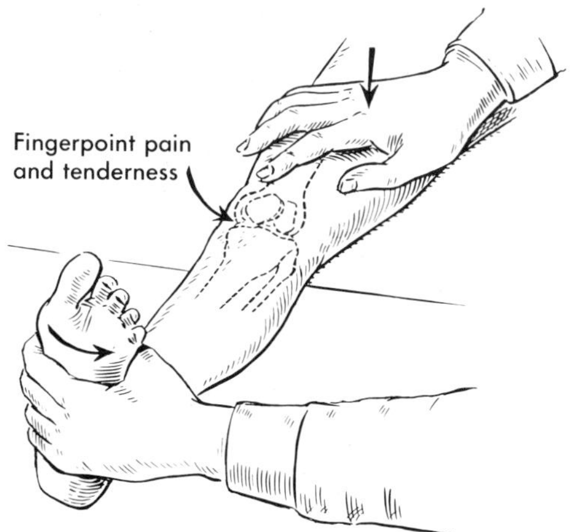

Fig. 6-16. Forced extension in external rotation causing finger point pain and tenderness anteriorly, therefore anterior horn tear. (From Helfet, A. J.: The management of internal derangement of the knee, Philadelphia, 1963, J. B. Lippincott Co.)

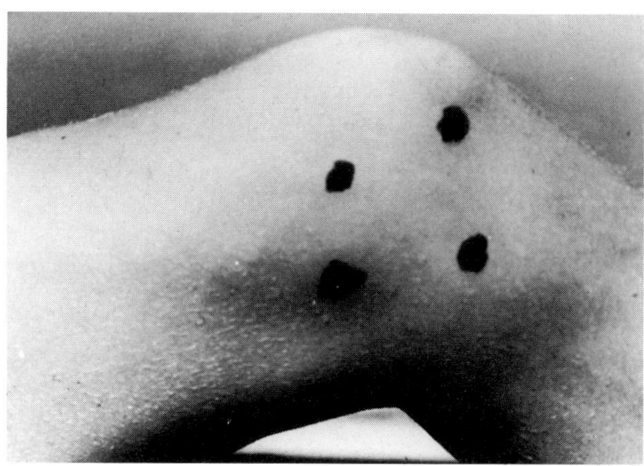

Fig. 6-17. The points of tenderness—meniscal or ligamentous. (From Helfet, A. J.: The management of internal derangement of the knee, Philadelphia, 1963, J. B. Lippincott Co.)

points are at right angles to the joint (Fig. 6-17).

Loss of rotation may be detected by asking the patient to sit with his knee flexed over the edge of the examination table. The tibial tubercle of the abnormal knee will be seen opposite the medial part of the patella. Extending the knee reveals that the tibia no longer rotates outward. The knee has been converted to a hinge or roller joint, and the tibial tubercle will remain opposite the medial part of the patella (Fig. 6-18). The distinction between this and a normal knee will be apparent.

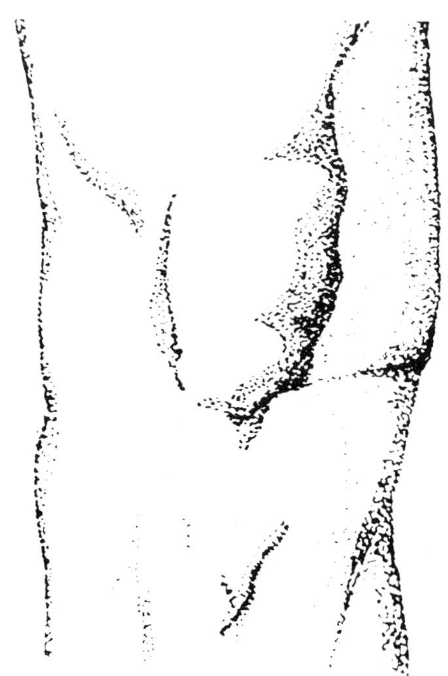

Fig. 6-18. Diagram showing tibial tubercle opposite medial part of the patella in the extended knee.

A meniscal lesion in the anterior compartment of the knee joint usually blocks extension and external rotation, whereas a posterior horn tear limits flexion and internal rotation of the tibia. A bowstrung tear usually limits both. With an anterior horn tear it is painful to straighten the knee. The patient with a tear at the back of the knee cannot squat or kneel. Finger point pain and tenderness confirm the side and site of the lesion. The McMurray click, when present, defines it exactly.

Moreover, in the normal knee the medial tibial and femoral condyles are so shaped that when extension and synchronous external rotation are complete, they fit snugly together with excellent congruity. The medial side of the knee thus presents a smooth, rounded surface. If external rotation has been prevented, they will not fit congruously. The tibial condyle remains behind its partner, and the edge of the medial femoral condyle projects forward. There will thus be a transverse bony step at the medial side of the joint line. It may usually be seen, but it is always easily felt by the examining hand. Neither obesity nor effusion will mask it. These two signs will often be present at the beginning of an operation, but when meniscectomy has been performed, they are no longer there. Congruity has been restored. The lack of external rotation of the tibia and the protrusion of the medial femoral condyle are immediately obvious (Fig. 6-19). The same physical signs are present in the older patient with what is often called an osteoarthritic knee.

A block to external rotation means that the patella can no longer follow its accustomed path into the trochlear groove. During extension, its medial edge is forced to impinge against the lateral surface of the medial condyle. If the abnormal movement is allowed to continue, trauma to the articular cartilage in this area occurs, with sur-

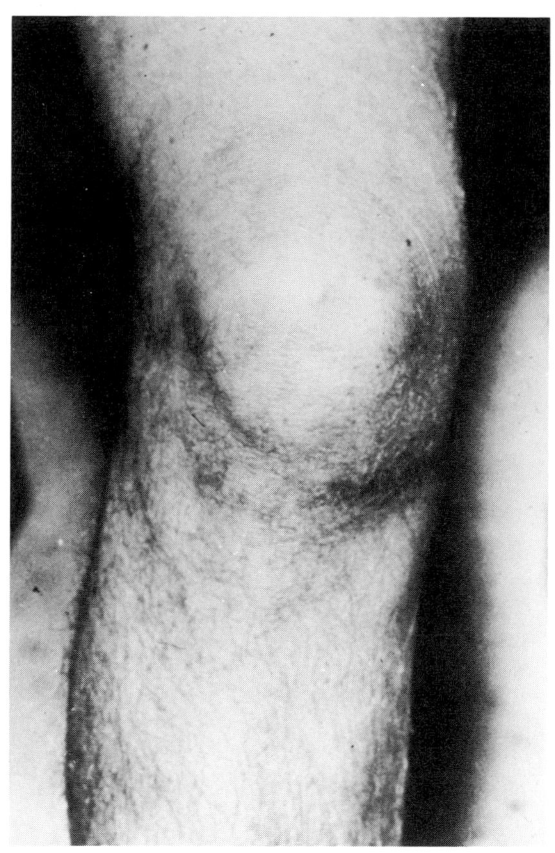

Fig. 6-19. The knee of a young athlete with a recent meniscal injury. (From Helfet, A. J.: The management of internal derangement of the knee, Philadelphia, 1963, J. B. Lippincott Co.)

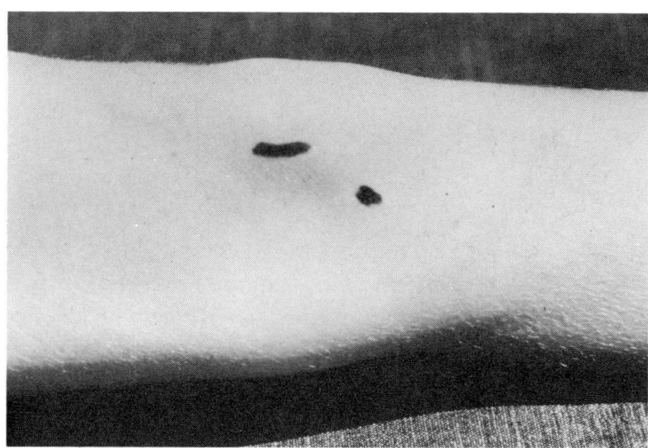

Fig. 6-20. Tenderness along medial border of patella. (From Helfet, A. J.: The management of internal derangement of the knee, Philadelphia, 1963, J. B. Lippincott Co.)

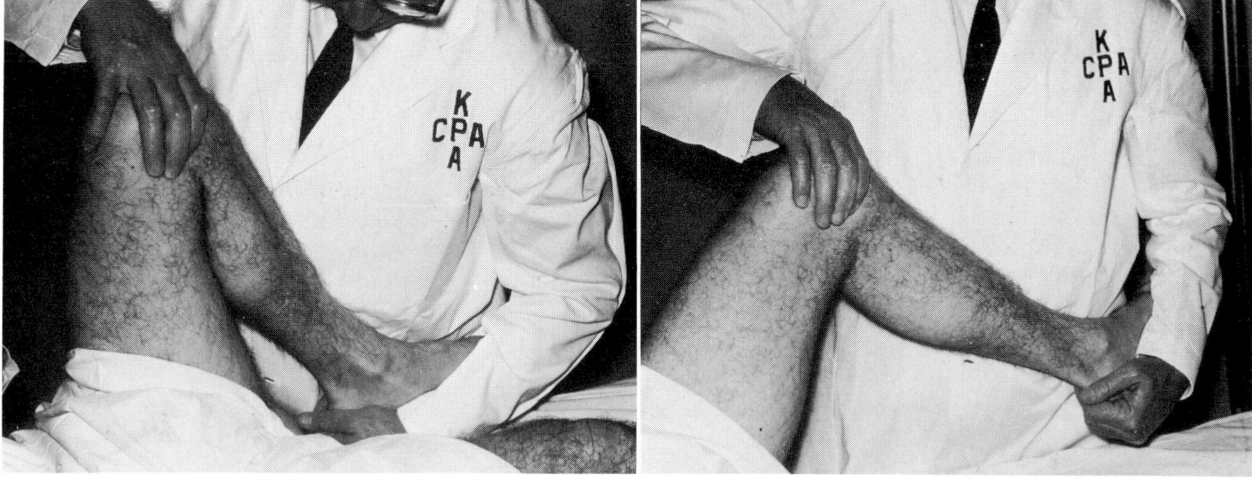

Fig. 6-21. Eliciting the McMurray click.

rounding inflammatory reaction. Tenderness appears, therefore, along the medial border of the patella (Fig. 6-20). This contrasts sharply with the recurrent subluxation of the patella, when tenderness is always along the lateral border. So in this knee finger point tenderness would be determined over the anteromedial joint line and along the medial border of the patella.

If there is a disturbance in the volume of the spiral due to a mobile segment of the meniscus, one can perform a maneuver in which the loose piece is made to jump or "click," as we traditionally describe it. This is called the McMurray click.[4]

The test cannot be performed adequately by taking the patient's foot in one's hand and attempting to rotate and maneuver what may be a heavy limb, often that of an athlete. The correct procedure is to control the limb with one's trunk (Fig. 6-21). The foot is placed against the examiner's body with his arm along the inner surface. The fingers of the other hand are placed over the joint line, where a click may be expected to be palpated. The knee is first flexed fully. Then the tibia is rotated outward and, while being forced into abduction, the knee is straightened.

A click will be felt at the portion of the meniscus that is torn or unstable and that slips during the test.

Occasionally the opposite maneuver will elicit the click, the leg being internally rotated and adducted during extension. This should also always be attempted.

Another maneuver produces what may be called the *reducing click*. Especially in the older patient with an unstable tear, occasionally it is possible for the surgeon to reduce the meniscus. The examiner flexes the knee fully and rotates it in and out. A little "jump" is felt, and the block to rotation disappears. One can tell the patient at this point, "You can get up now and walk without pain" because the meniscus has been reduced. The condition is, of course, likely to recur at any time, and one can put the meniscus out by doing the opposite maneuver. The test thus has a diagnostic value.

The patient can be taught to reduce the meniscus himself, and the maneuver has a second virtue in allowing the patient to overcome his symptoms while awaiting operation.

The patient is taught to sit and fully flex the knee passively and then rotate it externally. Often

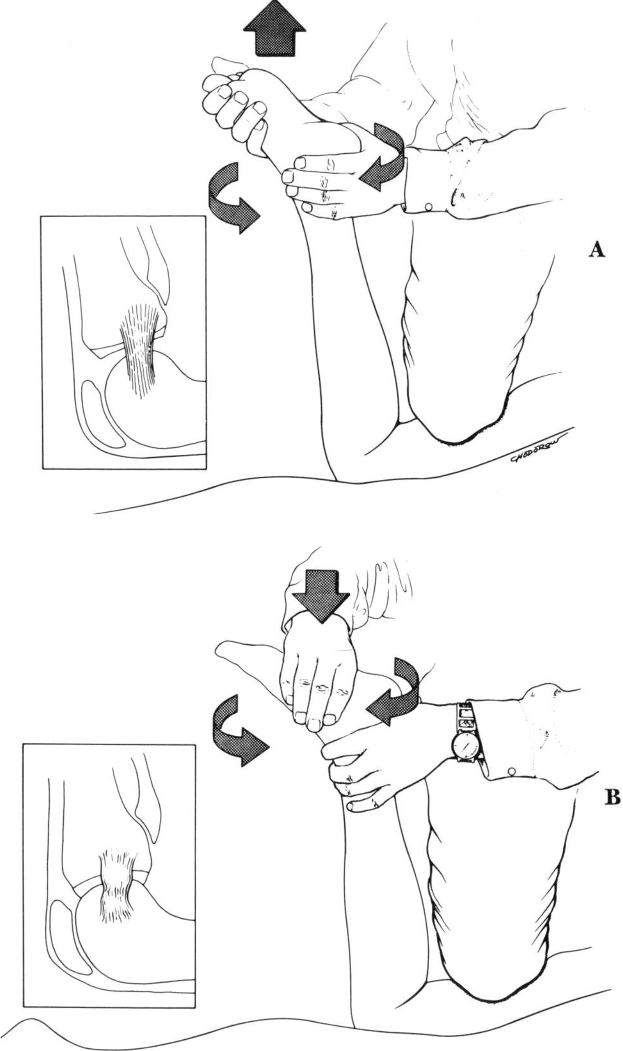

Fig. 6-22. A and **B,** The Apley test.

the meniscus is reduced at this point, but to make certain, the patient kicks the leg straight as though to kick a ball. In this manner the patient, who, while walking may suddenly "lock" the knee, is able to overcome the symptoms.

The Apley test[1] is designed to differentiate between ligamentous and meniscal injury. The patient lies prone with his knee flexed to 90°. The examiner grasps the leg and, applying his weight to the foot, rotates the tibia internally and externally (Fig. 6-22, *A*). Local pain is present if the meniscus has been injured. Then the examiner kneels on the back of the patient's thigh, and while pulling the tibia to distract the knee joint, again rotates the tibia (Fig. 6-22, *B*). If local pain is present on this maneuver, it indicates injury to

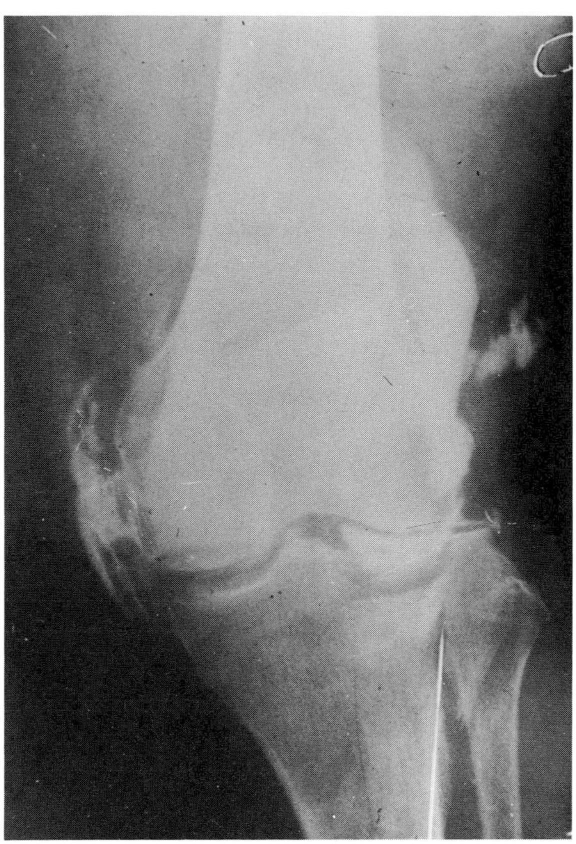

Fig. 6-23. Arthrogram—rupture of the medial collateral ligament and fracture of the lateral tibial condyle.

the collateral ligaments. The integrity of the ligaments of the knee joints is tested by putting stress on the injured side.

Rupture of the cruciate ligaments in themselves does not cause undue instability, but if the capsule of the knee joint has also been weakened, it is possible to slide the tibia forward or backward on the femur.

Arthrography is a difficult procedure to do well, requiring many views of the joint. Interpretation is difficult, and despite its elegance, I believe it to have little place in the diagnosis of most internal derangements. Careful attention to the clinical signs in the joint allows a precise diagnosis to be made.

Arthrography, however, is useful in certain conditions. In the presence of a ruptured ligament, for example, it is necessary to know whether the meniscus also has been ruptured or detached.

In impacted fractures of the lateral tibial condyle, although many people doubt it, the medial collateral ligament may well have been torn. Arthrography will reveal such a tear by a spillover of the radiopaque material through the capsule (Fig. 6-23).

The key to successful surgery of the knee is accurate preoperative diagnosis. There is no case for which the surgeon should use the phrase "open up the joint to have a look." This leads not only to unnecessary surgery but also to inadequate operations.

The operation itself should be performed gently and carefully and should be followed by adequate reablement. The operation should be regarded as an incident in the treatment of the derangement. Restoration of power and movement is the main factor.

Isometrics should begin the day before operation. Postoperatively the patient remains in bed for 10 days in a compression bandage, which allows only a jog of movement and which is applied to keep the knee straight. After 10 days, when the wound is healed, the compression bandage is taken off. After removal of the sutures, an ACE bandage is applied in a figure-of-eight. Active bending exercises are then encouraged. At this stage the patient can get out of bed and walk. Crutches are unnecessary, and there is no reason for him to limp. He continues to exercise within the power of his *muscles,* that is, he does not fatigue the knee and consequently does not develop an effusion in the joint. In young people reablement is usually complete in 5 to 6 weeks as this seems to be the time needed for them to return to active participation in games.

REFERENCES

1. Apley, A. G.: The diagnosis of meniscus injuries, J. Bone Joint Surg. **29**:78, 1947.
2. Bristow, W. R.: Injuries and displacements of the semilunar cartilage, Postgrad. Med. J. **13**:366, 1937.
3. Helfet, A. J.: The management of internal derangements of the knee, Philadelphia, 1963, J. B. Lippincott Co.
4. McMurray, T. P.: The semilunar cartilages, Brit. J. Surg. **29**:407, 1942.

Chapter 7

Orthopaedic management of muscular dystrophy and related disorders

BURR H. CURTIS, M.D.
Newington, Connecticut

Myopathies, dystrophies, and congenital neurologic defects are encountered frequently in the practice of children's orthopaedics. In most of this large group of disorders, there is at present very little that can be done to arrest progression of the disease, let alone cure it. This in no way should imply a passive attitude in management. Lack of understanding can lead to postponement or to the withholding of definitive assistance to which the patient is entitled. Treatment of these diseases requires knowledge of the signs and symptoms, pathology, neurophysiology and expected course, as well as applicable technical skills.

The slowly progressive nature of most of these diseases and their combined neurologic, musculoskeletal, and psychosocial aspects require a continuing team effort by medical and paramedical specialists (orthopaedists, pediatricians, neurologists, physiatrists, psychiatrists, physical therapists, occupational therapists, social workers, psychologists, and teachers).

In all these conditions, gradual loss of upper and lower extremity function with actual commitment to chair or bed has too often been accepted as the natural course of the disease by both physicians and families. Unfortunately, this has led to a certain degree of apathy in regard to the medical and surgical management. These patients deserve a more realistic approach to their problems. As orthopaedists, it is our responsibility to maintain independence, not only for its own sake but also because of the possibility that specific therapy to alter or arrest the course of these diseases may emerge from research before current cases have run their functional span. It is essential that patients and their families be given support in meeting their physical, psychologic and social needs.

FREQUENCY OF THESE DISORDERS IN A CHILDREN'S HOSPITAL

The necessity for orthopaedists to be knowledgeable about these disorders is obvious when the

Table 7-1. Statistical summary of muscular dystrophy and related disorders

Type	*1962 review*	*1962-1966*	*Total*
Childhood muscular dystrophy (Duchenne)	51	26	77
Fascioscapulohumeral muscular dystrophy	4	—	4
Adult muscular dystrophy	4	—	4
Ophthalmoplegic muscular dystrophy	1	—	1
Myotonic dystrophy	1	1	2
Amyotonia congenita	22	13	35
Kugelberg-Welander	1	—	1
Polymyositis	—	5	5
Charcot–Marie–Tooth	16	13	29
Muscle disease–unclassified	26	8	34
	126	66	192

experience at Newington Children's Hospital is reviewed. A 1962 study included 126 cases. Since then, sixty-six cases have been added to the study (Table 7-1). Most of these patients were first seen in the Orthopaedic Clinic, but they have been followed by several specialists, specifically a pediatrician, a physiatrist, a physical therapist, an occupational therapist, and a social worker, with consultation from a neurologist and from other specialists as needed.

Charcot-Marie-Tooth syndrome and amyotonia congenita are the principal congenital neurologic disorders, and muscular dystrophy of the Duchenne type comprises the largest group of myopathies.

Charcot-Marie-Tooth syndrome

Twenty-nine patients, who manifested a positive family history and slow progression of their disease, are included in this study. Initial signs and symptoms involve peculiar gait, high arches, fatigability, inability to fit shoes, toeing in, and among the older patients, weakness of the hands. The initial orthopaedic examination frequently revealed the following findings, which led to the appropriate diagnosis: steppage gait, cavus feet, claw toes, weakness of the peroneal and anterior tibial muscles, adduction of the forefoot, and diminished ankle reflexes. Weakness in the distribution of the ulnar nerve, the so-called "stork leg," and severe cavus deformities of the feet appear late in the disease. The majority of these patients ultimately require foot surgery and suitable bracing of the leg and foot.

Amyotonia congenita

Amyotonia congenita was diagnosed in thirty-five patients of the combined series. Early signs and symptoms of the Werdnig-Hoffmann type are limping, floppiness, a failure to thrive, and diffuse motor weakness. Most of these patients came to us between the ages of 3 and 6. Their physical state deteriorated rather rapidly.

In the Oppenheim group, seen also at an early age, deterioration does not occur as rapidly in spite of extensive muscle involvement. In contrast to the Werdnig-Hoffmann patients, they seemed to be

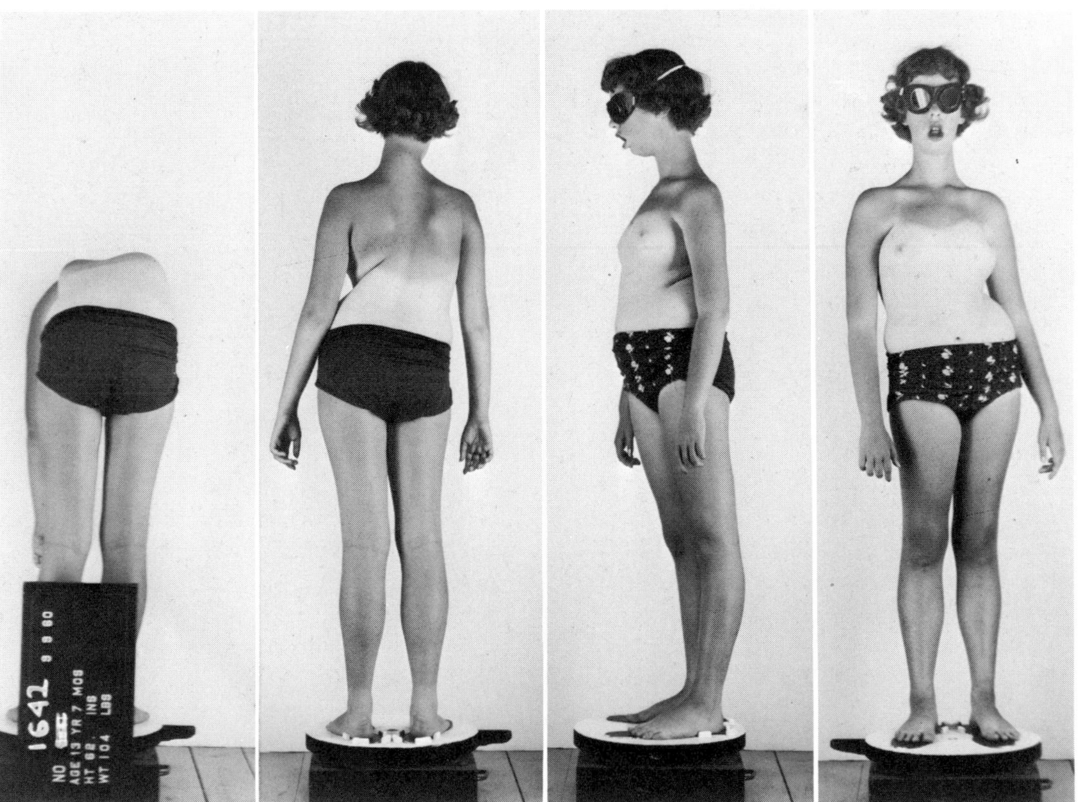

Fig. 7-1. Amyotonia congenita discovered in scoliosis clinic.

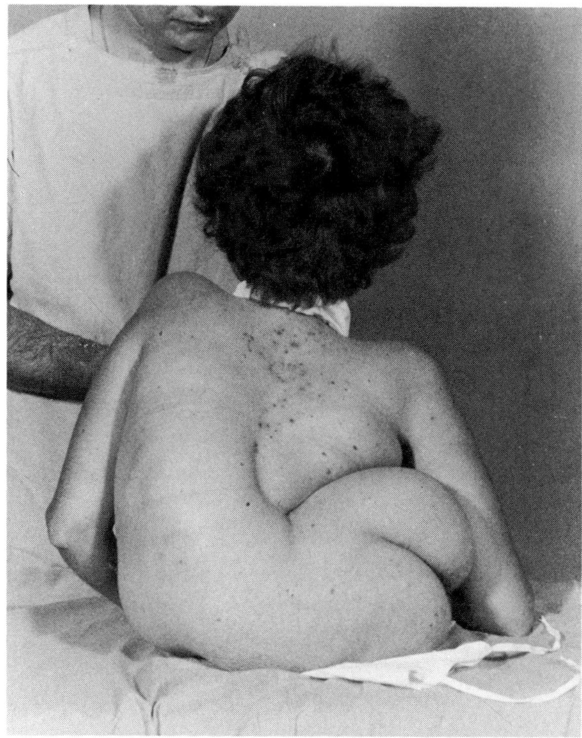

Fig. 7-2. Dystrophy with advanced scoliosis.

able to substitute spared muscles in a manner similar to that seen in a patient with chronic poliomyelitis. These children live longer, progress less rapidly, but ultimately develop respiratory difficulty. Some of these patients are first seen in the scoliosis clinic (Fig. 7-1). In the later stages of their disease, they demonstrate marked spinal deformity with severe collapse, which contributes to respiratory insufficiency (Fig. 7-2).

Progressive muscular dystrophy

Progressive muscular dystrophy is first seen in our clinic in children between the ages of 3 and 6. The presenting complaints are an inability to keep up with children of comparable age, frequent falls, a tendency to walk on the toes, and inability to arise from the floor or to climb stairs. Physical signs such as increased lumbar lordosis, enlargement of the calf, and waddling gait are noted later. If the family history is positive, the child is often seen at an earlier age. In afflicted families, the parents usually describe a tendency to fall frequently as the earliest sign in their affected child. The Gower, slip-through, boost, and stoop tests become positive late in the disease, usually long after the diagnosis has become apparent.

Of sixty-one children with progressive muscular dystrophy reviewed at the Newington Clinic in 1962, fifty-one were of the childhood (Duchenne) type. These patients were followed for an average of 10 years, and the usual interval from diagnosis until becoming bed and chair dependent was approximately 4 years. Death usually occurred by the age of 17. From 1962 to 1966, twenty-six more cases were added. (See Table 7-1.) In this latter period we benefited from improved diagnostic acumen. For some of these patients, especially those with polymyositis, specific therapy is now available.

Patients with muscular dystrophy at the Newington Hospital are now being followed in a combined study with Massachusetts Institute of Technology and with the University of Chicago under the direction of Dr. R. M. Dowben. A more aggressive approach to this disease, including earlier tenotomy, more active physical therapy, and the use of certain experimental drugs, has been undertaken with this group. It is too early to determine the effect of drugs versus other methods being employed. The activity span of the patients in this study and their level of activity are believed to be appreciably better since instituting a more aggressive regime.

In our clinic myotonic dystrophy is not common probably because of the late age of onset. The fascioscapulohumeral type is rare, and only a single case of ophthalmoplegic dystrophy has been recorded.

TOTAL MANAGEMENT

Differential diagnosis

Care should be taken to differentiate among diseases with different prognoses. Some are amenable to therapy, others have greater promise for longevity, and all are the subjects of research that may hold future promise for the patient and his family. Confirmatory laboratory studies, as well as careful observation of progress, should be made before a patient's family is confronted with an unfavorable prognosis. We should be prepared to prognosticate to patients' families and to include them as active participants in the therapeutic team. Even faced with a poor prognosis, a great deal can be done to maintain the independence of these children and to prolong their functional span.

Understanding parents can help to prevent contractures, to avoid obesity, and to assure continuance of observation and treatment. They can be directed in the appropriate care of the physical and psychosocial needs of these children.

The differential diagnosis of these disorders is difficult even for those working closely with them. Of the lower motor neuron lesions, poliomyelitis is usually not difficult to diagnose because of the pattern of typically scattered muscle involvement. Furthermore, the disease has an acute onset and is not progressive after the early stages. Another anterior horn cell disease, the Charcot-Marie-Tooth syndrome, includes changes in the posterior columns and dorsal root ganglia as well. It is an inherited disease that is slowly progressive and therefore is not likely to be confused with poliomyelitis. However, it can be confused with myopathies in the early stages. Certain upper motor neuron lesions cause hypotonia and generalized weakness, but ordinarily these lesions have some element of spasticity that is often intermittent and can usually be differentiated by observation. In the older child a diagnosis of myasthenia gravis must be considered; weakness of the facial, ocular, and pharyngeal muscles is typical. Electromyography, a favorable response to cholinergic drugs, and progressive weakness when muscles are repetitively tested will aid in the diagnosis. There are several other less common disorders associated with muscle weakness that appear in infancy and childhood. Differential diagnosis in depth is not the purpose of this presentation. It is useful, however, to separate diseases into groups identified by the primary source of difficulty, that is, lower motor neuron, upper motor neuron, upper and lower motor neuron, motor end-plate, altered sensitivity of muscle fibers, and metabolic diseases with muscle weakness (Table 7-2).

Table 7-2. Principal differential diagnoses confused with progressive muscular dystrophy

Lower motor neuron	Progressive muscular atrophy
	Amyotonia congenita syndrome:
	Werdnig-Hoffmann disease
	Oppenheim disease
	Benign congenital hypotonia (Walton)
	Peroneal muscular atrophy (Charcot–Marie–Tooth)
	Poliomyelitis
Upper motor neuron	Certain types of cerebral palsy
Upper and lower motor neuron	Amyotrophic lateral sclerosis
	Friedreich's ataxia
Motor end-plate	Myasthenia gravis
Altered sensitivity of muscle fibers	Thomsen's disease (myotonia congenita)
	Myotonic dystrophy
	Paramyotonia
	Polymyositis
Metabolic diseases with muscle weakness	

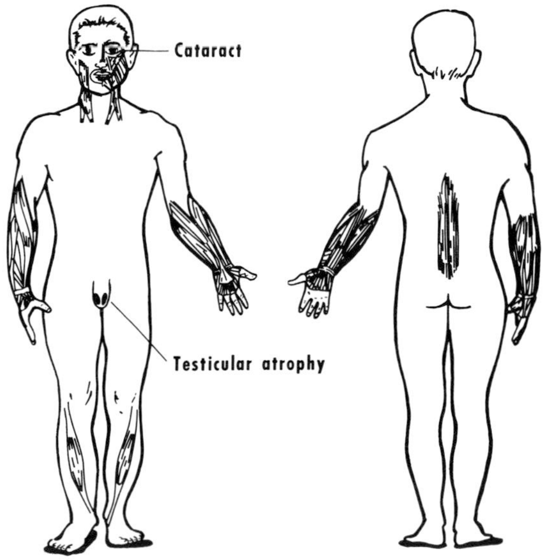

Fig. 7-3. Myotonic dystrophy.[2,9,11] (From Swinyard, C. A.: Pediat. Clin. N. Amer. **7**:703, 1960.)

To arrive at a working diagnosis of myopathies requires a knowledge of the patterns these diseases follow, combined with the use of serum enzyme determinations, electromyography, and muscle biopsy. The patterns of weakness in the principal forms of dystrophy are not as clear as we would like, but all the primary myopathies seen in a children's hospital start with proximal muscle weakness except myotonic dystrophy, which begins distally. For reference, the progression of various muscular dystrophies has been schematized in Table 7-3 and in Figs. 7-3 to 7-6 (modified from Swinyard, Deaver, and Greenspan).[11,12]

Laboratory tests have proved valuable in establishing a differential diagnosis, in recording the course of the disease, and in evaluating results of therapy. Electromyography helps to distinguish neuropathies from myopathies (Table 7-4) but is not diagnostic of specific disease. During voluntary contraction, myopathies show a relative in-

Table 7-3. Four major clinical forms of muscular dystrophy

	Type of muscular dystrophy			
	Duchenne or childhood	*Limb-girdle*	*Facioscapulohumeral*	*Myotonic*
Age of onset	2–10	10–40	10–18	15–80
Sex	Male	Male or female	Male or female	Male or female
Area of muscle weakness	Pelvic girdle	Pelvic or shoulder girdle	Shoulder girdle	Peripheral
Progression	Rapid; death by 20	Intermediate; death in middle age	Slow and abortive	Slow

Table 7-4. Major electromyographic criteria

	Myelopathy	*Myopathy*	*Polymyositis*	*Peripherial neuritis*
Fibrillation; fasciculation; spikes	All common	Occasional fibrillation	Common fibrillation	Fibrillation and spikes
Voluntary; amplitude	Normal or reduced	Reduced	Reduced or normal	Normal
Shape of units	Normal	Polyphasic	Polyphasic and normal	Polyphasic
Number of units	Reduced	Normal	Normal	Normal or reduced
Duration of units	Normal to increased	Decreased	Normal and decreased	Normal or increased
Nerve conduction	Decreased	Normal	Normal	Decreased

crease in the number and rate of unit firings and decrease in the size of the individual motor unit potential, with only occasional fibrillation. Neurogenic disease may reveal the opposite with more evidence of fibrillation and loss of motor units.

In the dystrophies there is evidence that cellular membrane permeability is altered, allowing leakage of cellular enzymes, affording the physician a diagnostic aid in the differentiation of muscular dystrophies and polymyositis from neurogenic disorders. Certain types of experimental therapy are directed toward prevention of this leakage or toward replacement of cellular enzymes. To date these methods have not been proved, but serum enzyme levels afford one means of testing the effectiveness of treatment, especially when correlated with serial muscle evaluation and with functional activity studies.

Repeated studies of several enzymes serve as appropriate checks of results and as an aid in differential diagnosis and in charting the progression of muscle wasting. Serum enzyme studies that have been most useful include serum aldolase (Ald. normal 1 to 10 Sibley-Lehringer units), creatin-phospho-kinase (C.P.K. normal 1 to 5 International units), lactic acid dehydrogenase (L.D.H. normal 100 to 600 Berger-Broida units), and serum glutamic oxaloacetic transaminase (S.G.O.T. normal 8 to 40 Sigma Frankel units). Muscle enzymes in the serum can vary with diet, exercise, fatigue, red cells in the specimen, liver damage, muscle wasting, etc.

In childhood dystrophy of the Duchenne type, our patients have shown marked elevation of serum Ald., C.P.K., and L.D.H.; S.G.O.T. is less specific. Serum C.P.K. is the most sensitive test, and the elevation of this enzyme in the mother of a dystrophic child is strong evidence that she is a carrier. Two thirds of carriers have abnormally elevated serum C.P.K. levels.[7] If muscle mass is reduced greatly, as in advanced stages of the disease, the C.P.K. has an advantage over Ald. because of its greater sensitivity. However, this test is more subject to error, so that the experience of the laboratory is important in evaluating reported results.

Daily output of urinary creatine can be used to determine the advancement of muscle wasting, but this test has largely been discontinued because it provides no information that cannot be determined by serial assessment of functional activity.

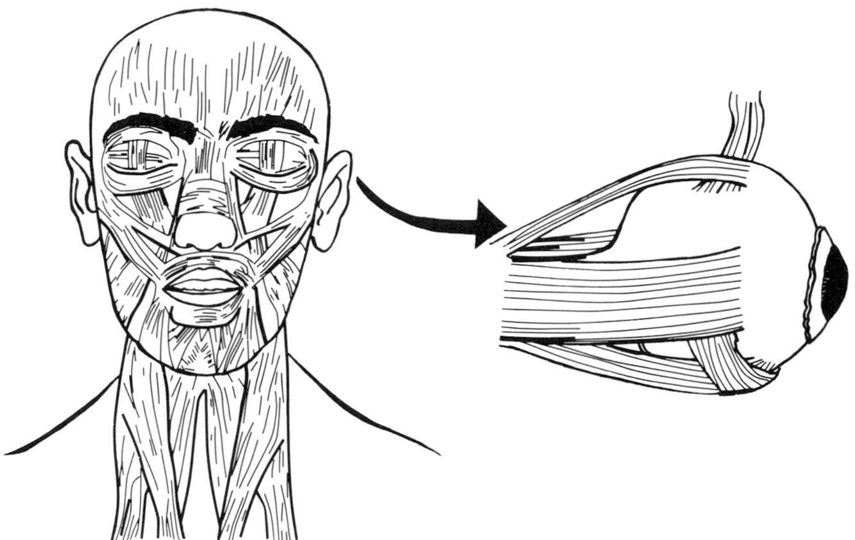

Fig. 7-4. Ophthalmoplegic dystrophy.[2,9,11] (From Swinyard, C. A.: Pediat. Clin. N. Amer. **7**:703, 1960.)

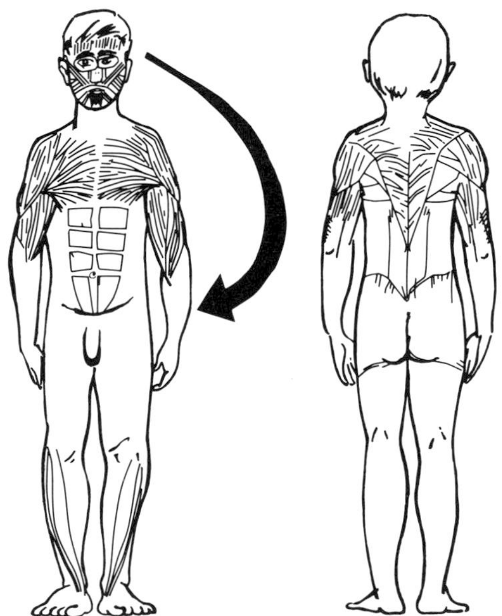

Fig. 7-5. Fascioscapulohumeral dystrophy.[2,9,11] (From Swinyard, C. A.: Pediat. Clin. N. Amer. **7**:703, 1960.)

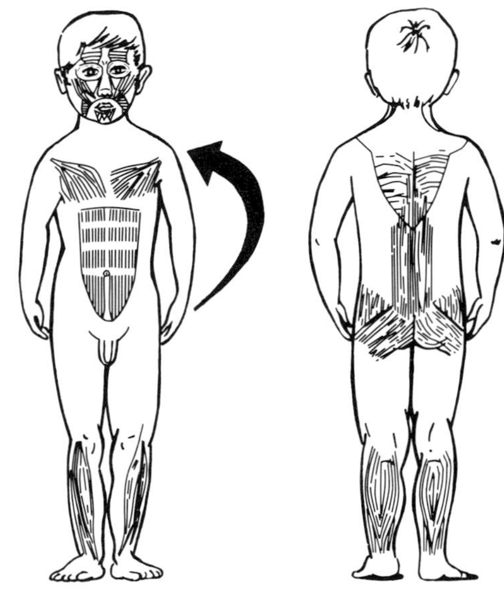

Fig. 7-6. Childhood muscular dystrophy (Duchenne).[2,9,11] (From Swinyard, C. A.: Pediat. Clin. N. Amer. **7**:703, 1960.)

Muscle biopsies are useful if performed properly. The selection of appropriate muscles for biopsy and careful technique are prerequisites. Biopsy has been found especially valuable in differentiating polymyositis from muscular dystrophy. Polymyositis has a relatively good prognosis if properly treated. The classical findings of fever, rash, elevated sedimentation rate, and abnormal gamma globulin may not be present or may have subsided before muscle weakness became troublesome. Since both polymyositis and muscular dystrophy cause elevation in serum enzymes, muscle biopsy will differentiate these diseases and lower motor neuron disease. The orthopaedic surgeon must perform a biopsy properly so that the pathologist receives an adequate specimen. The following criteria, similar to those described by Cohen,[3] should be followed carefully:

1. Choose a muscle that is known by test to be involved, but selection should avoid a

muscle that is in the end state of fatty infiltration and fibrosis. A recently involved muscle is best. In spite of good care, biopsy may lead to pain, contracture, and disuse, with permanent reduction in strength. For physical and psychologic reasons, a nonweight bearing and noncritical muscle should be used whenever possible. Biopsy of the rectus abdominis or any moderately involved proximal muscle can be done successfully. The gastrocnemius, selected so frequently, may be a poor choice.

2. Use adequate regional or general anesthesia, less often local infiltration. Since these patients often have respiratory difficulty, general anesthesia should be used cautiously.

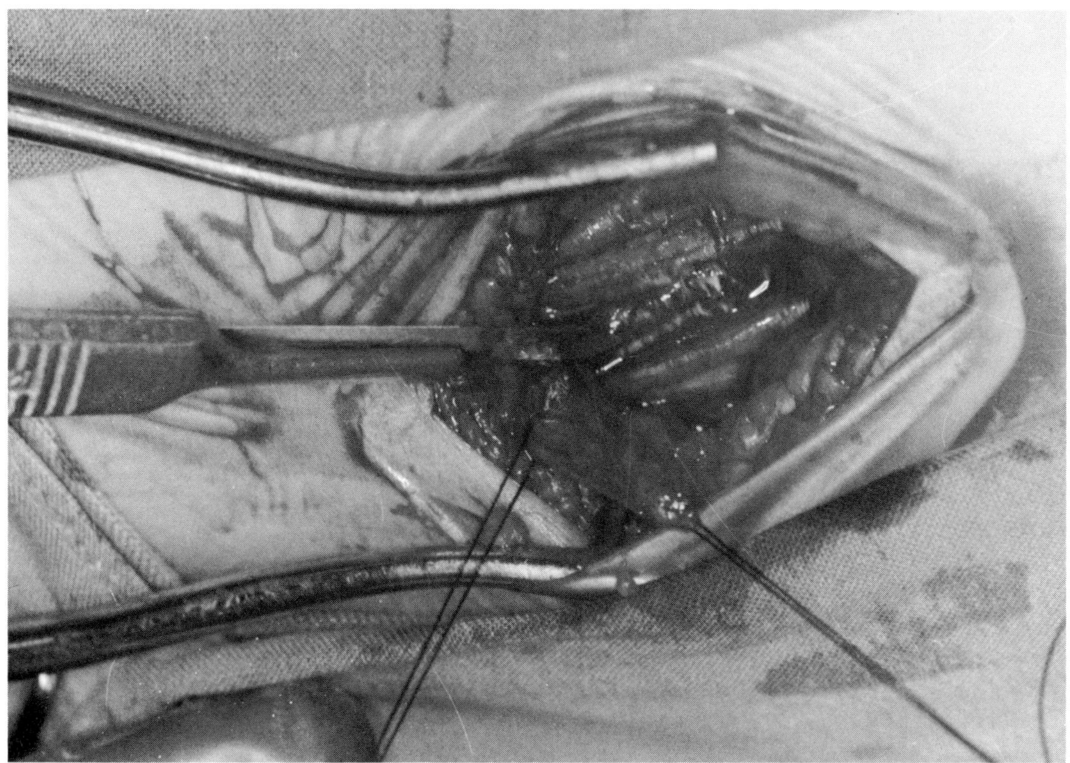

Fig. 7-7. Sutures set to prevent contraction of specimen.

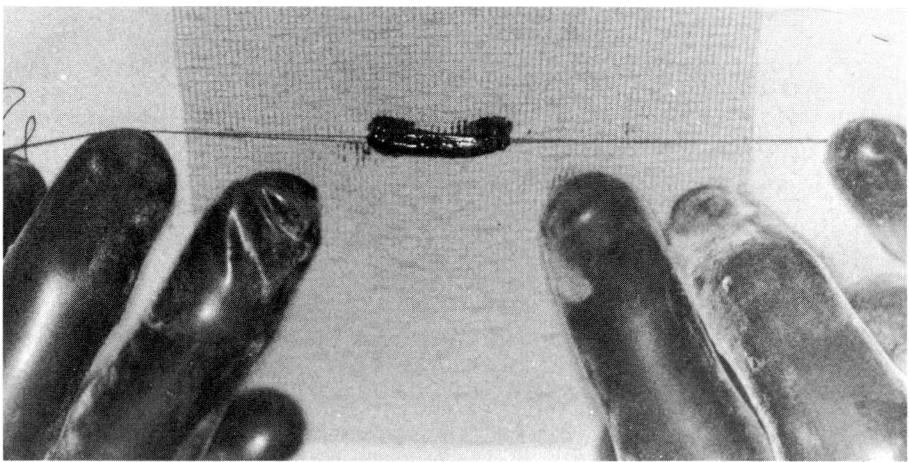

Fig. 7-8. Maintain "normal" length of tissue.

3. Make an adequate incision to permit gentle retraction.
4. Stay sutures should be set at either end of tissue to be removed. This allows the operator to keep the muscle stretched to the same degree after removal as it was in situ (Fig. 7-7).
5. Mobilize the muscle step by step and wait after each cut so that it has not contracted when excised.
6. Handle the specimen gently. Pin the specimen to sterile crepe paper or allow it to dry slightly and adhere to the paper in order to preserve length (Fig. 7-8).
7. To prevent contraction, which would occur in an acid fixative, place the specimen in neutral formalin or Bouin's solution without removing the biopsy from the paper.
8. Mobilize the patient early postoperatively to minimize functional loss.

The pathologist should cut longitudinal and cross sections of the specimen (not tangential sections) and may wish to use special stains as well as standard hematoxylin and eosin preparations.

BASELINE AND SERIAL ASSESSMENT

Baseline and regular serial assessments of physical status are important. The dystrophies are slow to progress and, therefore, difficult to chart. Ordinary muscle testing has some value for diagnosis, but a system of functional testing based upon abilities to carry out useful acts is better. Such techniques have been described by Swinyard, Deaver, and Greenspan[11] and Vignos, Spencer, and Archibald.[13] These methods of functional evaluation are extensions of the clinical observation used by all physicians in practice. This is not as simple as it would seem and requires familiarity with technique and consideration of strength and endurance. Careful recording by trained personnel and testing by the same persons each time provide greater validity. Repeated voluntary muscle testing of the conventional type has been largely discarded because it provides less information than functional testing. Furthermore, direct testing may produce a psychologic hazard to the patient and to his family by pointing out physical deterioration too vividly.

A chart should include weight, height, number of hours walking per day, and the time required to perform certain standard tests. A careful record of joint motion and the tendency to contracture is extremely important. Only with careful use of such repeated testing techniques can we sharpen our ability to recognize, prevent, and correct early contractures that interfere with balance or lead to premature commitment to chair or bed.

SPECIFIC OBJECTIVES

The use of androgenic steroids and prednisone in the treatment of polymyositis provides specific benefits. Myasthenia gravis responds to the use of Prostigmin. Myotonic dystrophy with a low basal metabolism may be helped by thyroid replacement. Preliminary reports on the use of anabolic steroids and digitoxin to retard progression are of interest, but further evaluation of this treatment is necessary before conclusions can be reached.[4,6]

Research may produce new drugs that will benefit some of the dystrophies, but it is likely that slowing of progression or arrest of the disease will be the most that can be expected from pharmacologic therapy unless drugs can be started before irreversible destruction occurs.

Preservation of strength in involved muscle is important. Some of the weakness in any of these disorders is related to disuse. Active contraction of musculature through the greatest possible range against gravity, the maintenance of contraction for several seconds, and exercise to the limits of tolerance should be carried out daily. This requires parental cooperation with constant supervision to maintain balance between the advantages of exercise and the disadvantages of excessive fatigue. With a more aggressive approach, we have extended the activity of our patients.

Prevention of contracture can best be accomplished by maintenance of strength and function. The use of stretching to prevent contracture has been advocated. What is meant by stretching requires clarification. If maintenance of range of motion is meant, there can be little argument. However, if vigorous stretching is implied, it can be harmful. Vigorous passive stretching is damaging, probably because it causes active resistance to avoid pain by contraction of antagonistic groups of muscles and by tearing of tissue. Night splints and braces are helpful in preventing contractures. Bracing and surgery and useful in the treatment of neuropathies such as Charcot-Marie-Tooth disease, which are more limited in extent, more gradual in progression, and tend to reach a relatively static state of muscle imbalance. In these diseases, the principles of bracing and of surgery are well known.

Reluctance to apply braces and to undertake surgery in the treatment of the myopathies and dystrophies is understandable. In these patients, tenotomies have to be combined with bracing. Short leg braces have questionable value. Long leg braces with knee locks help prevent knee joint contracture. With good follow-up and an active home exercise program, proper bracing need not reduce muscular strength. We agree with Spencer and Vignos,[9] who pointed out that "patients who continue to walk in braces maintain better alignment of weight bearing joints and probably have less disuse atrophy of muscles and less osteoporosis." Limited bracing, if applied early, may postpone the patient's confinement to a wheelchair. The brace should be of the simplest and lightest design obtainable.

The decision to use a brace or to perform surgery in the myopathies and dystrophies requires careful evaluation of possible advantages and disadvantages. Experience convinces one of the benefits to be derived from the early release of contractures followed by bracing. Relatively simple surgical procedures can be performed with minimal immobilization of the patient.

Minor degrees of contracture in weight bearing joints interfere with balance and reduce ability to ambulate. Judicious choice of surgery and bracing prolong independent ambulation. If the patient's ability to walk independently and if his tolerance for walking and standing diminish, the orthopaedist must determine whether this is the effect of contracture or a progressive weakness, so that appropriate steps can be taken. Early lengthening of the tendo Achilles under local infiltration anesthesia, followed by ambulation in a brace rather than a cast on the first or second postoperative day, is recommended. Tenotomy of the heel cord should be performed bilaterally so that the patient retains a symmetric posture. Simple subcutaneous tenotomies are preferred if done early. Sectioning of the iliotibial band is simple and may be advantageous if there is no response to physical therapy. More extensive contractures of the hip and knee may be corrected surgically with success if the patient is ambulated as promptly as possible, with appropriate bracing. A decision to perform extensive surgery must be based upon thoughtful observation and experience and must be implemented by a program of intensive convalescent rehabilitation. Before general anesthesia is administered, a careful evaluation of the patient's respiratory status should be made.

Adult dystrophies progress more slowly. Bracing will do much to prolong activity, and early surgical correction of joint contracture protects independence. Surgical stabilization of joints is not carried out to any extent in the dystrophies and myopathies because of the long period of immobilization required. In Charcot-Marie-Tooth syndrome, osteotomy of the os calcis, as described by Dwyer,[5] may be indicated to correct deformity. However, because of muscle imbalance the deformity of the heel will usually recur, and ultimately triple arthrodesis is required when the patient has attained sufficient skeletal maturity. Tendon transfers are not reliable because of a changing neurologic pattern.

Progressive scoliosis due to muscle imbalance or paralysis occurs in amyotonia congenita and in progressive muscular dystrophy. The use of corsets and braces is of limited value. In amyotonia congenita, longevity may be considerable; here a spinal fusion to control scoliosis is indicated in order to maintain ambulation, to improve ability to sit, and to preserve vital capacity. Death in these patients is usually caused by respiratory decompensation. Early treatment should be undertaken to minimize the degree of scoliosis and the attendant risk of surgical correction. The patient should be managed as though he had a progressive paralytic scoliosis; the risk of surgery will be less if deformity and general deterioration have not been allowed to progress too far (Fig. 7-9). Spinal instrumentation and Milwaukee bracing have facilitated postoperative management in those patients who do not tolerate casts well. A period of recumbency on a turning bed is utilized, as well as a Milwaukee brace for external support and Harrington instruments for internal bracing of the spine.

Life expectancy with and without surgery should be discussed frankly with the families of these patients, for they must participate in decisions as to whether to accept or reject the risks of surgery. With spinal fusion, the life-span of patients with amyotonia congenita has been extended, and patients who have been chair-bound have been able to return to an ambulatory status. This is in contrast to the chair-bound patient with muscular dystrophy, who can rarely be returned to activity

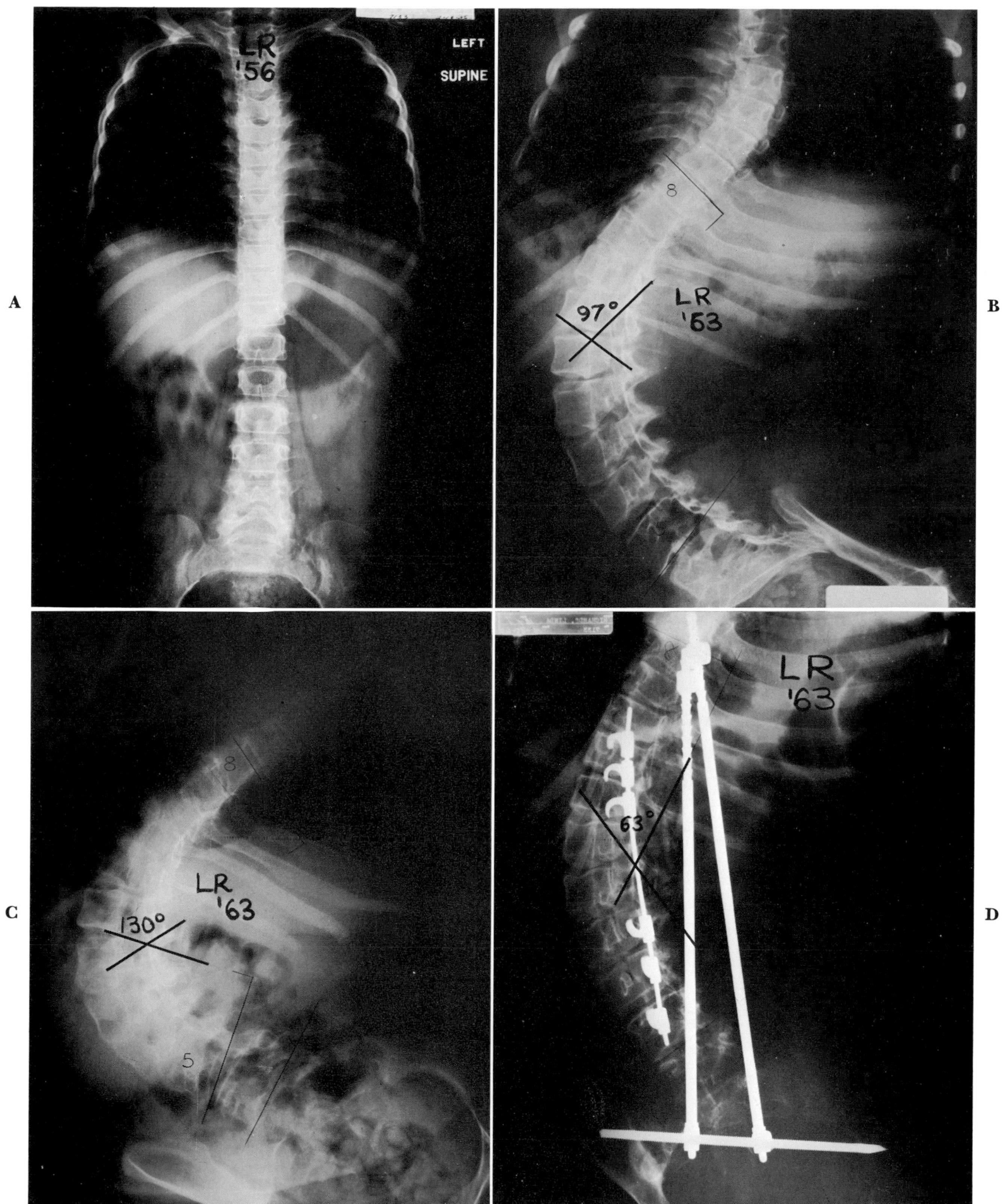

Fig. 7-9. A, Amyotonia congenita, straight spine. **B,** 97° in 5 years. **C,** 130° in 5½ years. **D,** 63° after correction and return to ambulation.

after prolonged recumbent therapy. Spinal arthrodesis is not advised in muscular dystrophy.

Obesity in the later stages of the disease, particularly in myopathies and dystrophies, becomes a great problem. These patients gain weight from inactivity. Some of their obesity is exogenous, resulting from excessive eating, but in any circumstance it handicaps mobility and independence. The better the rapport between physician, family, and patient, the less serious the problem of weight control.

COMPREHENSIVE CARE

The physician must be ever mindful that these patients should be encouraged to live as normal lives as possible by maintaining independence and social contacts through ambulation. If the patient is immobile, educational, vocation, and social opportunities are lost. The wheelchair must be avoided as long as possible in order to postpone the isolation of the patient (Fig. 7-10).[8,12] As weakness progresses, falls become more frequent—fractures become a greater problem. Trauma, illness, or surgery in the patient with muscular dystrophy is a serious occurrence and can lead to rapid deterioration.

A skilled social service worker is vital to support the family. Psychiatric help is often needed. Hospitalization should be avoided if possible, particularly in patients with myopathies and dystrophies, not only for physical reasons but also to avoid abandonment of the patient by families after years of devotion and physical depletion. In our early group of sixty-one children with dystrophies, eighteen patients and eleven parents had psychiatric problems sufficiently severe to disturb adequate management of the child.

Deterioration of the intelligence quotient has been observed in muscular dystrophy.[14] Proof of this is difficult because exposure to education and to social contacts gradually decreases. Nevertheless, there is some evidence that true mental deterioration can occur. If these children are mentally retarded or autistic, they will not exercise, are unable to manage braces, and do not tolerate surgery.

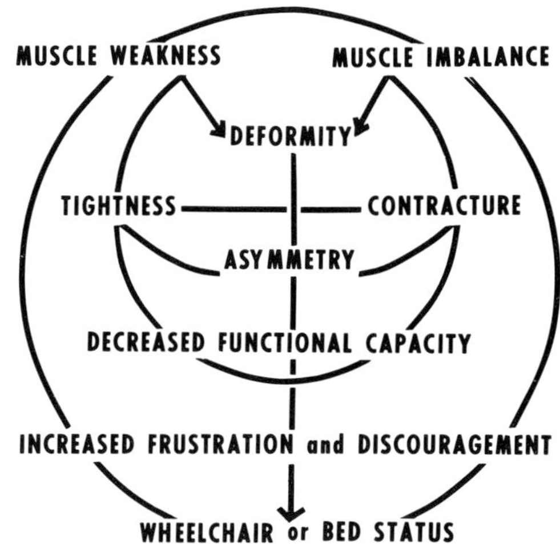

Fig. 7-10. The pernicious cycle of muscle deterioration.[2,11] (From Archibald, K. C., and Vignos, P. J., Jr.: Arch. Phys. Med. **40**:150, 1959.)

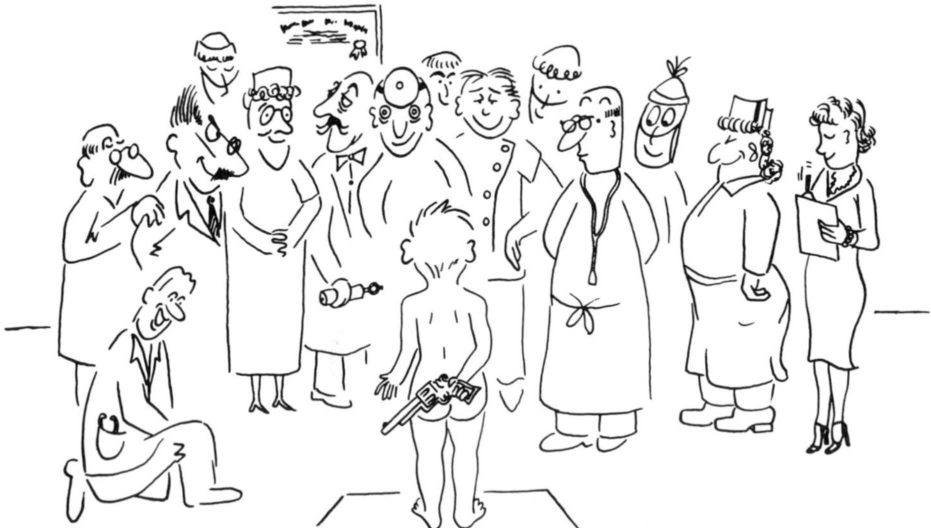

Fig. 7-11. The "team" approach.

Attendance at school with normal children should be continued as long as possible. Special education can be postponed until the patient is confined to home.

The combined effort of the orthopaedist, the pediatrician, physical and occupational therapists, social workers, teachers, and especially the families working together as a team (Fig. 7-11) is absolutely essential in the management of patients with these disorders. Orthopaedic surgeons are physicians first and surgeons next, so they should be prepared to work with other specialists and to assume leadership in developing a multidiscipline approach for comprehensive care of the patient.

I am indebted to Douglas Buchanan, M.D., Professor of Neurology, University of Chicago, and A. T. Milhorat, M.D., Clinical Professor of Medicine, Cornell University, for having participated in the presentation of this material in an instructional course at the American Academy of Orthopaedic Surgeons in 1963 to 1966. In the course, they elaborated extensively on the differential diagnosis and medical aspects of congenital neurologic disorders, the dystrophies, and the myopathies. Appreciation is also extended to Thomas T. Rizzo, M.D., of New York, who, as a resident at Newington Hospital for Crippled Children, assisted greatly in the review of our patients.

REFERENCES

1. Adams, R., Denny-Brown, D., and Pearson, C.: Diseases of muscle, ed. 2, New York, 1965, Harper & Row, Publishers, p. 710.
2. Archibald, K. C., and Vignos, P. J., Jr.: A study of contractures in muscular dystrophy, Arch. Phys. Med. **40**:150, 1959.
3. Cohen, Jonathan: Personal communication.
4. Dowben, R. M.: Treatment of muscular dystrophy with steroids. A preliminary report, New Eng. J. Med. **268**:912, 1963.
5. Dwyer, F. C.: Osteotomy of the calcaneum for pes cavus, J. Bone Joint Surg. **41B**:80, 1959.
6. Fowler, W. M., Jr., Pearson, C. M., Egstrom, G. H., and Gardner, G. W.: Ineffective treatment of muscular dystrophy with an anabolic steroid and other measures, New Eng. J. Med. **272**:875, 1965.
7. Pearce, J. M., Pennington, R. J., and Walton, J. N.: Serum enzyme study in muscle disease. III. Serum creatine kinase activity in relatives of patients with the Duchenne type muscular dystrophy, J. Neurol. Neurosurg. Psychiat. **27**:181, 1964.
8. Patterns of Disease. Detroit, August, 1962, Parke, Davis & Co. (Pamphlet.)
9. Spencer, G. E., Jr., and Vignos, P. J., Jr.: Bracing for ambulation in childhood progressive muscular dystrophy, J. Bone Joint Surg. **44A**:234, 1962.
10. Swinyard, C. A.: Progressive muscular dystrophy and atrophy and related conditions. Diagnosis and management, Pediat. Clin. N. Amer. **7**:703, 1960.
11. Swinyard, C. A., Deaver, G. G., and Greenspan, L.: Gradients of functional ability of importance in rehabilitation of patients with progressive muscular and neuromuscular diseases, Arch. Phys. Med. **38**:574, 1957.
12. Swinyard, C. A., Deaver, G. G., and Greenspan, L.: Progressive muscular dystrophy, diagnosis and problems of rehabilitation, New York, Muscular Dystrophy Associations of America, 1958. (Pamphlet.)
13. Vignos, P. J., Spencer, G. E., Jr., and Archibald, K. C.: Management of progressive muscular dystrophy in childhood, J.A.M.A. **184**:89, 1963.
14. Worden, D. K., and Vignos, P. J., Jr.: Intellectual function in childhood progressive muscular dystrophy, Pediatrics **29**:968, 1962.

Chapter 8

Unstable intertrochanteric fractures

Part I*

HENRY H. BANKS, M.D.
Boston, Massachusetts

During the last 25 years, the pendulum has swung from traction to internal fixation in the treatment of intertrochanteric fractures of the hip. This change is related to the reduction of morbidity, mortality (from 30% to 15%), and malunion (from 20% to 10%) with internal fixation. The cost of prolonged hospitalization also plays a role.

It has been clear for some time that some of these injuries are stable and others are unstable. The usual definition (Figs. 8-1 and 8-2) states that if the medial cortical buttress is intact or undisplaced or restored by reduction, the fracture is stable and the result inevitably good.[2] When there is cortical overlap that is not corrected or destruction that cannot be restored, the fracture is considered to be unstable. Obviously the degree of comminution is important here. Stability would then depend on the structural strength of the metallic fixation unless the fracture could be converted to a stable one.

Based on an analysis of 237 fractures in 234 patients treated at the Peter Bent Brigham Hospital in Boston from 1955 to 1966, we believe that there are more factors involved in stability than this definition recognizes. This belief is supported by a study of twenty-eight intertrochanteric fractures obtained at postmortem examination.

The definition of stability should include not only what is seen on the anteroposterior roentgenogram but also the appearance of the lateral roentgenogram. As noted in the lateral view of Fig. 8-3, *B*, it is clear that it is possible for the head-neck fragment to telescope into the shaft fragment. In Fig. 8-3, *C*, this complication was present 2 months postoperatively. Indeed, Fig. 8-4, *C* shows this happening within 3 weeks of the time of internal fixation, when the postmortem specimen of the hip was examined.

If there is significant posterior comminution even though there is apparent medial cortex contact on the anteroposterior roentgenograms, the fracture may well be unstable. Where this anatomic situation is not recognized, loss of valgus and penetration of the joint by the fixation may result as

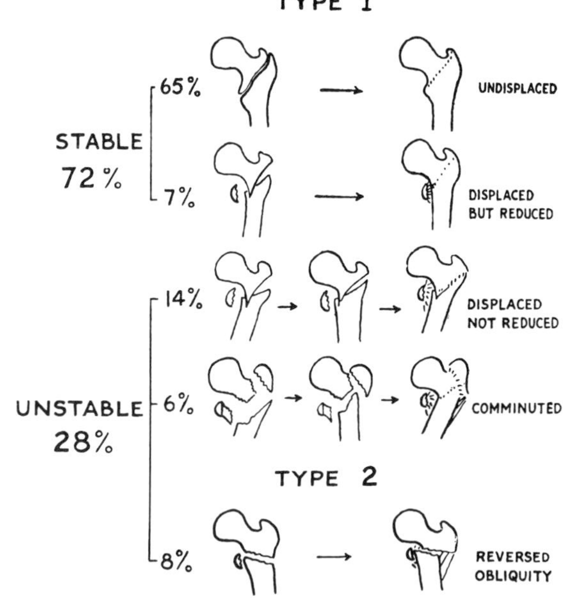

Fig. 8-1. Types of intertrochanteric fractures. (From Evans, E. M.: J. Bone Joint Surg. **31B**:190, 1949.)

*Supported by Easter Seal Research Foundation Grant, U.S.P.H.S. Grant AM-OO854-13, and U. S. Army Research Grant DA-49-193-MD2237.

in Fig. 8-5. Where this anatomic situation is recognized, it is possible that with rigid fixation and delayed weight bearing the fracture may heal without complications, as noted in Fig. 8-6. Hughston[4] and Dimon and Hughston[1] pointed out the importance of recognizing posterior comminution.

The degree of comminution present may not be seen clearly in either the anteroposterior or the lateral roentgenogram. In Fig. 8-7, the preoperative and postoperative roentgenograms showed only a small degree of comminution. Yet the roentgenogram of the postmortem specimen showed a very significant degree of comminution, obviously affecting stability.

Iatrogenic fractures may also contribute to instability. It is possible to create a subtrochanteric fracture during the insertion of the internal fixation. The shaft may then tend to shift medially in relation to the head-neck fragment. Such a situation is noted in Fig. 8-8.

Metal failure may also contribute to instability and nonunion. This complication is noted in Fig.

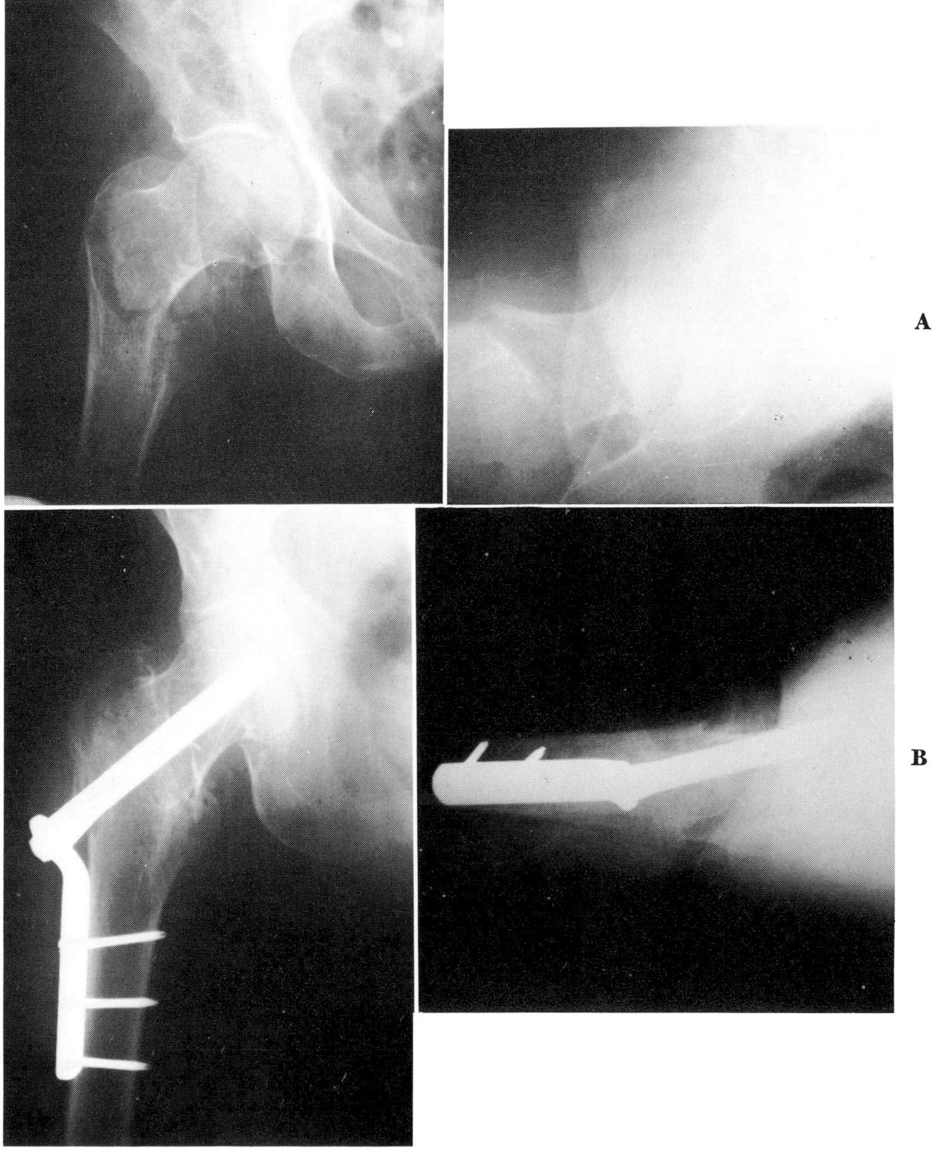

Fig. 8-2. A, Preoperative roentgenograms in an 85-year-old woman with an intertrochanteric fracture of her right hip. **B,** Postoperative roentgenograms. This would be considered to be a stable fracture.

Continued.

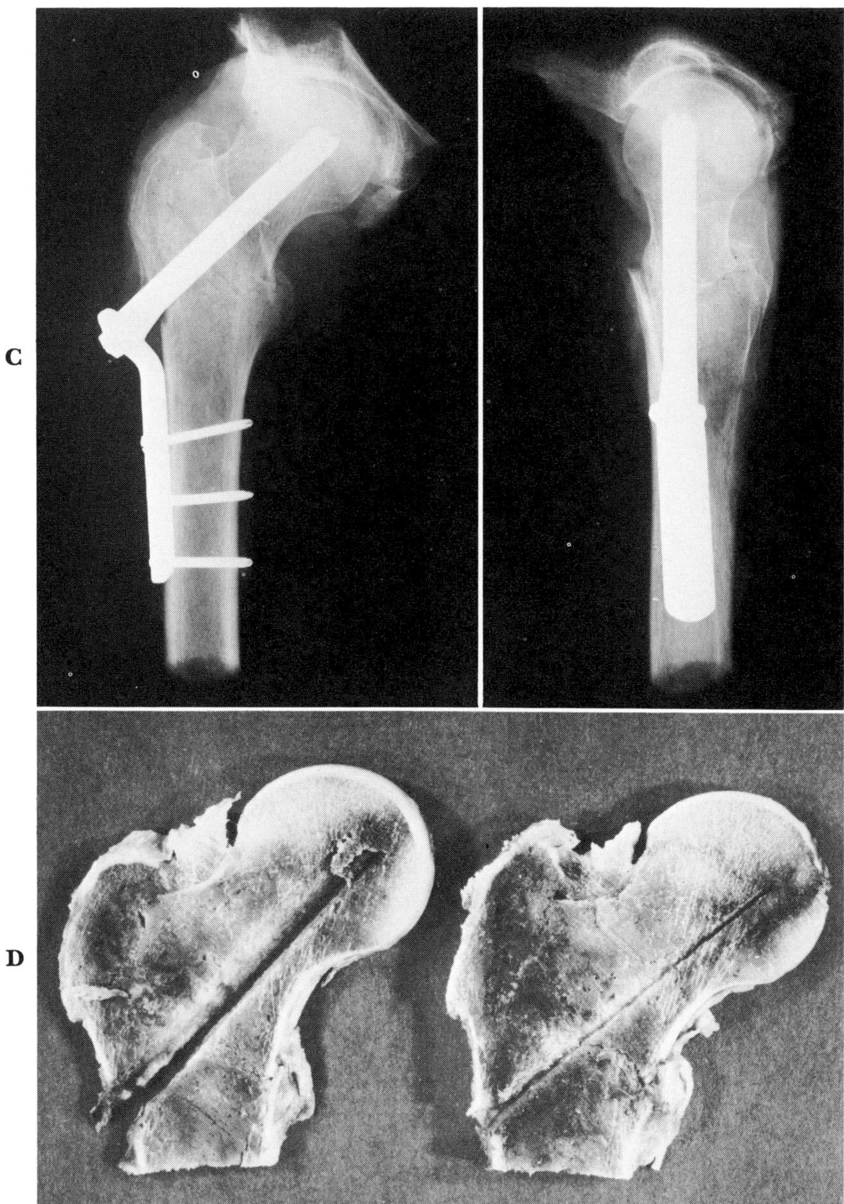

Fig. 8-2, cont'd. C, Roentgenograms of the postmortem specimen obtained 3 weeks postoperatively. Note evidence of stability. **D,** Sawed slabs of postmortem specimen. Note contact at medial cortical buttress.

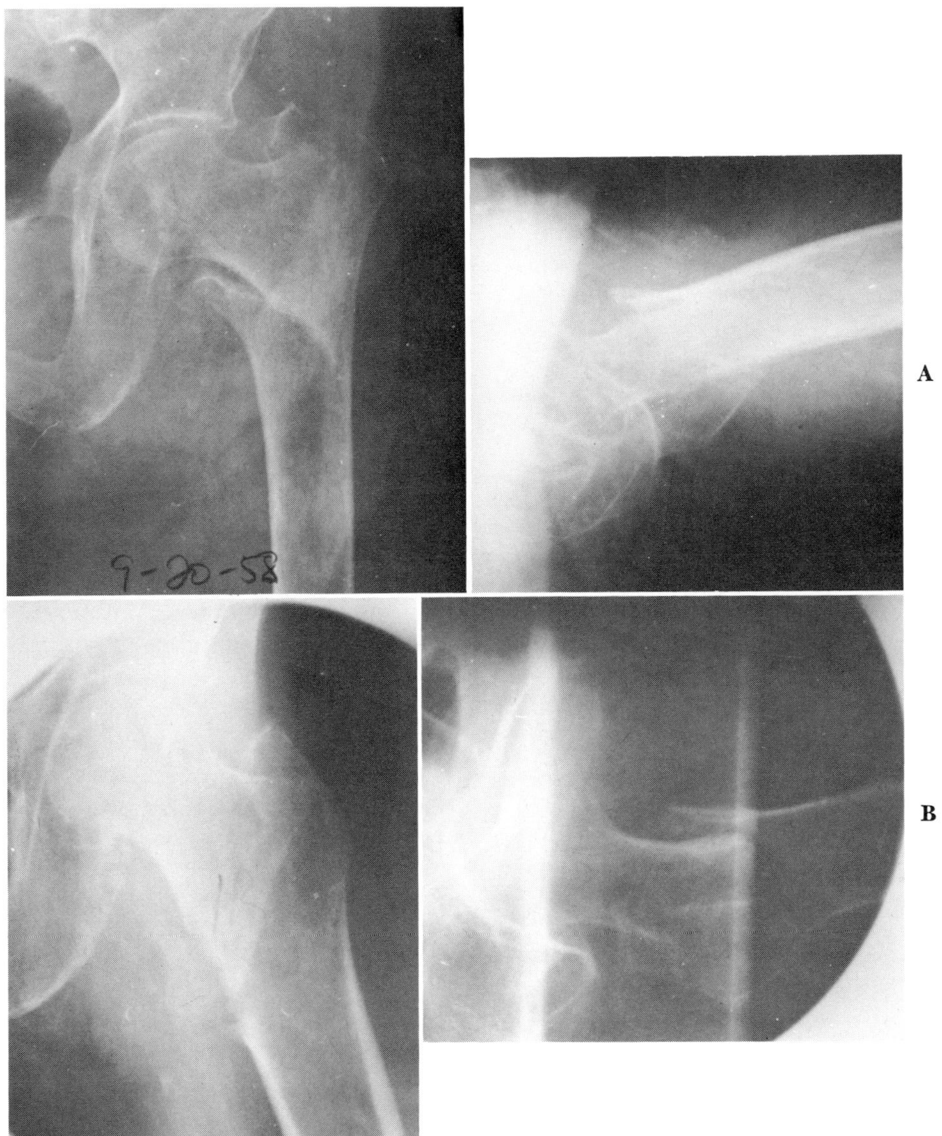

Fig. 8-3. A, Preoperative roentgenograms in an 86-year-old woman with an intertrochanteric fracture of her left hip. **B,** Reduction roentgenograms obtained in the operating room. Note, in the lateral view, the possibility of the head-neck fragment telescoping into the shaft.

Continued.

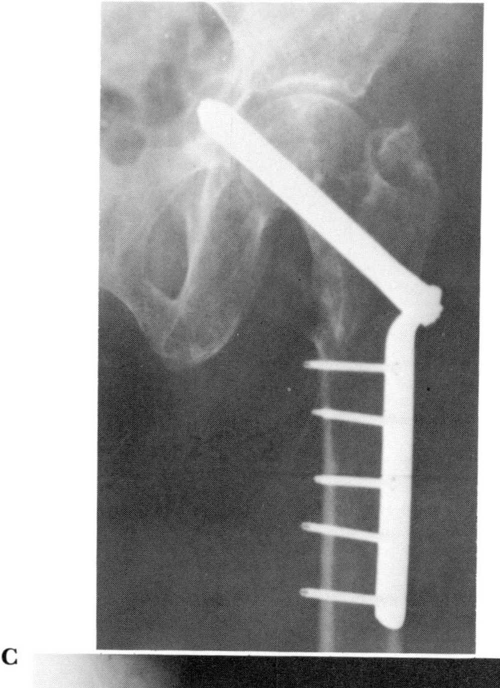

C

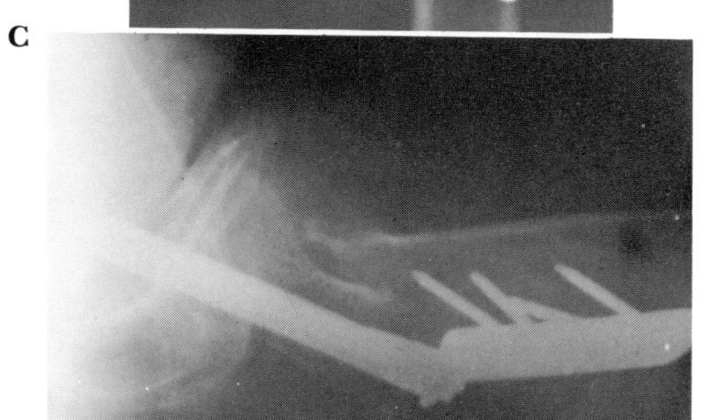

8-9, in which premature weight bearing was the leading factor. Twenty of the twenty-eight postmortem specimens were examined from 1 to 3 months after internal fixation with a cannulated Smith-Petersen nail and a Thornton plate. Nine of these twenty specimens showed motion at the fracture site. In each of these, the motion was due to lack of rigidity at the nail plate juncture when the cannulated Smith-Petersen nail and the Thornton plate were used.

Yet, it is entirely possible for a badly comminuted, potentially unstable fracture, if restored to good alignment and adequately immobilized, to heal with a good result. This was noted in twenty-seven of thirty such injuries and is illustrated in Fig. 8-10.

When the result (Table 8-1) in 121 intertrochanteric fractures assessed from 1 to 6 years after injury is analyzed, it is clear that the incidence of nonunion is small. Of the sixty injuries that were converted to stable fractures, fifteen of the fifty-eight healed fractures presented complications. In ten the nail advanced toward the joint surface, penetrating it in seven instances. In five there was loss of valgus, including a significant amount (more than 10°) in two. Of the thirty unstable fractures,

Fig. 8-3, cont'd. C, Roentgenograms obtained 2 months postoperatively. Note that the head-neck fragment has telescoped into the shaft fragment with nail penetration.

A

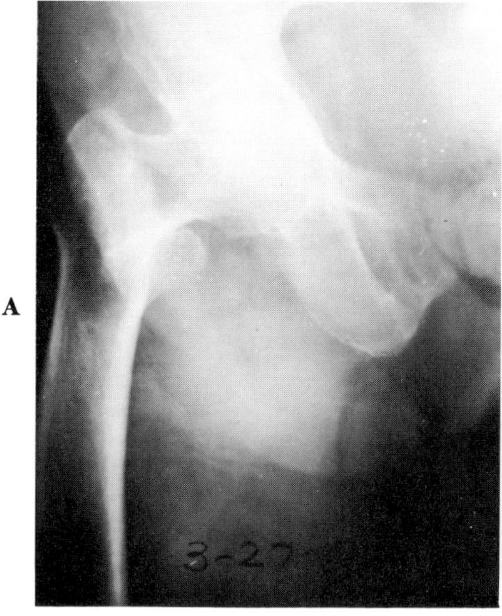

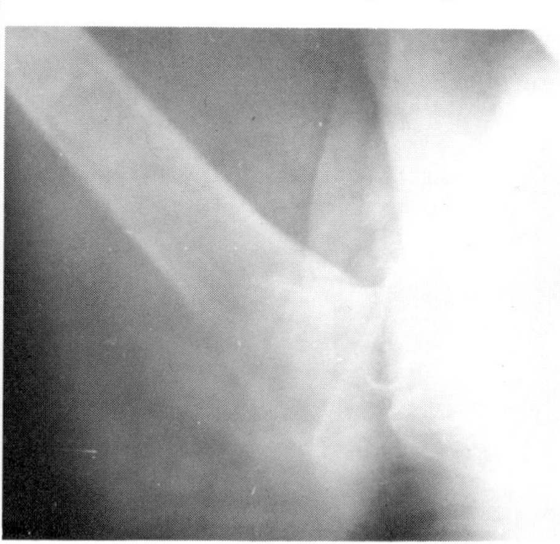

Fig. 8-4. A, Preoperative roentgenograms in a 94-year-old woman with an intertrochanteric fracture of her right hip.

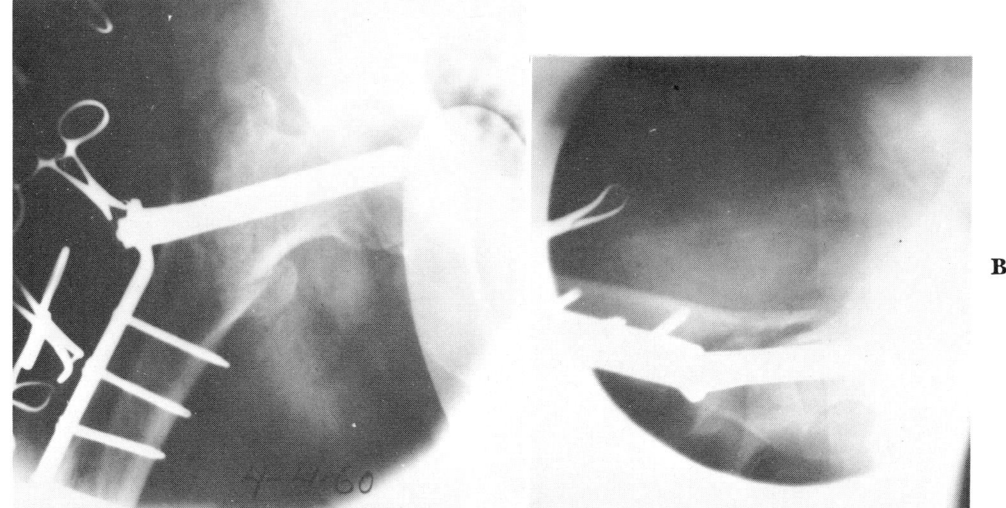

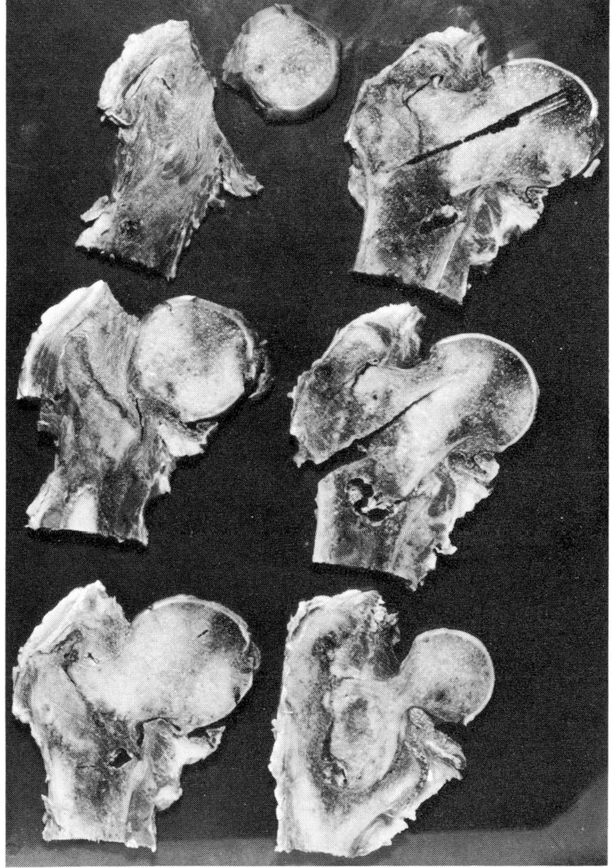

Fig. 8-4, cont'd. B, Roentgenograms obtained in the operating room. Note in the lateral view the possibility of the head-neck fragment telescoping into the shaft fragment. **C,** Sawed slabs of the postmortem specimen obtained 3 weeks postoperatively. Note the telescoping of the head-neck fragment into the shaft fragment.

there were twenty complications. Nail advancement occurred in nine, but in only one did the nail penetrate the joint. In eleven instances there was loss of valgus, including two with a significant degree (more than 10°).

Table 8-1. Result in 121 intertrochanteric fractures

Type	*Number*	*Healed*	*Nonunion*
Stable	31	31	0
Converted to stable	60	58	2
Unstable	30	27	3
Total	121	116	5

Of the five nonunions, metal failure was present in four instances, including two in which premature weight bearing was allowed prior to adequate healing. In one nonunion, multiple insertions of the fixation compromised its holding power.

A study of the twenty-eight postmortem specimens showed that these fractures healed like a shaft fracture with periosteal and endosteal response and not like a femoral neck fracture. These findings are illustrated in Fig. 8-11.

SUMMARY

There is an entity known as an unstable intertrochanteric fracture of the hip. Its definition should include additional factors, as noted previously.

Text continued on p. 110.

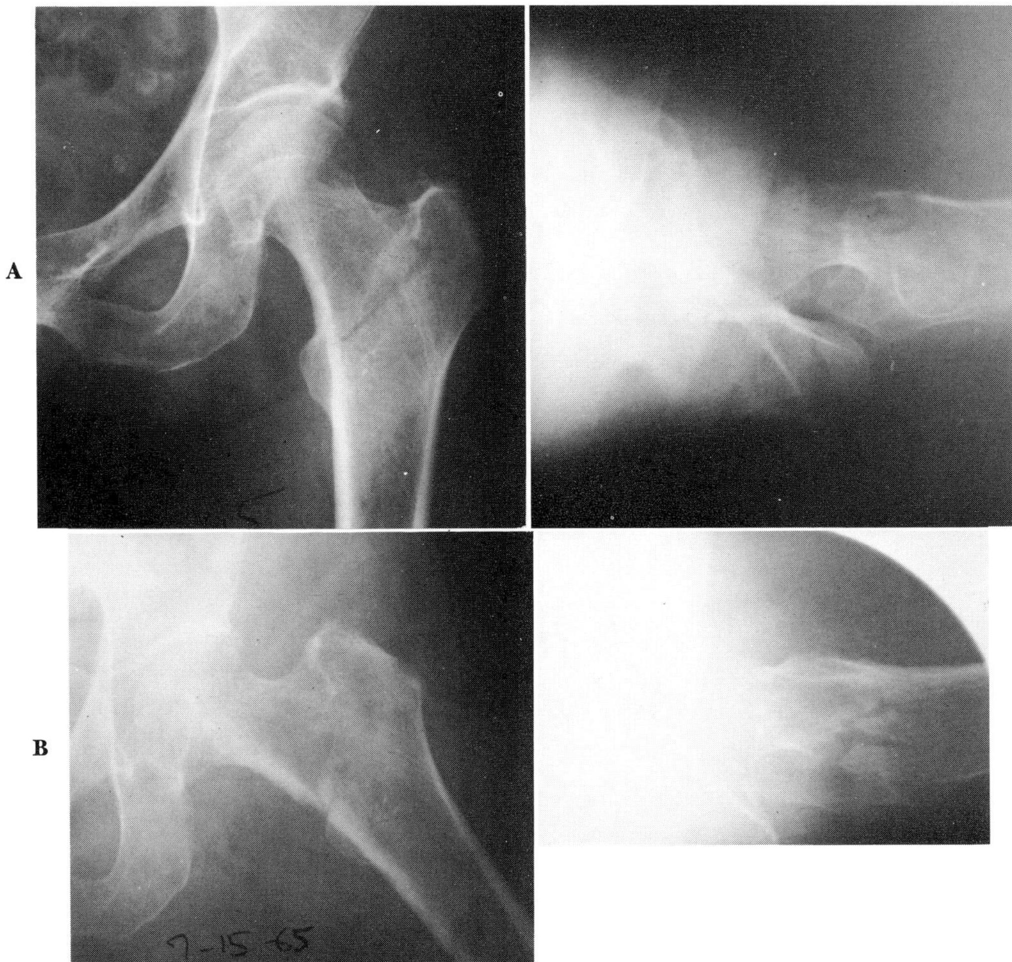

Fig. 8-5. A, Preoperative roentgenograms of a 56-year-old woman with what appears to be a classical "stable" intertrochanteric fracture of her left hip. **B,** Reduction roentgenograms obtained in the operating room. Note the "stability" of the anteroposterior roentgenogram. Note the posterior comminution seen in the lateral view. **C,** Postoperative roentgenograms (5 days). Note slight loss of valgus. **D,** Roentgenograms obtained 5 months postoperatively. Note loss of valgus and nail penetration. **E,** Roentgenograms obtained 15 months postoperatively. The fracture has healed with varus and posterior tilt of the head.

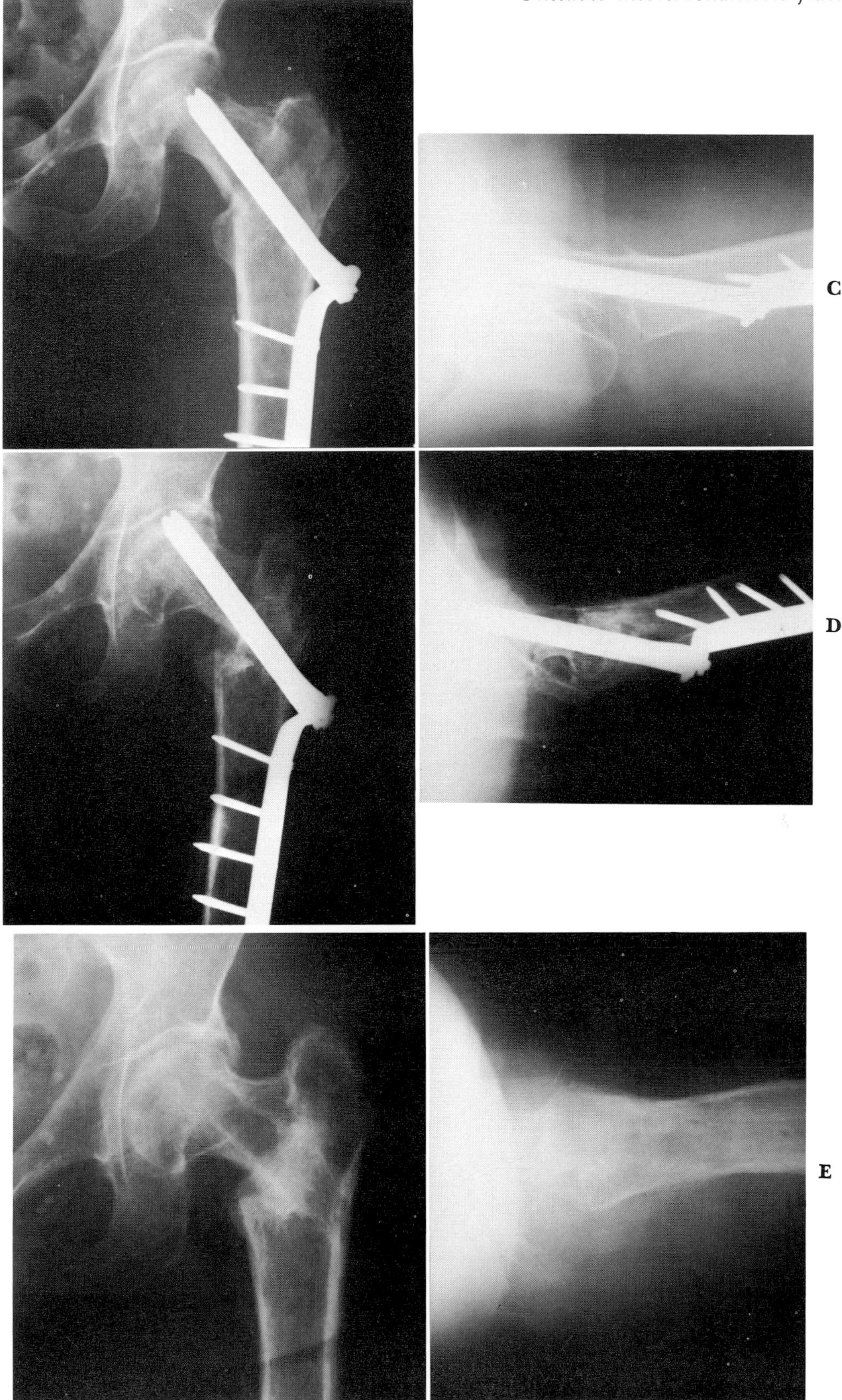

Fig. 8-5, cont'd. For legend see opposite page.

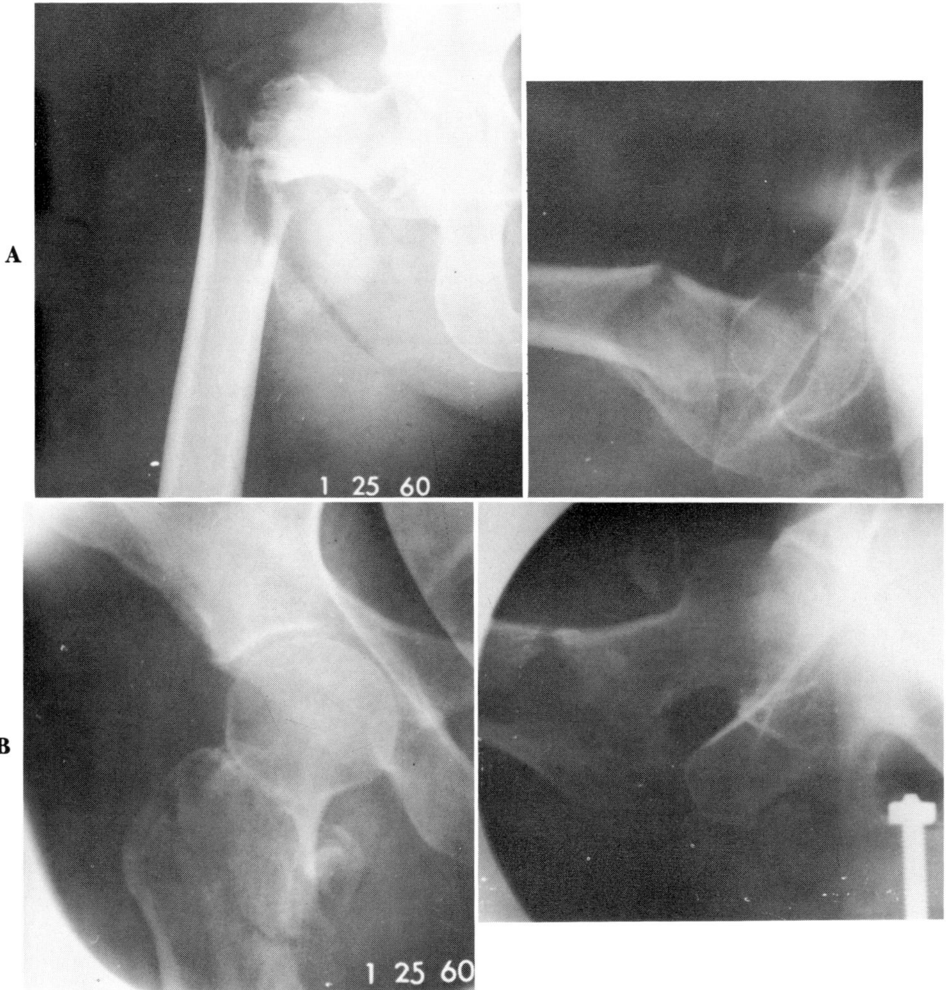

Fig. 8-6. A, Preoperative roentgenograms of a 53-year-old woman with an intertrochanteric fracture of her right hip. **B,** Roentgenograms obtained in the operating room. Note "stability" of the anteroposterior roentgenogram, but the severe comminution seen posteriorly in the lateral view.

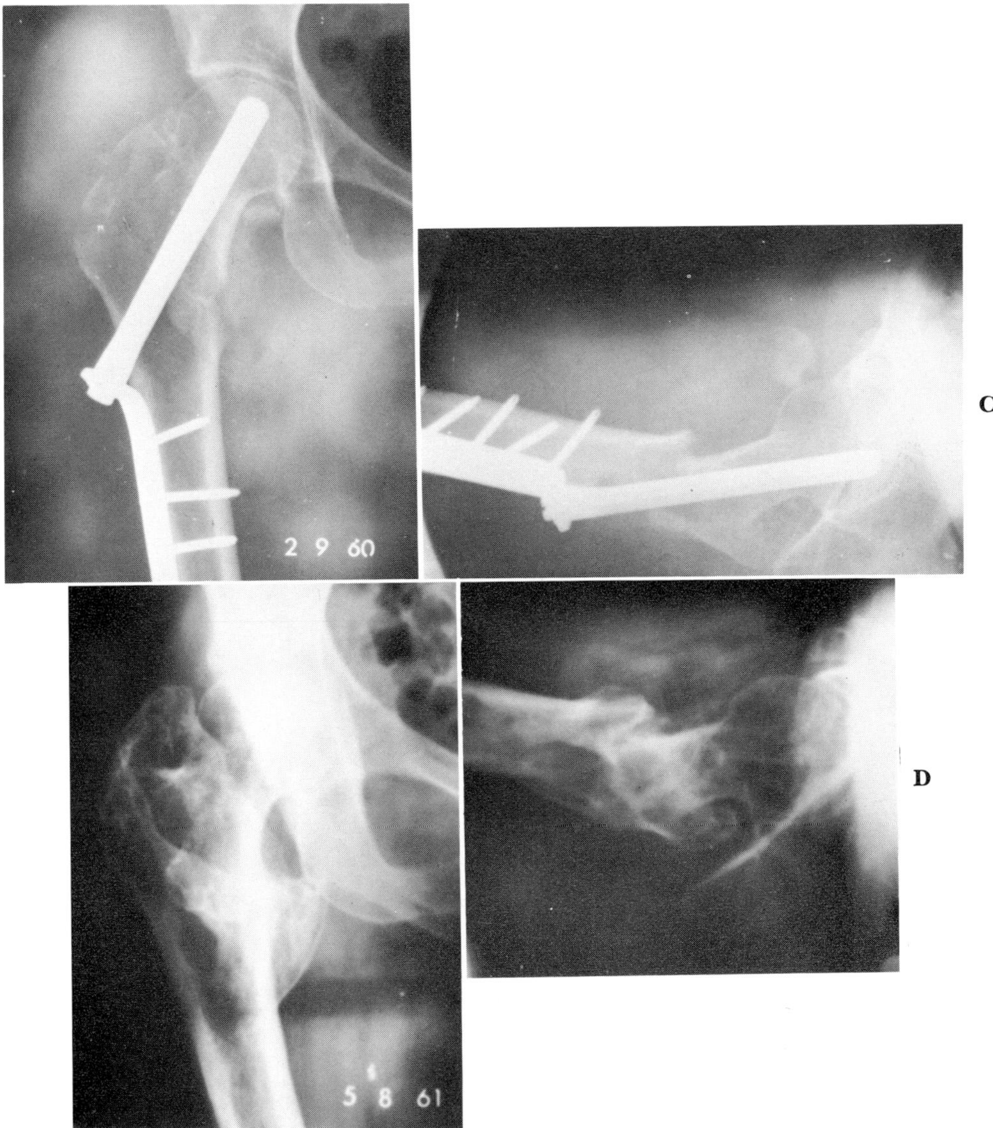

Fig. 8-6, cont'd. C, Roentgenograms obtained 2 weeks postoperatively. **D,** Roentgenograms obtained 16 months postoperatively. The internal fixation has been removed. The reduction has been maintained in a potentially unstable situation.

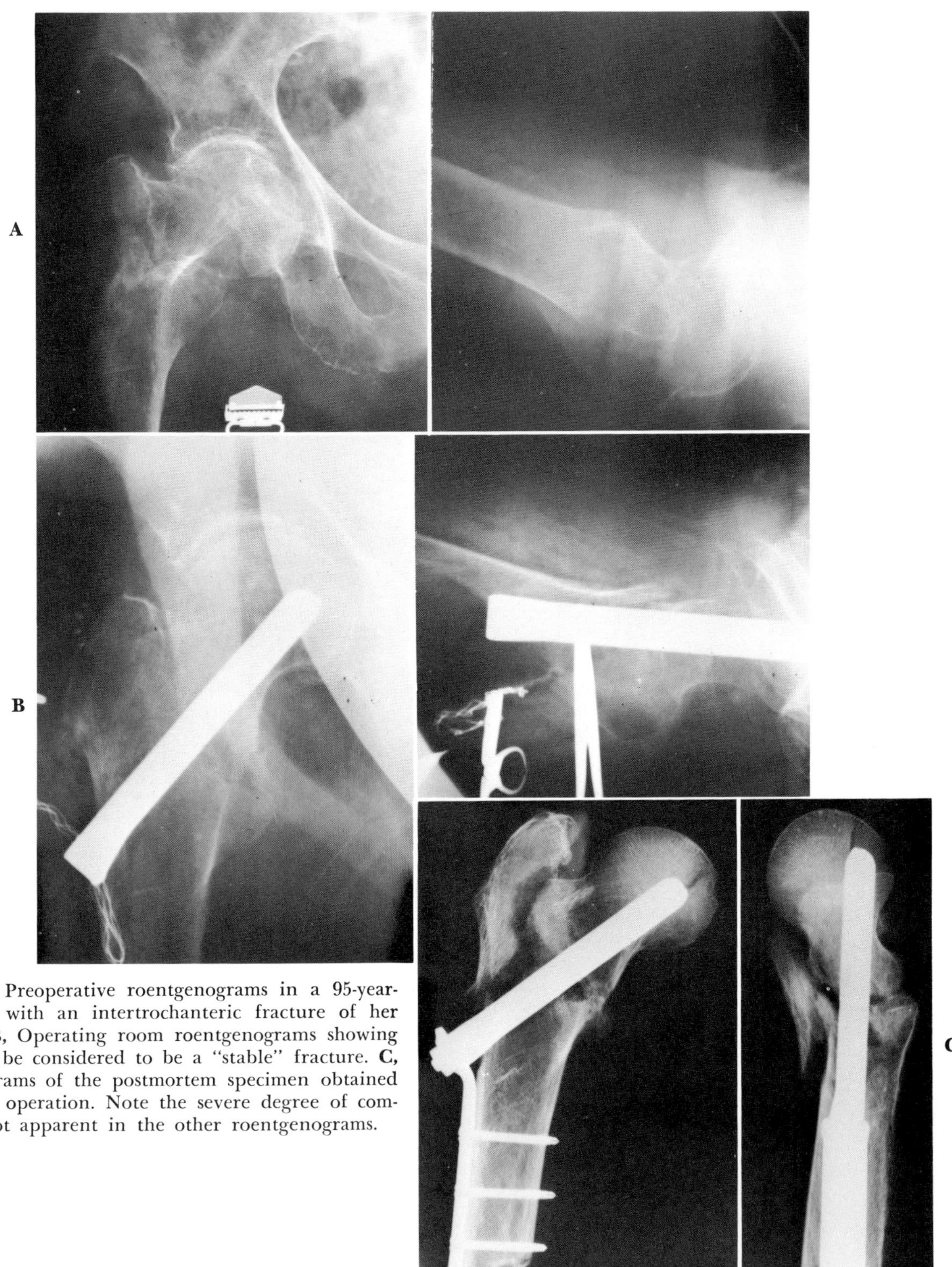

Fig. 8-7. A, Preoperative roentgenograms in a 95-year-old woman with an intertrochanteric fracture of her right hip. **B,** Operating room roentgenograms showing what might be considered to be a "stable" fracture. **C,** Roentgenograms of the postmortem specimen obtained 2 days after operation. Note the severe degree of comminution not apparent in the other roentgenograms.

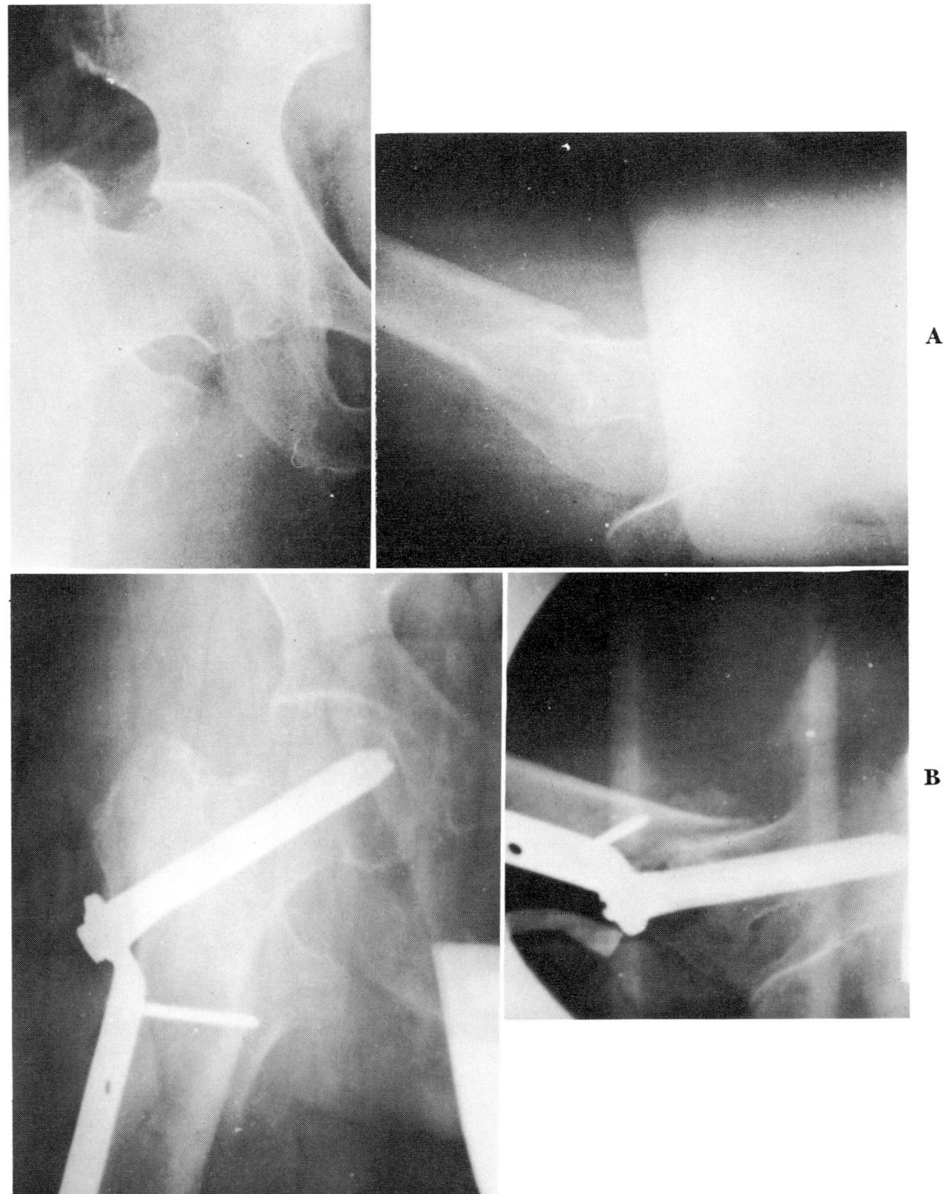

Fig. 8-8. A, Preoperative roentgenograms of a 76-year-old woman with an intertrochanteric fracture of her right hip. **B,** Operating room roentgenograms showing good alignment and internal fixation. Note subtrochanteric fracture line in the anteroposterior roentgenogram and the possibility of telescoping in the lateral view.

Continued.

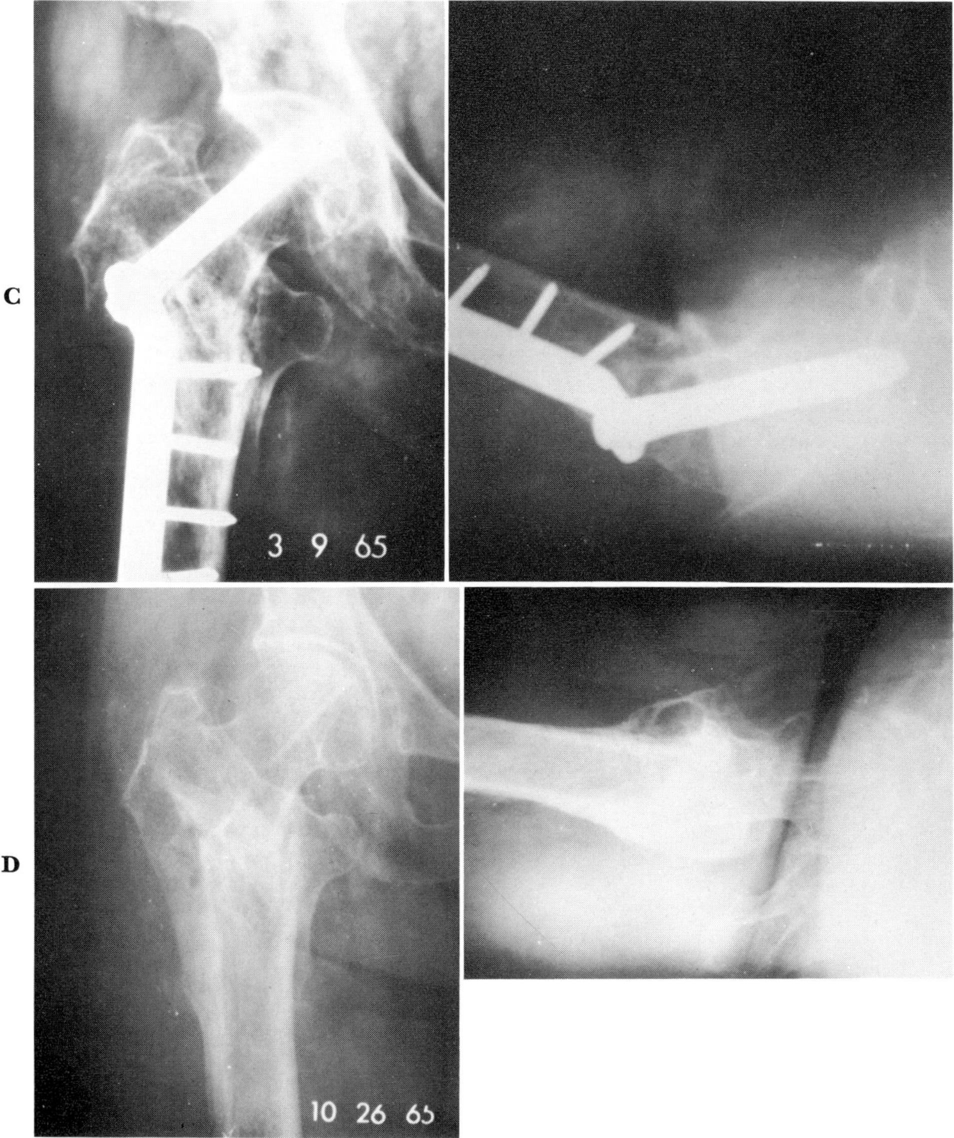

Fig. 8-8, cont'd. C, Roentgenograms obtained 6 months after internal fixation. Note the postoperative medial displacement of the shaft and the nail penetration. **D,** Roentgenograms obtained 1 year after operation. The internal fixation has been removed, and the fractures (intertrochanteric and subtrochanteric) have healed.

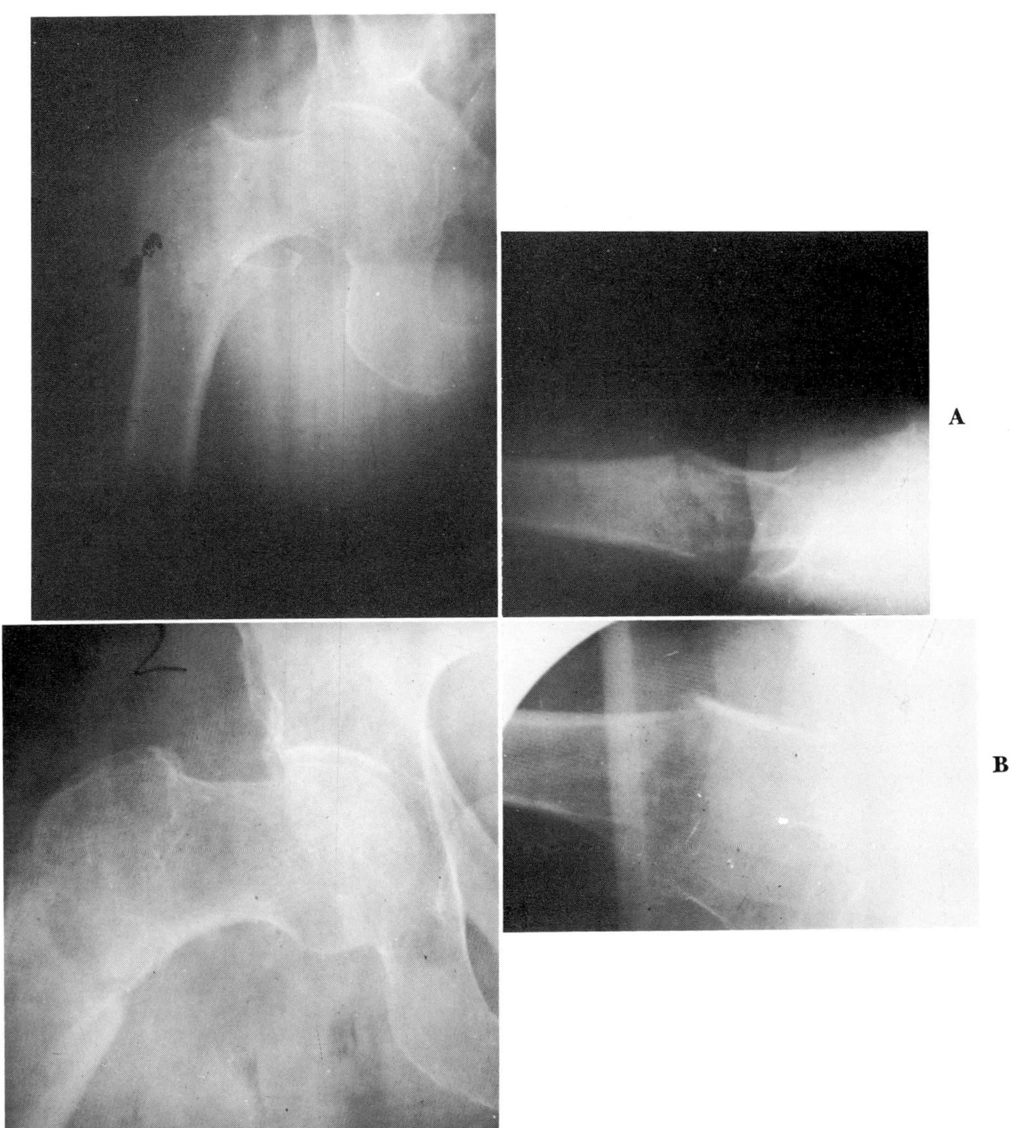

Fig. 8-9. A, Preoperative roentgenograms of a 73-year-old woman with an intertrochanteric fracture of her right hip. **B,** Roentgenograms obtained in the operating room. Note comminution of the medial cortex and posteriorly.

Continued.

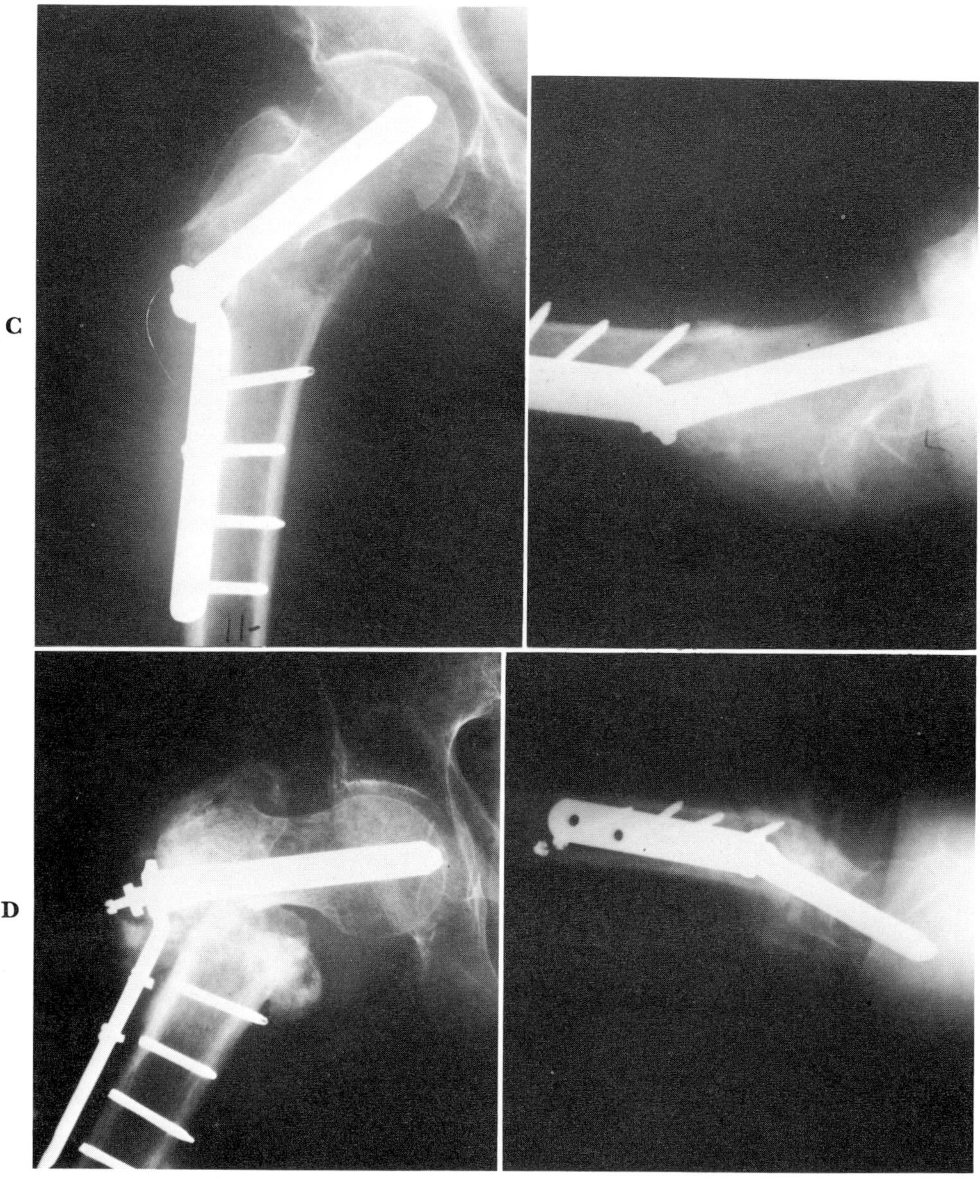

Fig. 8-9, cont'd. C, Roentgenograms obtained immediately after the operation. Note an iatrogenic subtrochanteric fracture with medial displacement of the shaft. **D,** Roentgenograms obtained 1 year after internal fixation. Ill-advised weight bearing began about a month after operation. Note metal failure and nonunion.

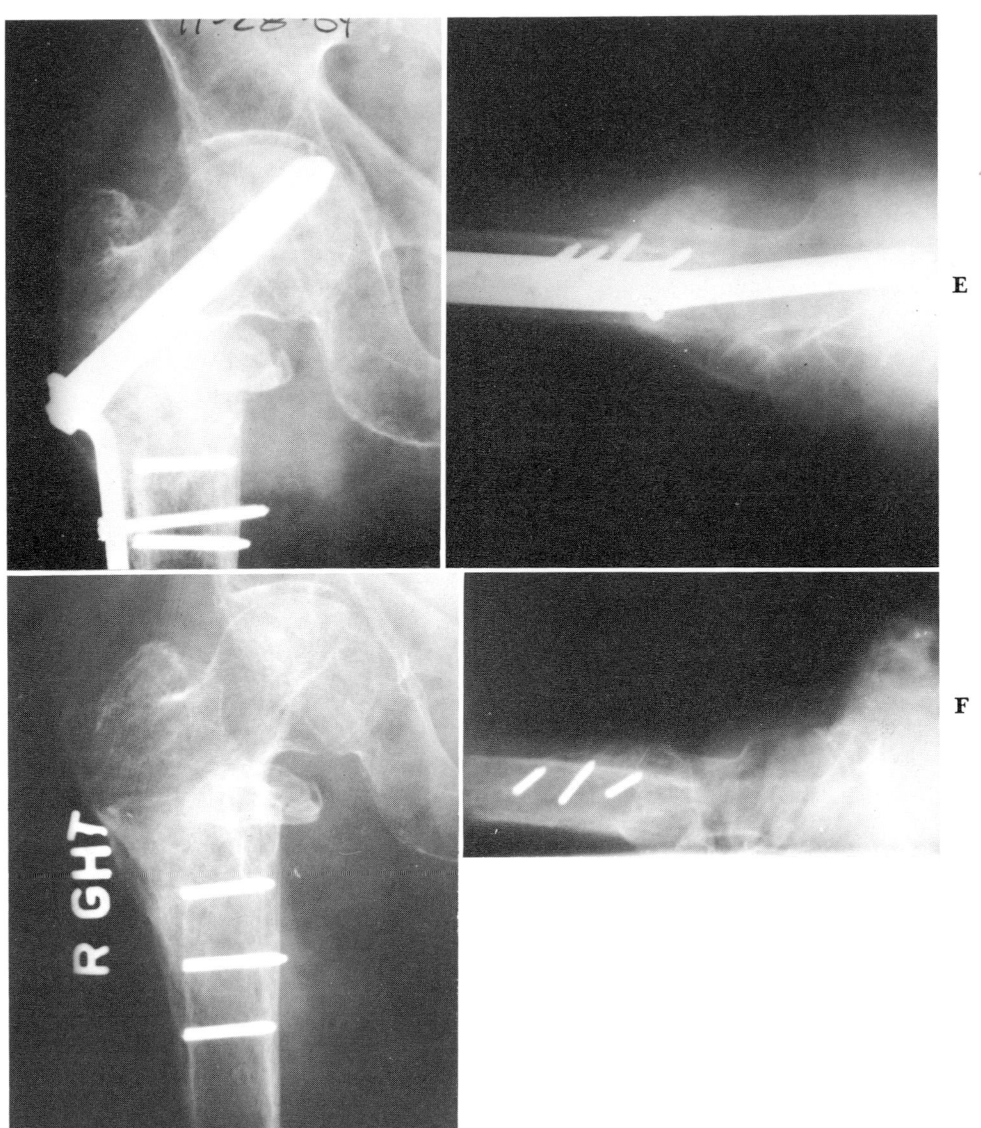

Fig. 8-9, cont'd. E, Roentgenograms obtained 2 years after the original injury and 1 year after new internal fixation and bone grafting. The displacement of the shaft medially was accepted at the second procedure. **F,** Roentgenograms obtained 4 years after the original injury and 3 years after the second operation. The internal fixation has been removed. The fracture has healed with an excellent functional result.

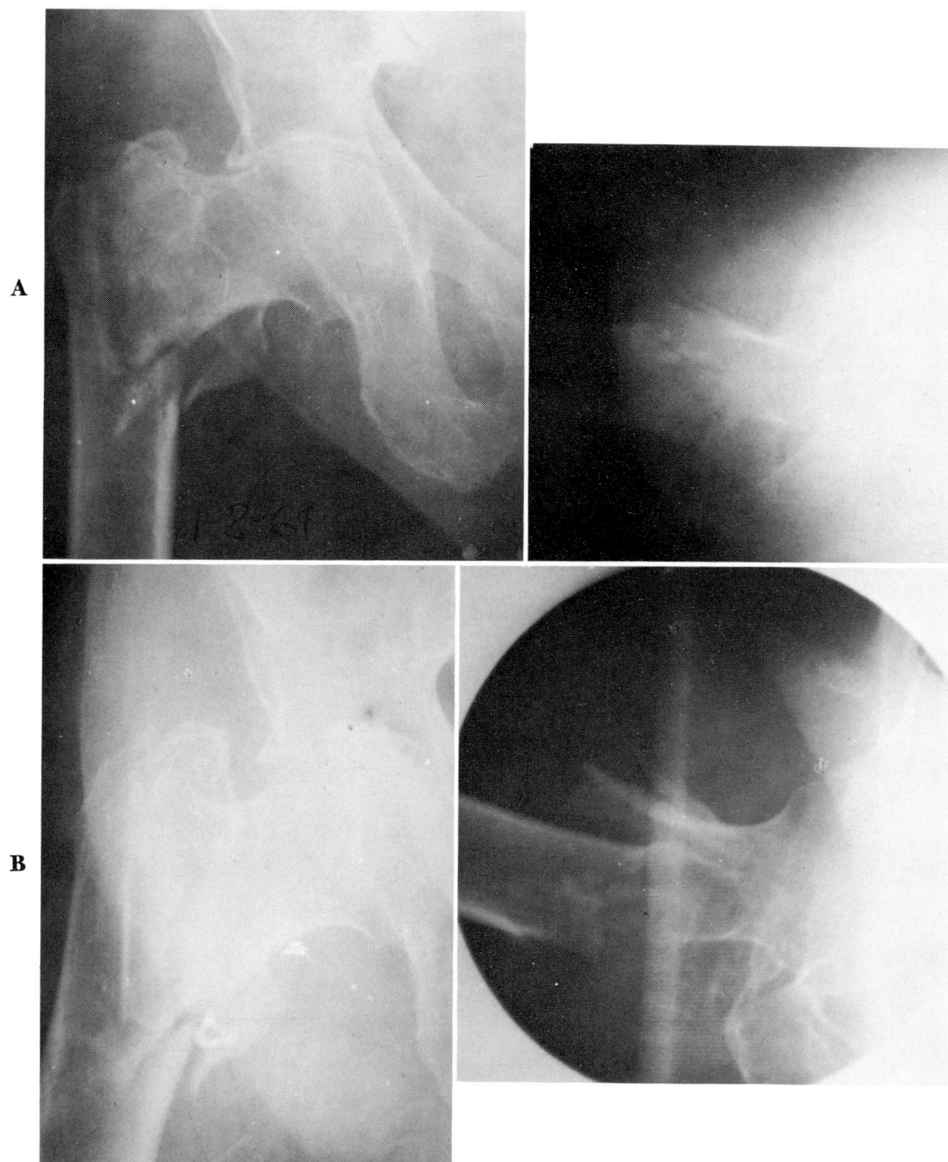

Fig. 8-10. A, Preoperative roentgenograms of a 73-year-old woman with a comminuted intertrochanteric fracture of her right hip. **B,** Operating room roentgenograms showing severe comminution. This fracture would certainly be classified as "unstable."

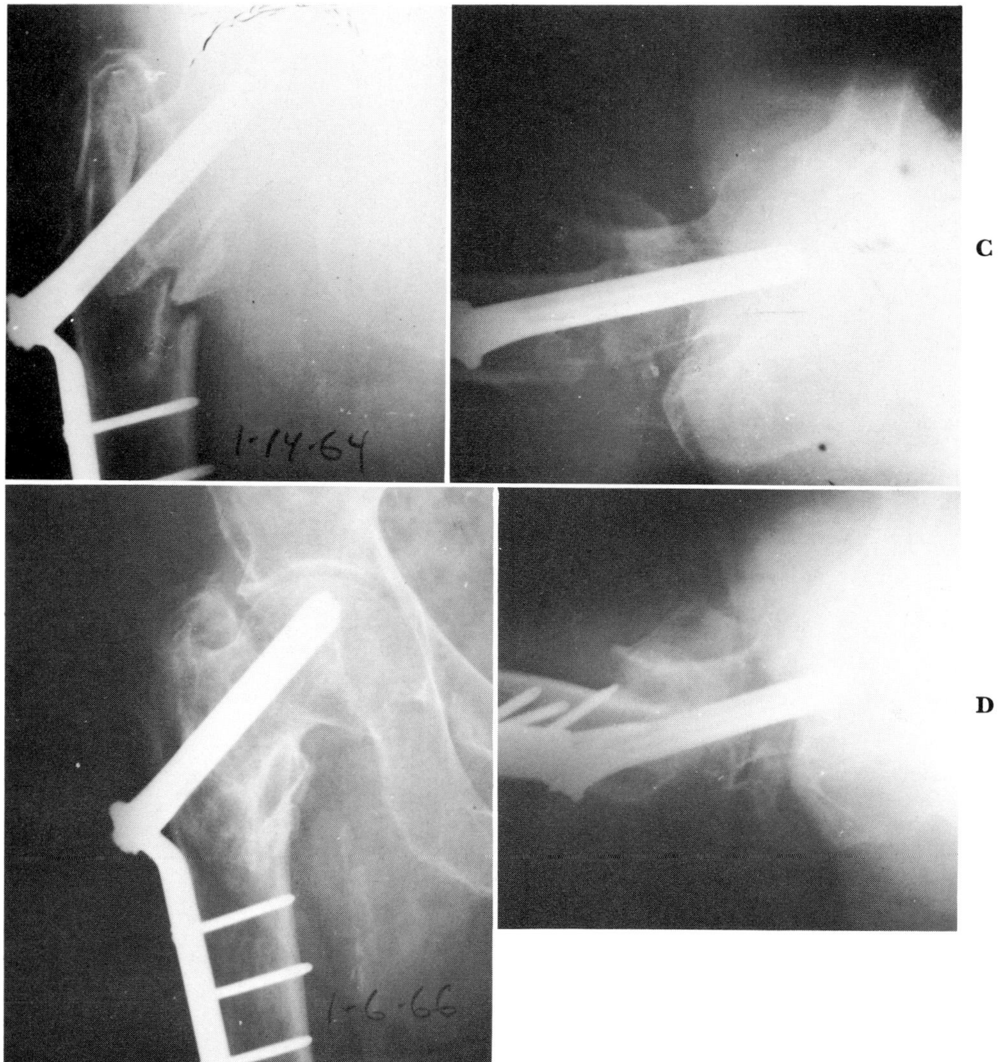

Fig. 8-10, cont'd. C, Roentgenograms obtained 5 days after operation. Bed rest with balanced suspension and skin traction were used for 1 month. Weight bearing was not allowed for more than 4 months. **D,** Roentgenograms obtained 2 years after internal fixation. The fractures healed with a good functional result. There has been some settling at the fracture site. The nail is apparently closer to the articular surface now than in the roentgenograms obtained soon after operation.

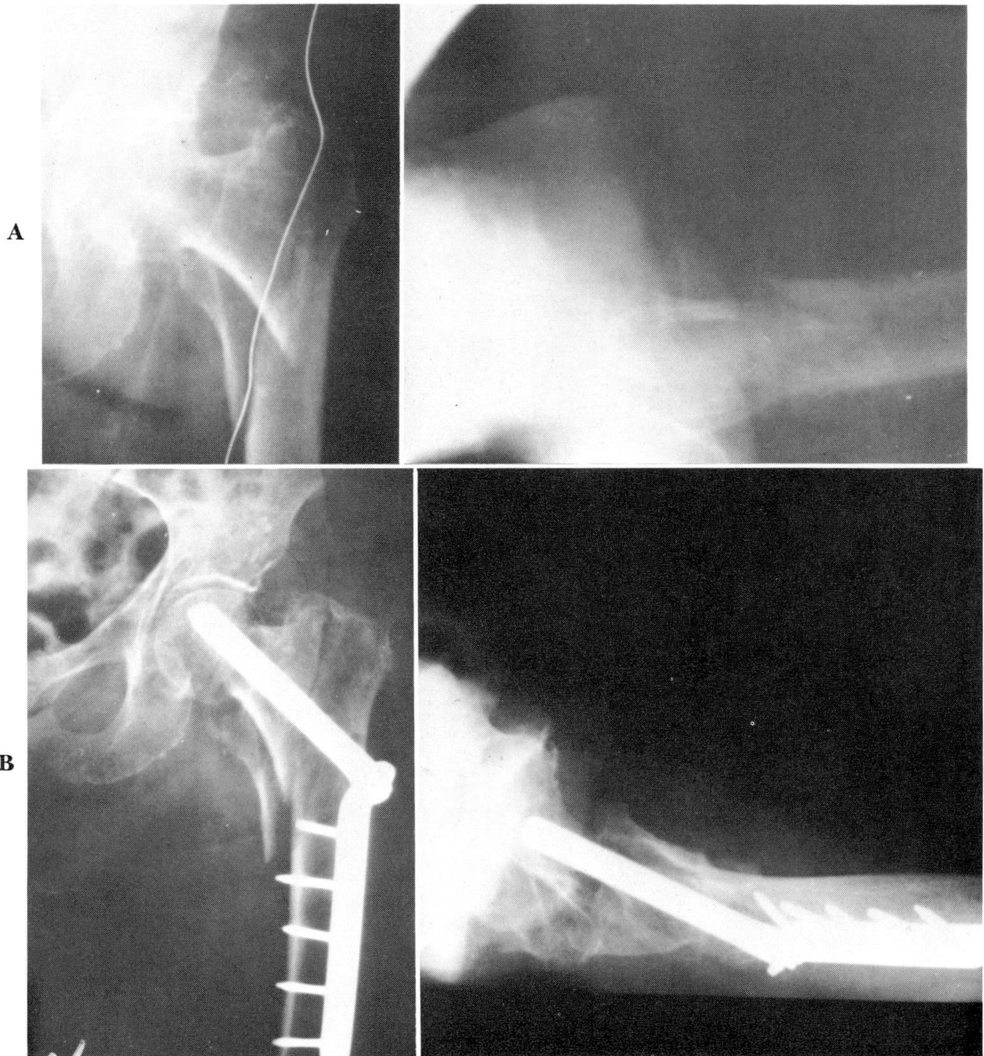

Fig. 8-11. A, Preoperative roentgenograms of a comminuted intertrochanteric fracture of the left hip of a 90-year-old woman. **B,** Roentgenograms obtained 1 week after internal fixation.

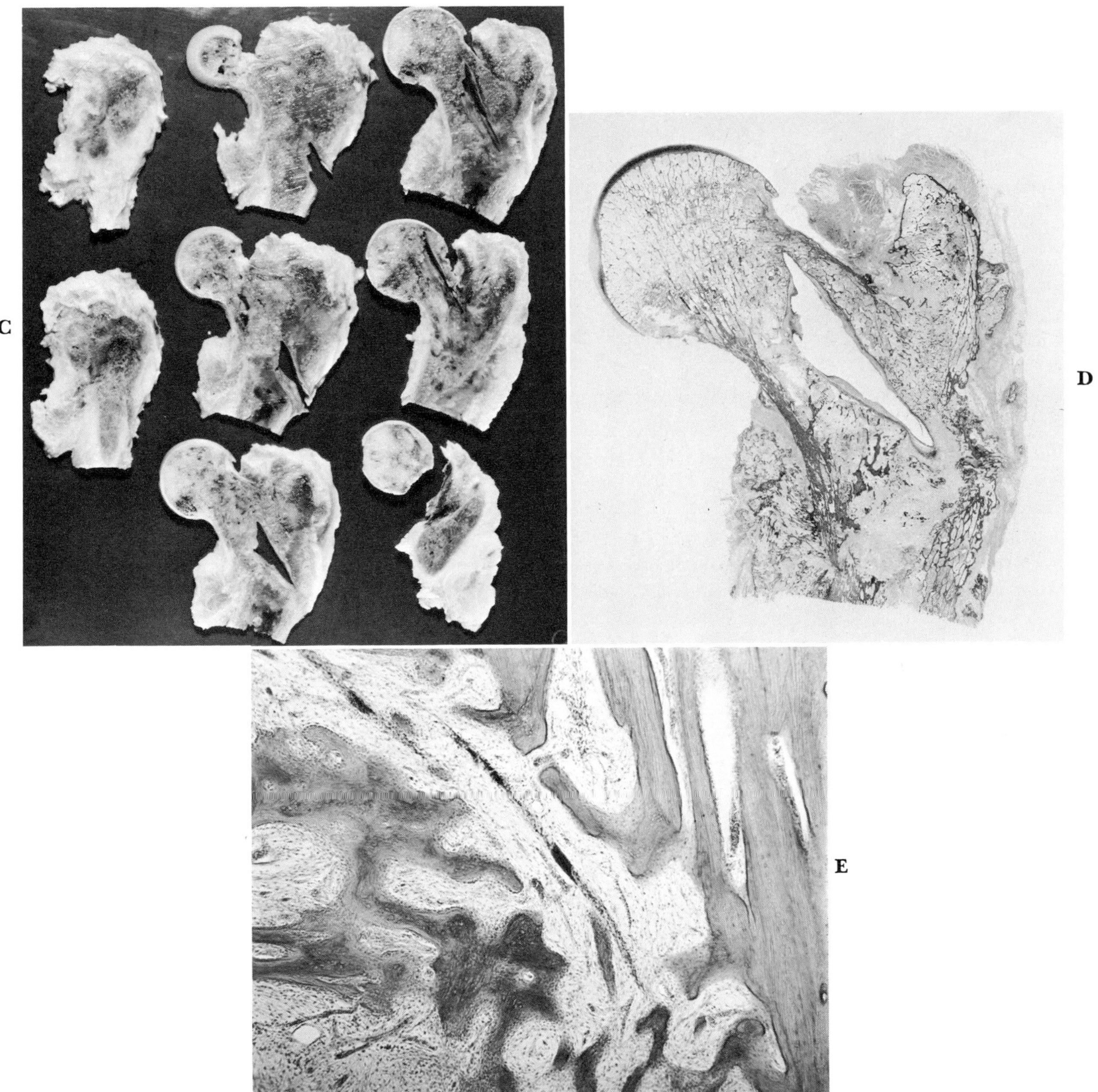

Fig. 8-11, cont'd. C, Sawed slabs of postmortem specimen obtained 8 weeks after injury and internal fixation. **D,** Photograph of celloidin section made from the middle sawed slab of the postmortem specimen. Note the abundant periosteal response to the injury, especially medial to the shaft. **E,** Photomicrograph (×109) of periosteal response medial to the shaft.

Restoration and proper internal fixation can maintain a potentially unstable fracture. The use of the cannulated Smith-Petersen nail and the Thornton plate is successful only if there is rigid fixation at their juncture. The intertrochanteric fracture heals as a shaft fracture, so that there is more leeway in reduction. The incidence of nonunion is low. Aseptic necrosis did not occur in this series.

REFERENCES

1. Dimon, J. H., and Hughston, J. C.: Unstable intertrochanteric fractures of the hip, J. Bone Joint Surg. **49A**:440, 1967.
2. Evans, E. M.: The treatment of trochanteric fractures of the femur, J. Bone Joint Surg. **31B**:190, 1949.
3. Hughston, J. C.: Unstable intertrochanteric fractures of the hip, J. Bone Joint Surg. **46A**:1145, 1964.

Part II

JOSEPH H. DIMON, III, M.D.
Atlanta, Georgia

JACK C. HUGHSTON, M.D.
Columbus, Georgia

We seek to emphasize the importance of recognizing and treating effectively the unstable intertrochanteric fractures of the hip.

In a previously published report,* we, in reviewing a consecutive series of 302 intertrochanteric fractures, documented the frequency of unstable intertrochanteric fractures, the complications that do occur with conventional nailing, and the marked improvement if the unstable intertrochanteric fracture is recognized and dealt with appropriately. Readers are referred to this article for specific figures.

A review of the literature indicates that recognition of instability as a possible component of intertrochanteric fractures is frequently overlooked. Most reports on intertrochanteric fractures give anatomic rather than functional end results and concern themselves primarily with various structural changes in the internal fixation apparatus in an attempt to decrease postoperative complications. Since Thornton[11] added the Thornton plate to the Smith-Petersen nail for internal fixation of the intertrochanteric hip fracture, gadgeteers and instrument companies have been trying to develop some form of device strong enough to hold this unrecognized, unstable fracture. The problem of instability and its importance, however, has been emphasized by some authors.

Evans[6] classified trochanteric fractures of the femur as stable and unstable. In order to gain stability and avoid complications occurring with unstable intertrochanteric fractures, he recommended fixing them in a position of deformity, that is, nail them in coxa vara. Moore,[8] Cram,[5] and Parker[9] noted the importance of comminution of the medial femoral cortex and its relationship to the subsequent collapse into varus of the intertrochanteric fracture. Clawson[4] referred to stable and unstable intertrochanteric fractures. After reviewing his cases, he advised a return to radical conservatism with continuous traction as the treatment of choice. Boyd and Lipinski[3] suggested additional internal fixation in managing this problem and pointed out that overlapping of cortices was sometimes helpful. Aufranc and Lowell,[1] as well as Boyd and Anderson,[2] pointed out the value of medial displacement and valgus fixation if medial drift and instability could be initially determined.

DEFINITION AND RECOGNITION OF THE UNSTABLE INTERTROCHANTERIC FRACTURE

An unstable intertrochanteric fracture lacks continuity of the bone cortex on the opposing surfaces of the proximal and distal fragments. This cortical deficit is due either to comminution on the medial aspect of the neck (calcar region) or to a large and separate posterior trochanteric fragment. Sometimes a combination of the two is present. The instability is generally unrecognized, and anatomic reduction does not restore stability. Unstable intertrochanteric fractures, upon careful review of the initial radiographs and the first anteroposterior and true lateral films made in the operating theater, have the following features in common: the presence of a major head and neck segment; the shaft; a large or comminuted medial lesser trochanter and medial cortical arch fragment; and a large posterior fragment (Fig. 8-12). The extent

*J. Bone Joint Surg. **49-A**:440, 1967.

of the large posterior fragment is frequently difficult to discern on the anteroposterior roentgenogram as it is sometimes covered by the head and neck fragment or by the trochanteric spike of the shaft fragment. On the lateral roentgenogram, however, this large posterior fragment can usually be identified by an oblique fracture line. This fragment causes the loss of stability at the fracture site.

FREQUENT COMPLICATIONS OF CONVENTIONAL FIXATION

The fracture components lend themselves to a seemingly anatomic reduction when the head and neck fragment is aligned with the distal shaft. Conventional fixation with a Jewett nail does not eliminate the structural loss of stability medially and posteriorly, secondary to the medial and posterior fragments (Fig. 8-13). The adductor pull tends to displace the shaft medially, and any type of longitudinal stress, such as muscle pull, weight bearing, or putting pressure on the foot, tends to collapse the fracture into varus position as there is a posterior and medial gap at the fracture site. Several complications occur in response to these forces, which attempt to create stability at the fracture site by closure of the posterior and medial gaps:

1. The nail penetrates the femoral head and enters the acetabulum as the distal fragment migrates medially and proximally (Fig. 8-14, *A*).
2. The nail or plate bends or breaks as the fracture collapses (Fig. 8-14, *B*).
3. The nail cuts through the head and neck as the fracture settles into varus deformity (Fig. 8-14, *C*).
4. The screw heads pull off as the plate pulls away from the femoral shaft (Fig. 8-14, *D*).

All of these complications occur as a result of the fracture fragments shifting into a more stable position. (See Figs. 8-15 to 8-18; Cases 1 to 4.)

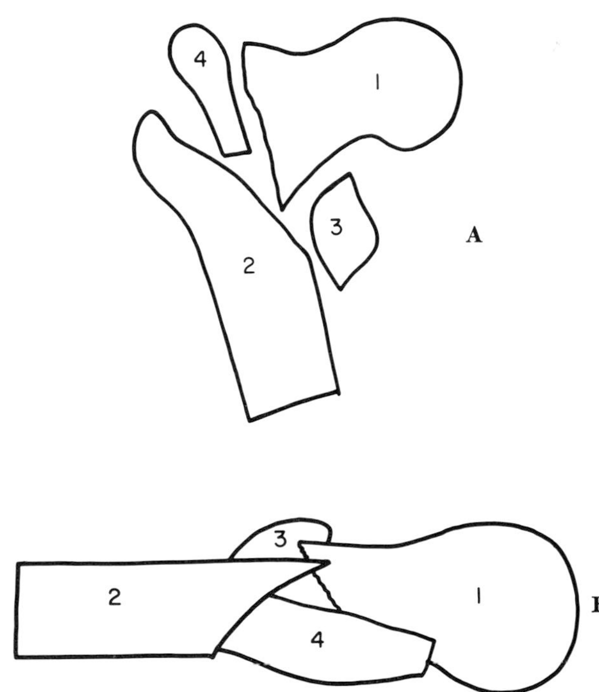

Fig. 8-12. A, Anteroposterior. **B,** Lateral. Drawings illustrating the major components of unstable intertrochanteric fractures: **1,** head and neck; **2,** shaft; **3,** medial fragment including the lesser trochanter; **4,** posterior fragment. (From Dimon, J. H., III, and Hughston, J. C.: J. Bone Joint Surg. **49A:**440, 1967.)

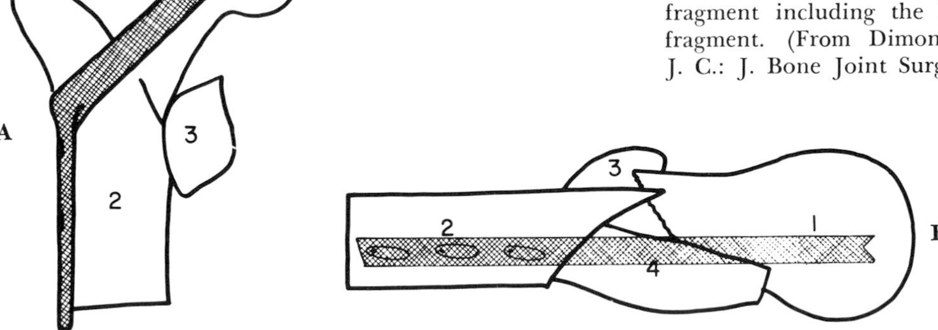

Fig. 8-13. A, Anteroposterior. **B,** Lateral. Drawing showing conventional anatomic fixation aligning head and neck fragment, **1,** with shaft, **2.** This does not restore stability due to fragments **3** and **4.** (From Dimon, J. H., III, and Hughston, J. C.: J. Bone Joint Surg. **49A:**440, 1967.)

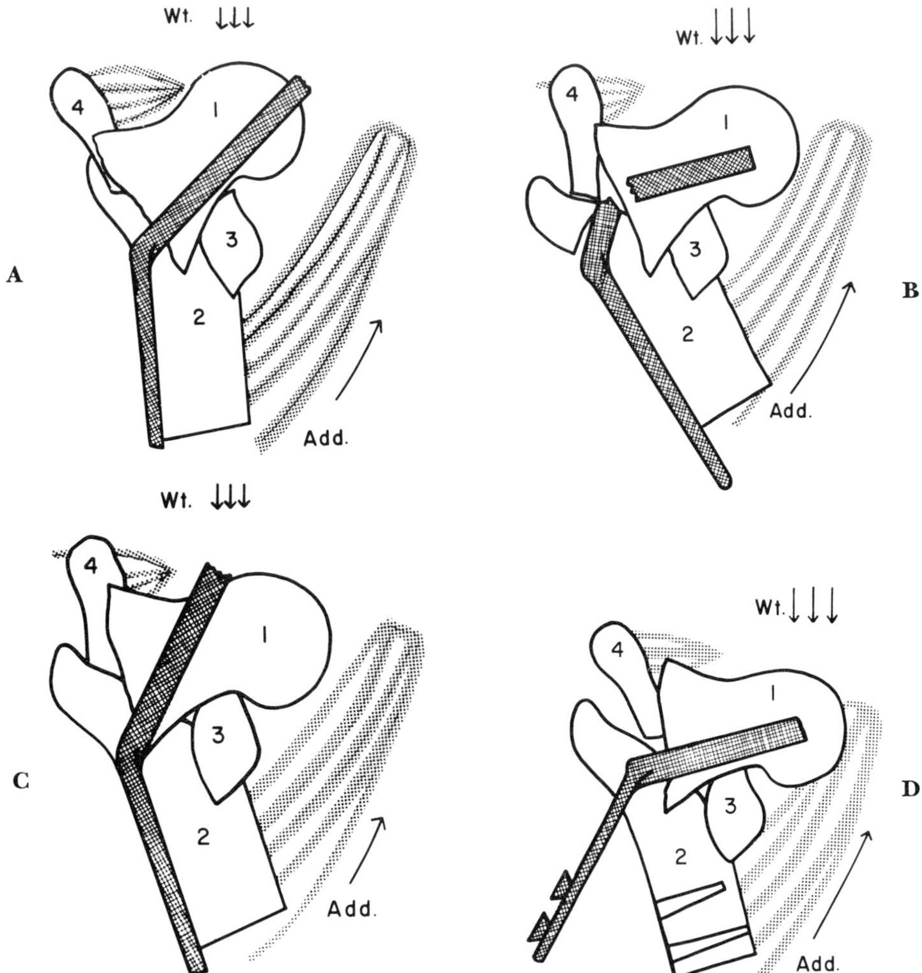

Fig. 8-14. Complications occurring as a result of the forces at work on the unstable conventionally fixed intertrochanteric fracture. **A,** Nail penetrates head into acetabulum. **B,** Nail bends or breaks. **C,** Nail cuts through the head and neck. **D,** Screws break off and plate migrates laterally with collapse of fracture into varus. (From Dimon, J. H., III, and Hughston, J. C.: J. Bone Joint Surg. **49A**:440, 1967.)

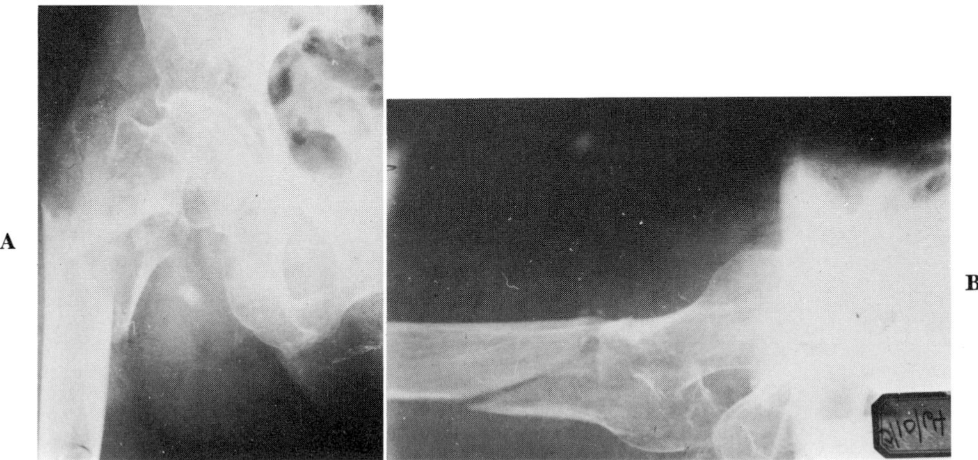

Fig. 8-15. For legend see opposite page.

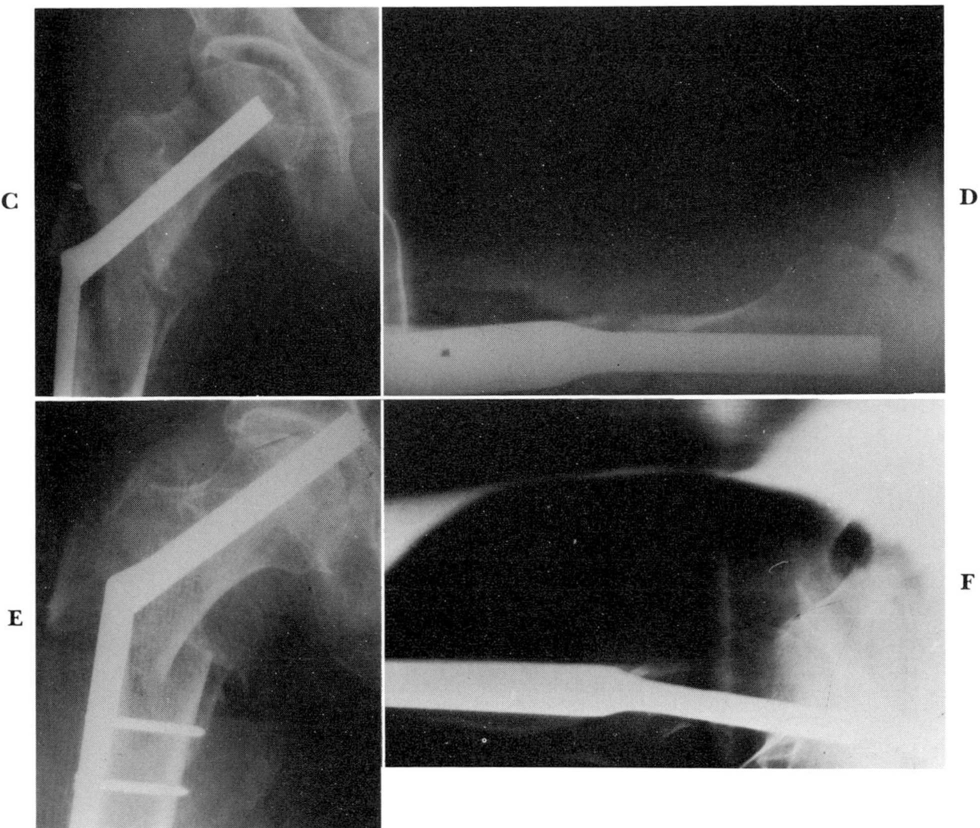

Fig. 8-15. Case 1. Unstable fracture nailed conventionally. Migration of nail through head into acetabulum by the fourth postoperative day on bed rest. **A** and **B,** Preoperative. **C** and **D,** at operation. **E** and **F,** Four days postoperative. (From Dimon, J. H., III, and Hughston, J. C.: J. Bone Joint Surg. **49A:**440, 1967.)

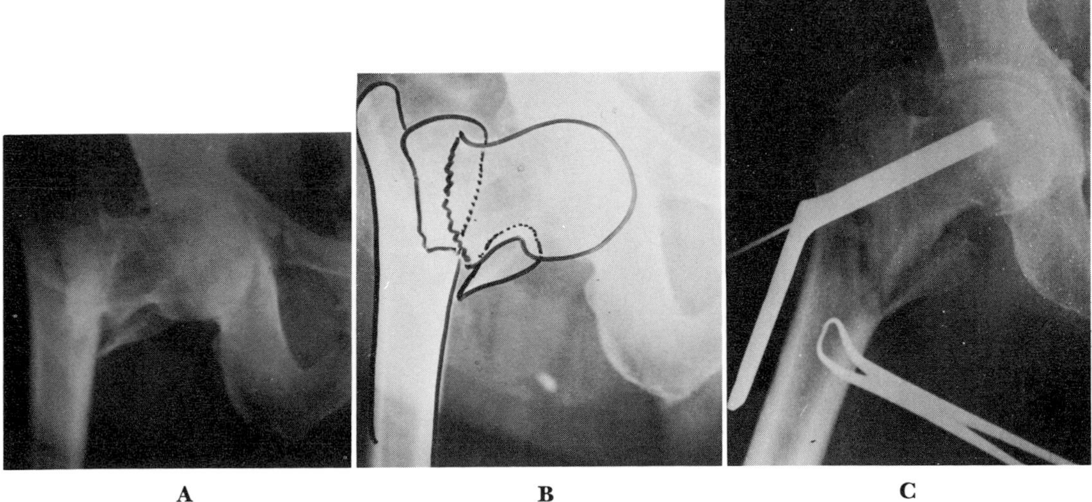

Fig. 8-16. Case 2. Screws pulled loose with varus collapse and nonunion after conventional fixation of unstable intertrochanteric fractures. **A** and **B,** Preoperative. **C** and **D,** At operation. **E,** Eight months postoperative. (From Dimon, J. H., III, and Hughston, J. C.: J. Bone Joint Surg. **49A:**440, 1967.)

Continued.

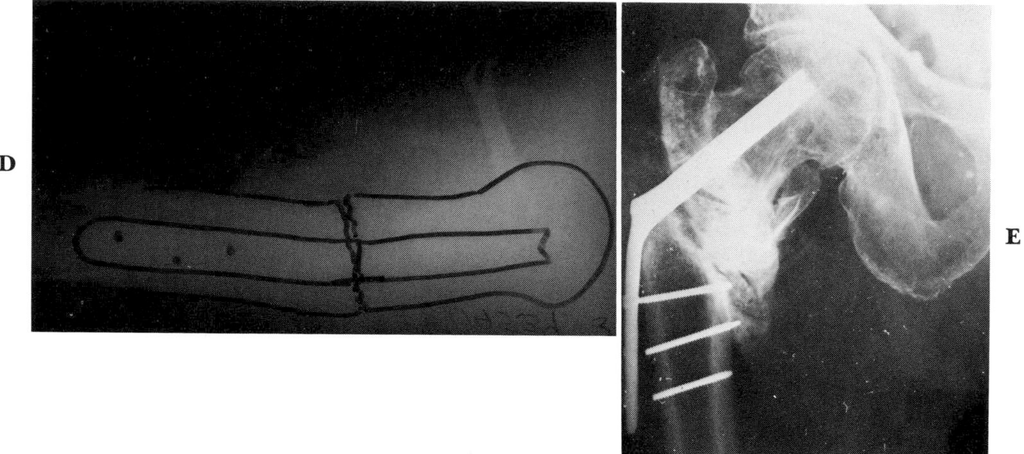

Fig. 8-16, cont'd. For legend see p. 113.

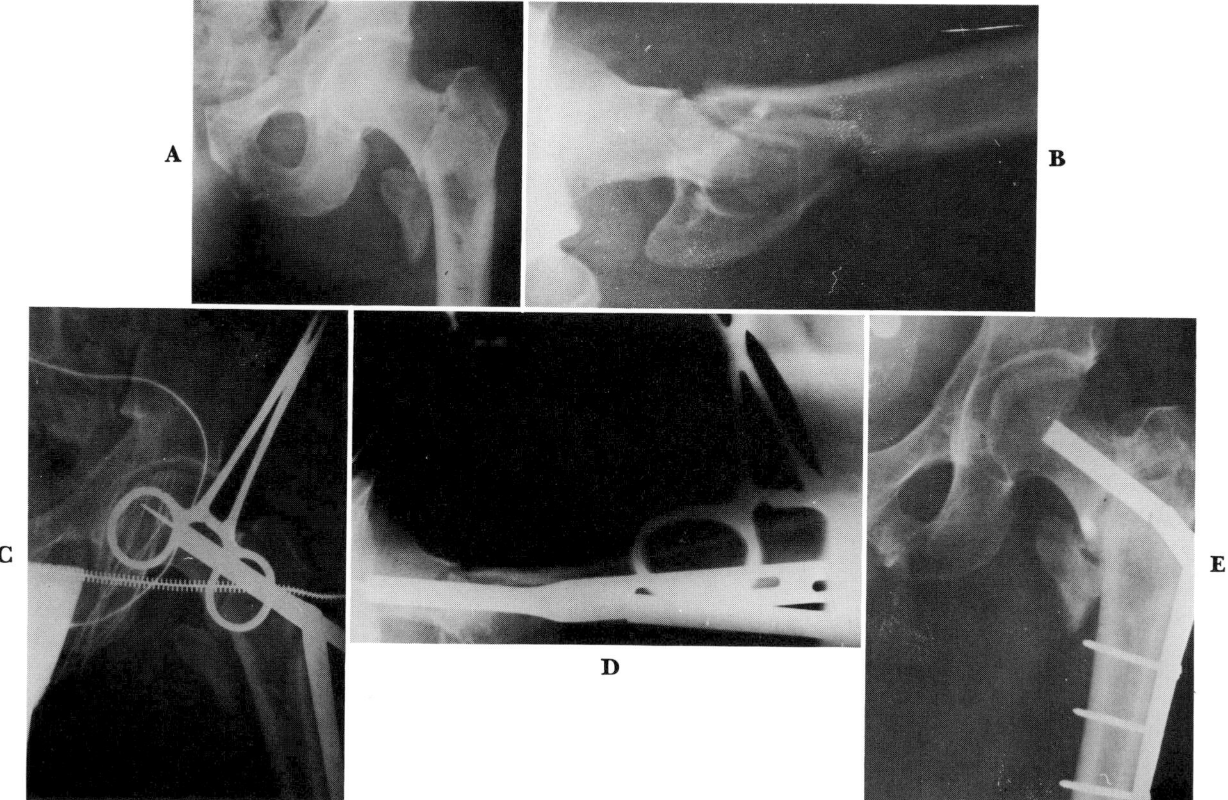

Fig. 8-17. Case 3. Breakage of Vitallium nail 4 months after conventional fixation of an unstable intertrochanteric fracture. **A** and **B,** Preoperative. **C** and **D,** At operation. **E,** Four months postoperative. (From Dimon, J. H., III, and Hughston, J. C.: J. Bone Joint Surg. **49A**:440, 1967.)

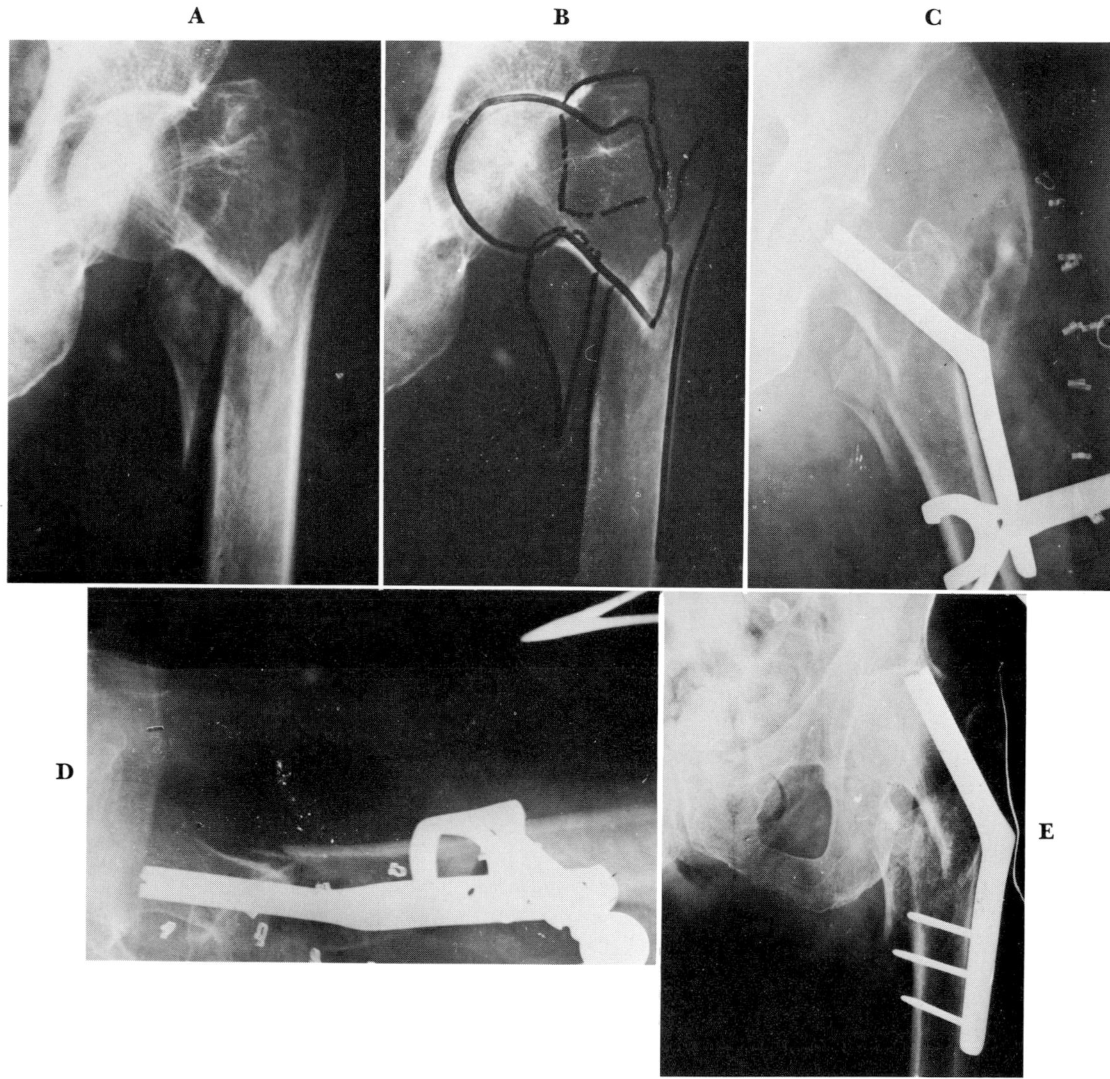

Fig. 8-18. Case 4. Nail cuts out of head and neck after conventional fixation of unstable intertrochanteric fracture. **A** and **B,** Preoperative. **C** and **D,** At operation. **E,** Three months postoperative. (From Dimon, J. H., III, and Hughston, J. C.: J. Bone Joint Surg. **49A:**440, 1967.)

FIXATION OF UNSTABLE INTERTROCHANTERIC FRACTURES BY PRIMARY MEDIAL DISPLACEMENT FIXATION

We have found that concentric stability can be obtained in the unstable intertrochanteric fracture. Anatomic reduction and achievement of a "good-looking x-ray" by alignment of the major head and neck segment with the shaft segment (Fig. 8-13) does not give bony stability and contact at the fracture site. By primary medial displacement fixation, the fracture can be impacted, and bony contact with resulting concentric stability can be accomplished by the following steps:

1. The thin greater trochanteric spike is osteotomized and left free, thus giving excellent end-on exposure to the fractured surface of the head and neck segment (Fig. 8-19, *A*).
2. A guide wire is placed in the head and neck segment (Fig. 8-19, *B*); anteroposterior and lateral roentgenograms are made to confirm this correct position. This is felt to be quite important to avoid the necessity for redriving

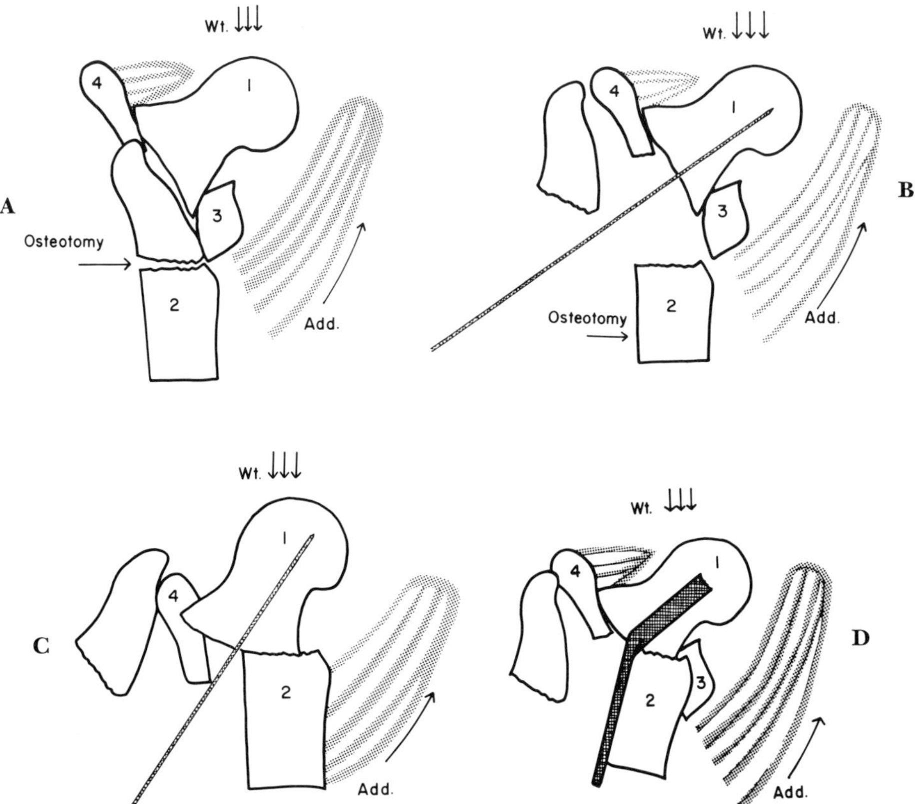

Fig. 8-19. Steps in primary medial displacement fixation. **A,** Osteotomy of spike on shaft fragment (when present). **B,** Placement of guide wire. **C,** Shaft displaced over the spike of the head and neck segment. **D,** Impaction of fracture and fixation with nail. (From Dimon, J. H., III, and Hughston, J. C.: J. Bone Joint Surg. **49A**:440, 1967.)

a Jewett nail in the head and neck. Reinsertion may shatter the posterior cortex of the neck and may destroy what stability the nail can have in the proximal fragment.

3. The shaft is then displaced medially under the spike of the head and neck fragment (Fig. 8-19, *C*).
4. Measurement of the guide wire will then indicate the necessity for placement of a short 2 to $2\frac{1}{2}$ inch nail in the head and neck portion. A standard 130° or 150° Jewett nail is used (slotted plate recommended). Correct rotation of the leg should be achieved, noting the position of the knee through the drapes and aligning it carefully with the head and neck segment.
5. The fracture site is thoroughly impacted after releasing traction, and the plate is then affixed to the shaft of the femur (Fig. 8-19, *D*). It should be noted that a normal or slight valgus neck-shaft angle should be obtained.

On occasion, with placement of the nail in the head and neck segment and with displacement and impaction of the distal shaft, the lateral cortex at the site of osteotomy may jam against the under edge of the nail, preventing desired impaction. If this occurs, a U-shaped trough should be rongeured in the lateral cortex, allowing the shaft segment to impact fully over the head and neck segment.

Fig. 8-20 illustrates a typical unstable fracture treated by this method. The slight shortening that can occur is of no clinical significance, nor is there any clinically significant diminution in abductor power.

DISCUSSION

Numerous complications may be seen in the management of unstable intertrochanteric frac-

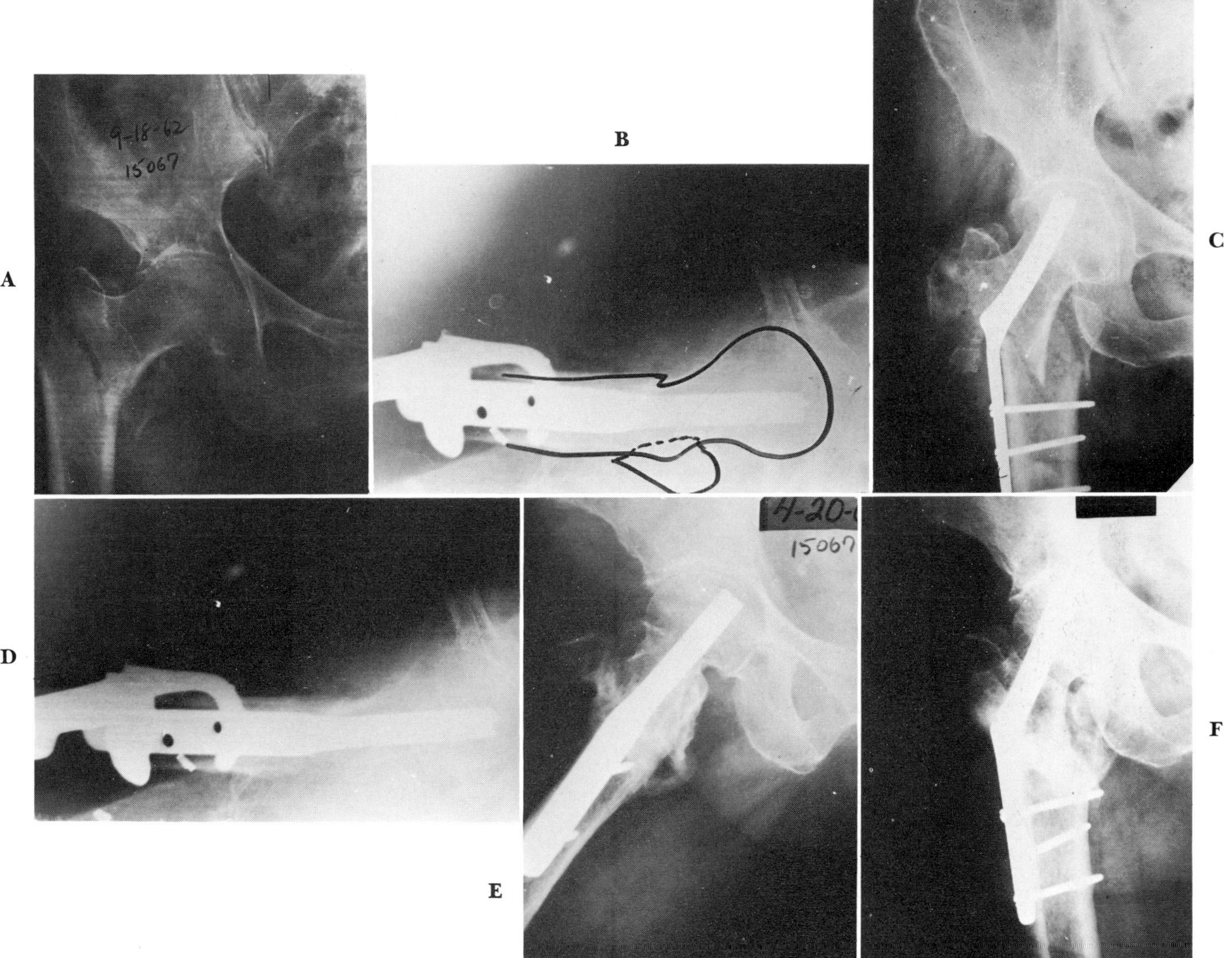

Fig. 8-20. Typical unstable fracture treated by medial displacement fixation. **A,** Preoperative. **B-D,** At operation. **E** and **F,** Seven months postoperative. (From Dimon, J. H., III, and Hughston, J. C.: J. Bone Joint Surg. **49A:**440, 1967.)

tures.[2-10] The most common cause of failure of fixation of the fracture is nailing of the unstable intertrochanteric fracture in the so-called anatomic position, aligning the head and neck segment with the shaft. This, however, leaves a posterior medial defect, and thereby stability is not achieved. If stability by primary medial displacement fixation is achieved initially, then it seems reasonable to expect the complication rate to decrease as the fracture no longer needs to settle and migrate into a position of stability. Although every fracture is unique, and long-term follow-up and comparison of individual cases is difficult in this age group, we continue to find a considerable reduction of complications in management of these unstable intertrochanteric fractures by primary medial displacement fixation.

CONCLUSIONS

1. By careful study of the preoperative and first reduction roentgenograms, an intertrochanteric fracture can usually be recognized as being stable or unstable.
2. The unstable fracture should not be treated so as to make the "x-ray look good," but it should be treated by primary medial displacement fixa-

tion in order to get good bony contact and concentric stability.

3. Primary medial displacement fixation has significantly reduced the postoperative tendency for these fractures to develop a varus deformity with attendant complications.

REFERENCES

1. Aufranc, O. E., and Lowell, J. D.: Massachusetts General Hospital, personal communication.
2. Boyd, H. B., and Anderson, L. D.: Management of unstable trochanteric fractures, Surg. Gynec. Obstet. **112**:633, 1961.
3. Boyd, H. B., and Lipinski, S. W.: Nonunion of trochanteric and subtrochanteric fractures, Surgery, Gynec. Obstet. **104**:463, 1957.
4. Clawson, D. K.: Intertrochanteric fracture of the hip, Amer. J. Surg. **93**:580, 1957.
5. Cram, R. H.: The unstable intertrochanteric fracture, Surg. Gynec. Obstet. **101**:15, 1955.
6. Evans, E. M.: The treatment of trochanteric fractures of the femur, J. Bone Joint Surg. **31B**:190, 1949.
7. Hughston, J. C.: Unstable intertrochanteric fractures of the hip, J. Bone Joint Surg. **46A**:1145, 1964.
8. Moore, M., Jr.: Treatment of trochanteric femoral fractures with special reference to complications, Amer. J. Surg. **84**:449, 1952.
9. Parker, S. G.: Analysis of one hundred fifty consecutive intertrochanteric fractures of the femur, J. Int. Coll. Surg. **24**:202, 1955.
10. Taylor, G. M., Neufeld, A. J., and Nickel, V. L.: Complications and failures in the operative treatment of intertrochanteric fractures of the femur, J. Bone Joint Surg. **37A**:306, 1955.
11. Thornton, Lawson: The treatment of trochanteric fractures of the femur: two new methods, Piedmont Hosp. Bull. **10**:21, 1937.

Part III

EARL P. HOLT, JR., M.D.
St. Louis, Missouri

First, it is understood that this subject may include any major fracture in the trochanteric area of the hip, leaving off proximally above the base of the femoral neck (Case 1) and below where one might better utilize an intramedullary nail; thus a comminuted, very high shaft fracture can be fixed with a trochanteric appliance (Case 2).

Second, we must agree, before going on, that internal fixation of these fractures in adults and in some older children is best. While homage is paid to Hugh Owen Thomas, M. G. Pearson, Fritz Steinman, Martin Kirschner, Gurdon Buck, Hamilton Russell, John Hodgen, and Roger Anderson, and despite the tremendous advancements of antibiotics, air mattresses, flotation mattresses, anticoagulants, and superior comprehensive nursing care, we believe operative management is better than balanced traction. And while the age group involved is getting older, anesthesiology, operative technique, and immediate postoperative care are improving. We have not found it necessary in recent years to rush elderly patients through a hip operation and "get them off the table." There is time for precise work.

Third, all trochanteric fractures do not need to be nailed. There is a small percentage of incomplete or complete but minimally displaced trochanteric fractures that need only brief skin traction or bed rest or even bed-chair management, and occasionally a healthy patient from any age group may go directly to nonweight bearing crutch or walker ambulation. Union in such cases is swift, and costs can be admirably small.

On the other side of the coin are trochanteric fractures of chronically ill, debilitated, nonambulatory patients, sometimes with pathologic fractures from metastatic disease. In these, attempts at nailing are no more than an expensive exercise. In fact, if a patient was not ambulatory prior to hip fracture and has no real prospect of being ambulatory afterward, there is little excuse for operative fixation. If such a patient was living a bed-chair existence, he can soon continue to do so without the need of hip nailing. Two to three weeks of scar fixation about his fracture, and he can be lifted onto his wheelchair again. We are not talking about such cases in this discussion.

But if a patient, no matter how elderly, was usefully ambulatory prior to his fracture and there is no reason to think he could not be so again, he is a candidate for operative fixation. There remains only a decision about the method and the device. This is where Drs. Hughston and Dimon and I split off into camps and begin watching each other for areas of vulnerability.

Lawson Thornton logically extended the Smith-Petersen nail with a screw-on plate in 1937. In 1941,

Earl Jewett made a one-piece tri-flanged cannulated nail by welding plate to nail. As years have gone by, fabrication of this nail and design has been vastly improved. Alonzo Neufeld presented a simple and easy-to-apply nail in 1944. Harrison McLaughlin attacked the problem of nail application by pursuing the variable angle principle in 1947. This, too, has gone through revolutionary stages. Telescoping nails appeared first in 1955 (Pugh) for the problem of "the unsolved fracture" or femoral necks. Almost immediately they were used in trochanteric fractures as well. Carl Badgley has one of his own design. Most are of conventional angles. Improved engineering, but more difficult application, is noted in William Massie's wide-angled telescoping nail (1962). It has been shown that any of the telescoping nails may allow medial shaft migration without advancement or penetration of the acetabulum by the nail. If medial shaft migration is really the great problem of unstable intertrochanteric fractures, I am surprised that Drs. Hughston and Dimon have not utilized this remedy, or have not turned to the supplemental trochanter extension plate available for conventional nails, or to the one-piece Higley nail.

We were taught and have continued to teach that portions of the greater trochanter unbroken from the shaft were to be zealously guarded, and breaking them off during drilling, nailing, etc. was grounds for suggestion that the operating house officer go into obstetrics or dermatology. We speak of this as converting a simple intertrochanteric fracture into a comminuted subtrochanteric fracture, vastly complicating the problem.

But, another equally dreadful complication of trochanteric nail fixation is nail failure by bending or breaking. The operator's first impulse is to blame the patient for bearing weight against advice or to blame personnel for rough handling. Only a more critical analyst may see inadequacy of the implant as the fault, especially when there are trochanteric nails still marketed today that can be bent with the bare hands!

A third problem common to neck and trochanteric fractures alike is plowing of the nail in or through the femoral head. The operator, having recovered all possible stability with his reduction and having used a strong rigid-angled Vitallium or stainless steel nail securely fixed to the shaft, may give the "Oriental shrug" on seeing his nail plow through the head as it drifts into varus or the assembly disrupt altogether. "I have done all I could. I cannot be blamed for this poor protoplasm."

On finding that many intertrochanteric fractures cannot be fixed satisfactorily with conventional nails and anatomic reductions, Dimon and Hughston classify these as unstable fractures and treat by primary medial shaft displacement. The steps are as follows:

1. Osteotomize the trochanteric site
2. Place guide wire in the proximal segment
3. Displace the shaft medially
4. Use short 2 or 2½, 135°-155° Jewett nail
5. Impact the fracture site before plate fixation

To me, it has never seemed important to classify intertrochanteric fractures except, as mentioned before, into those in which operation is justifiable at all and into those in which it is not. Beyond that, the entire concept has been to recover what stability the bone fragments offer by reduction (anatomic) and bridging and anchoring the femoral head at topside to the shaft below, paying no attention to the number of fragments between. Can any nail be fixed into the femoral head and any plate be so secure to the shaft that it will withstand the accidental step prior to some degree of union? And in more favorable cases, will such an implant allow intentional weight bearing when the surgical wound is healing? Will end results in these fractures be better with such an approach, or should we take another look at medial shaft displacement? You must judge for yourselves.

Work was begun on a stronger trochanteric appliance in 1956, presented at the American Association of Orthopaedic Surgeons meeting in Chicago in 1960, and the first one hundred cases were summarized in the *Journal of Bone and Joint Surgery* in 1963. The work included stress testing of twenty-eight stock versions of nine types of angled hip nail plates, and their weaknesses and inadequacies were reported (Table 8-2). The modern Holt nail design with three Barr bolts will bear end loading of above eight hundred pounds. It is designed to provide sufficient strength for early ambulation of patients with trochanteric fractures. It is not recommended in patients who were not previously ambulatory. Comminution in trochanteric fractures is not a contraindication to its use, but it may defer the day when weight may be borne. It is useful in basal neck as well as subtrochanteric fractures, and it is probably in the latter

Table 8-2. Stress tests

3½″ nails		*Average (lb.)*
SP–Thornton plate,	ss*†	77
Original Jewett	ss	33
Neufeld	ss	61
Key	ss	241
McLaughlin VI, Vitallium		133
Modern Jewett, Vitallium		183
Modern Jewett, 316L, ss		311
Holt nail		
Original, 1956	ss	240
Model I, Vitallium		300
316L	ss	391
Titanium		444
A–286	ss	769
Model II, Vitallium		845

*A variety of stainless steel.
†All nails end loaded to failure.

group that its great strength is most advantageous.

The technique of application varies only slightly from conventional hip nailing. A traction table and biplane roentgen-ray control are needed. The approach is strictly lateral, but most of the vastus lateralis is reflected anteriorly. Reduction must be precisely anatomic, except in the occasional case in which there is considerable comminution, and it seems advisable to allow some telescoping of fragments to ensure earlier and more certain union. An angled guide set to the exact angle of the nail is used; a takeoff point is chosen, so that a 3/32″ guide wire may pass into the head somewhat below dead center, or bull's-eye position, as seen in anteroposterior projection, but midline or bull's-eye, as seen in the lateral view. It is desirable for the nail to penetrate two thirds to three quarters of the way into the femoral head. A ½″ cannulated and calibrated drill, attached to a Hudson type brace, is used to drill to a sufficient depth within the head. *Overdrilling is to be avoided.* A few bites with a rongeur at the inferior margin of the hole in the outer cortex serve to allow flush adaptation of the plate to the shaft. Fixation is with three Barr bolts, 5/32″ in diameter and penetrating the deep cortex sufficiently to allow putting on the plastic stop nuts. The bolts should not be excessively tightened, since this wastes strength of the bolts by applying useless stress. The wound must be slightly longer than usual, and the quadriceps muscle must be stripped more completely anteriorly and medially to allow placement of the nuts and securing with a 150°-angled hexagonal wrench. As in any hip nailing, it is important not to have distraction of the fragments at the time the plate is bolted to the shaft.

Postoperative management is conventional, except that the patient may put weight on the extremity immediately, as in getting out of bed on the first day, but no ambulatory efforts are urged until a few days have passed and benign wound healing is anticipated. This seems to be similar to the program most orthopedists use with hip prosthesis for fresh fractures of the neck of the femur.

The complication rate should be low and does not differ from nailings with other devices, except that failures of the implant have been virtually eliminated. The fractures seem to heal surprisingly rapidly, and motion and muscle tone are better preserved. There seems to be no tendency for the proximal fragments to rotate around the nail, probably because of engagement of the fracture fragments and anchorage by ligamentous and capsular attachments.

After 14 years of use, the Holt nail has proved to offer distinct advantages in management of trochanteric fractures in patients young or old—it has inevitably shortened hospitalization and reduced disability.

Some additional examples of the method follow:

Case 1. M. Mc., a 90-year-old woman fell and sustained a low basal neck fracture (Fig. 8-21, *A*) that was promptly bolted. Heart disease limited ambulation, but ambulation was started within a few days after surgery. Sound union was seen 3 months later (Fig. 8-21, *B* and *C*).

Case 2. J. L., a 71-year-old man fell from a ladder. His severely comminuted left subtrochanteric fracture (Fig. 8-22, *A* and *B*) was fixed with a Holt nail. Weight bearing was deferred for 2 months but was allowed thereafter. Union was seen at 6 months (Fig. 8-22, *C* and *D*). His gait was excellent.

Case 3. C. L., a 77-year-old woman, was blown down by the wind. Her right comminuted trochanteric fracture (Fig. 8-23, *A*) was fixed with an A-286 stainless steel Holt nail. She used a walker for several months but bore weight all the while. Her united fracture was seen 6½ years later (Fig. 8-23, *B* and *C*). A small, persistent sinus developed spontaneously 6 years after operation, and the nail was removed. Cultures were negative. A-286 steel

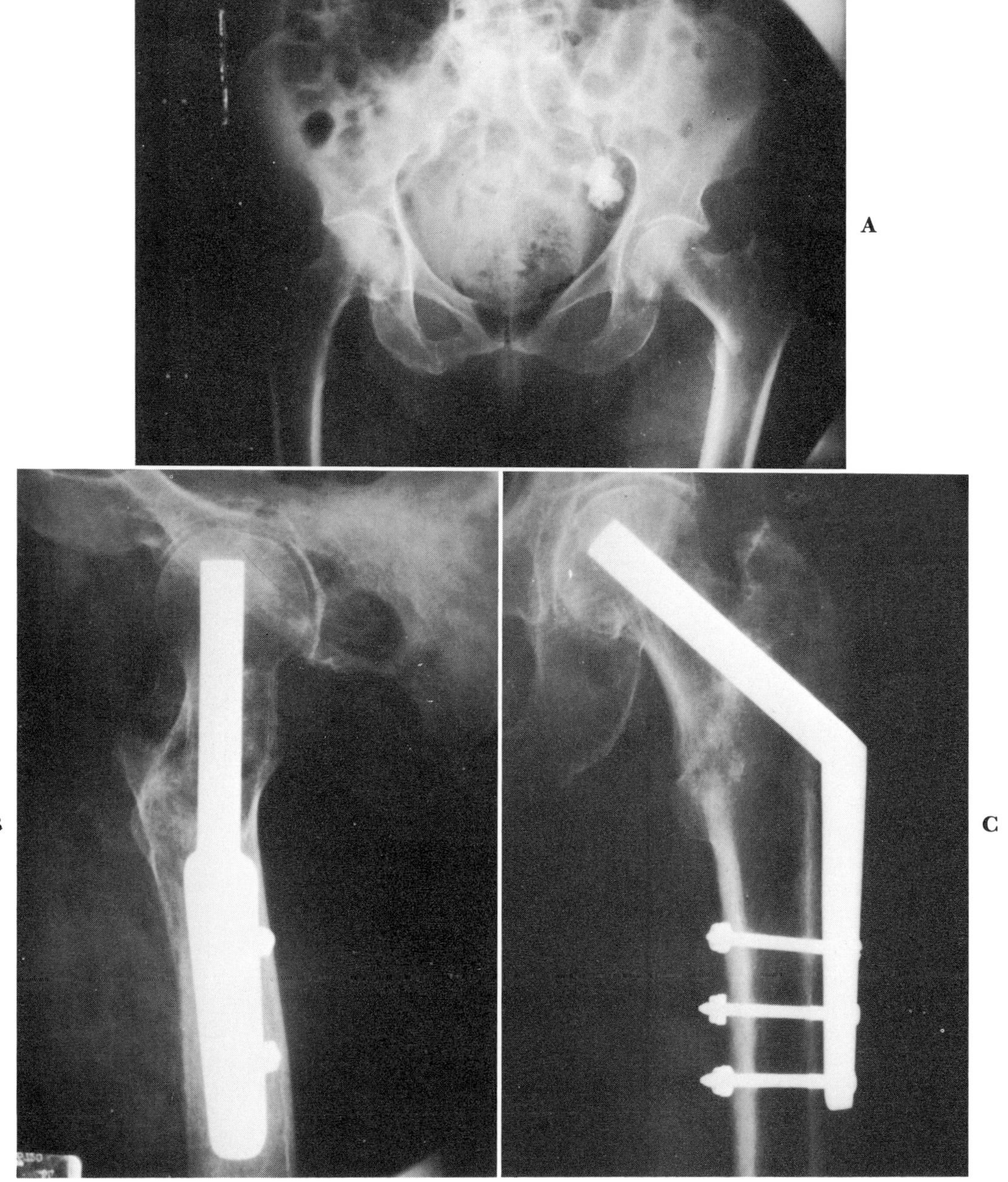

Fig. 8-21. See text.

is still experimental. The nail and bolts were not corroded and were normal in appearance. Looseness and resorption around the penetrating portion of the nail were noted.

Case 4. S. H., a 77-year-old woman, fell. Her intertrochanteric fracture (Fig. 8-24, *A*) of the left hip was bolted. She bore weight with a walker in a few days and was discharged healed in 2 months, using only a cane (Fig. 8-24, *B* and *C*).

Case 5. E. G., a 65-year-old man, fell (Fig. 8-25, *A*). His right intertrochanteric fracture was bolted, and he bore weight promptly. He walked well with a cane in 2 months with the fracture united. He was discharged (Fig. 8-25, *B* and *C*).

Case 6. R. A., a 55-year-old high school teacher, was hit by a student's car (Fig. 8-26, *A*). His hip was bolted, and he left the hospital in 2 weeks on crutches (Fig. 8-26, *B*). He bore weight

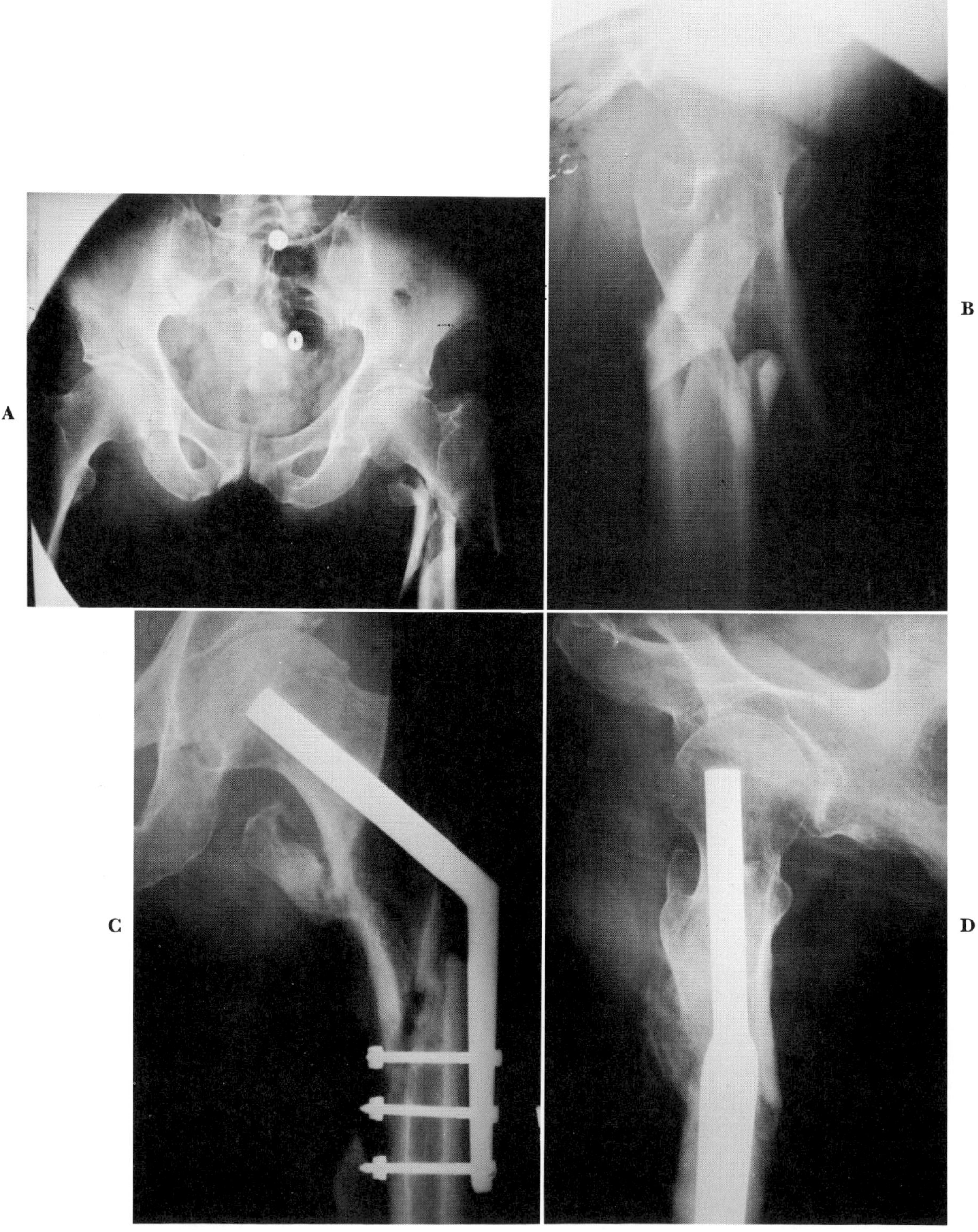

Fig. 8-22. See text.

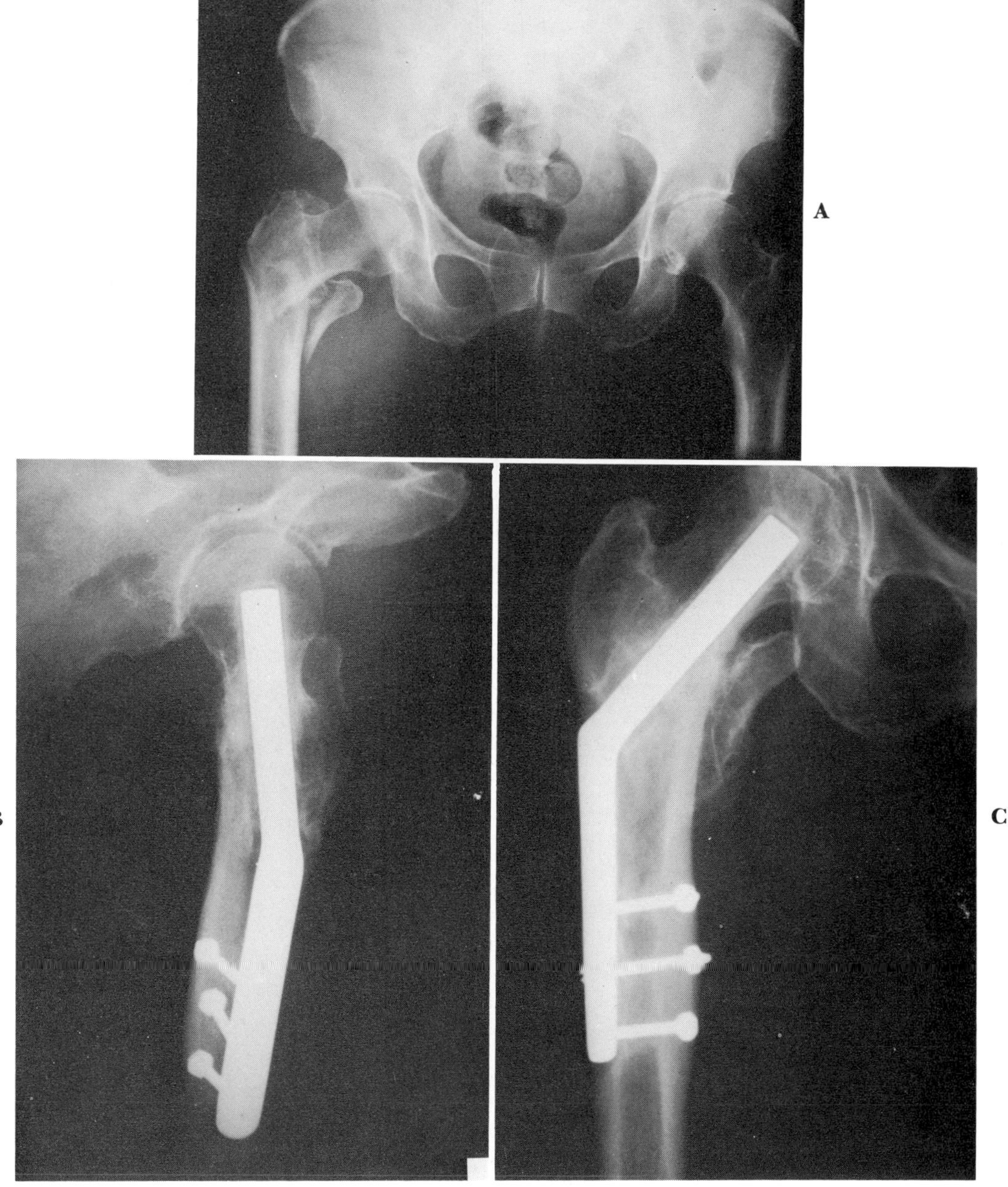

Fig. 8-23. See text.

after a month and used a cane after 3 months. Solid union was seen at 9 months (Fig. 8-26, *C* and *D*).

Case 7. A. C., a 58-year-old man with stroke residuals on the left, fell (Fig. 8-27, *A*). His displaced left intertrochanteric fracture was fixed with a steel Jewett (Fig. 8-27, *B*). All screws broke 10 months later (Fig. 8-27, *C*). Reoperation with a Vitallium Jewett and using Barr bolts to attach the plate, along with iliac bone grafting, was done (Fig. 8-27, *D*). This nail punched through the head within 2 or 3 months but was tolerable (Fig. 8-27, *E*). Three and one-half years later the plate broke when he fell (Fig. 8-27, *F*). Reoperation confirmed lack of union in the major fracture. A Holt nail and bone grafting resulted in solid union and relief of his prior pain and stiffness (Fig. 8-27, *G* and *H*).

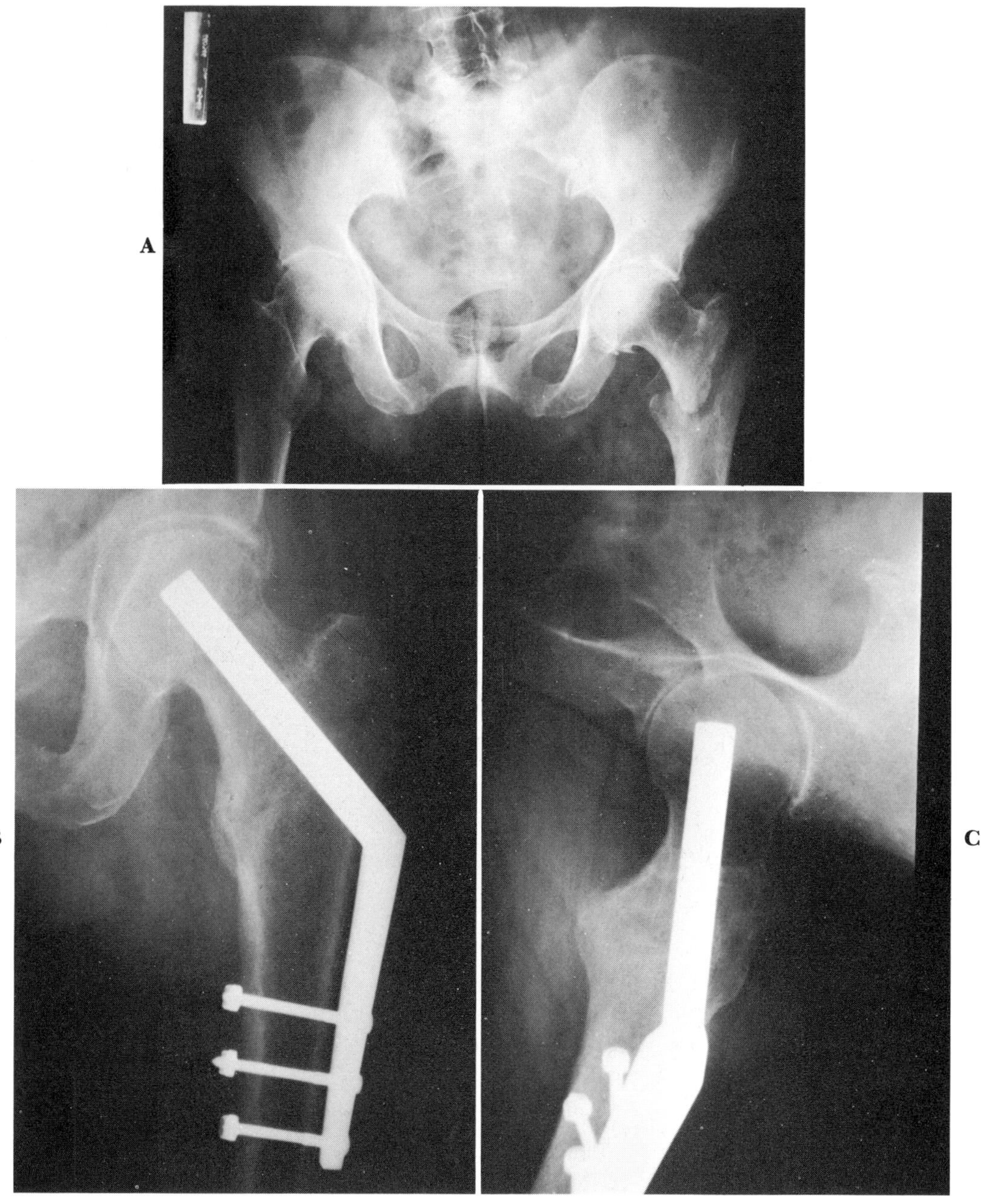

Fig. 8-24. See text.

DISCUSSION

These cases have served to illustrate what can be accomplished by conventional reduction of trochanteric fractures when fixed with an unconventional bolt or nail. They are a cross section of my own series of 62-odd hips operated since the published series of 100 that ended January, 1961. Advantages seem many; complications were few (five in the original 100, and four of these sixty-two). It is obvious that Drs. Hughston and Dimon have solved many problems of unstable trochanteric fractures with their method and have strikingly reduced the complication rate (thirty-eight in seventy-five hips conventionally nailed versus five in sixty-five hips treated by primary medial displacement fixation). Johnson, Lottes, and Arnot, found twenty-two complications in 148 Holt nailings, which could be blamed on the method (discount-

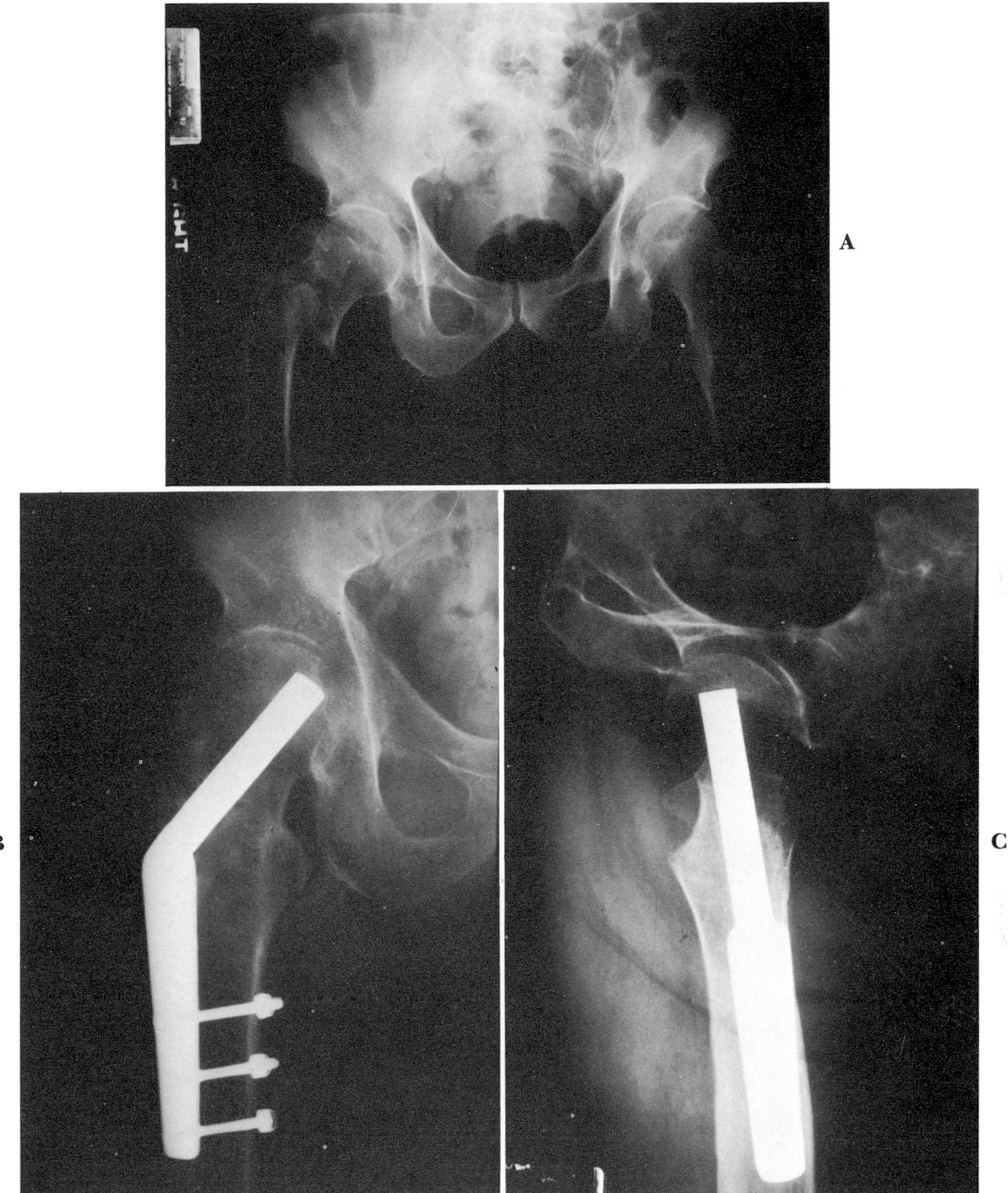

Fig. 8-25. See text.

ing wound infections and deaths prior to union from other causes). They pointed out that fifteen different residents did half of the operations on house services. In my original 100, seventy were done by twenty-four residents on four house services, but in almost every instance I scrubbed to assist and was able to demand a higher standard of technique. Nine of the complications in Johnson's report were broken bolts. I would like to emphasize the improvement of the $\frac{5}{32}''$ Barr bolts since 1966. Their ductility and shear strength have been nearly doubled by fabrication from wrought Vitallium. Bolt fracture has not been observed since that time. It is also interesting to note that of twelve penetrations of the femoral head by the nail, eight declined removal or replacement. Five such penetrations by the short nails used by Hughston and Dimon that penetrated the

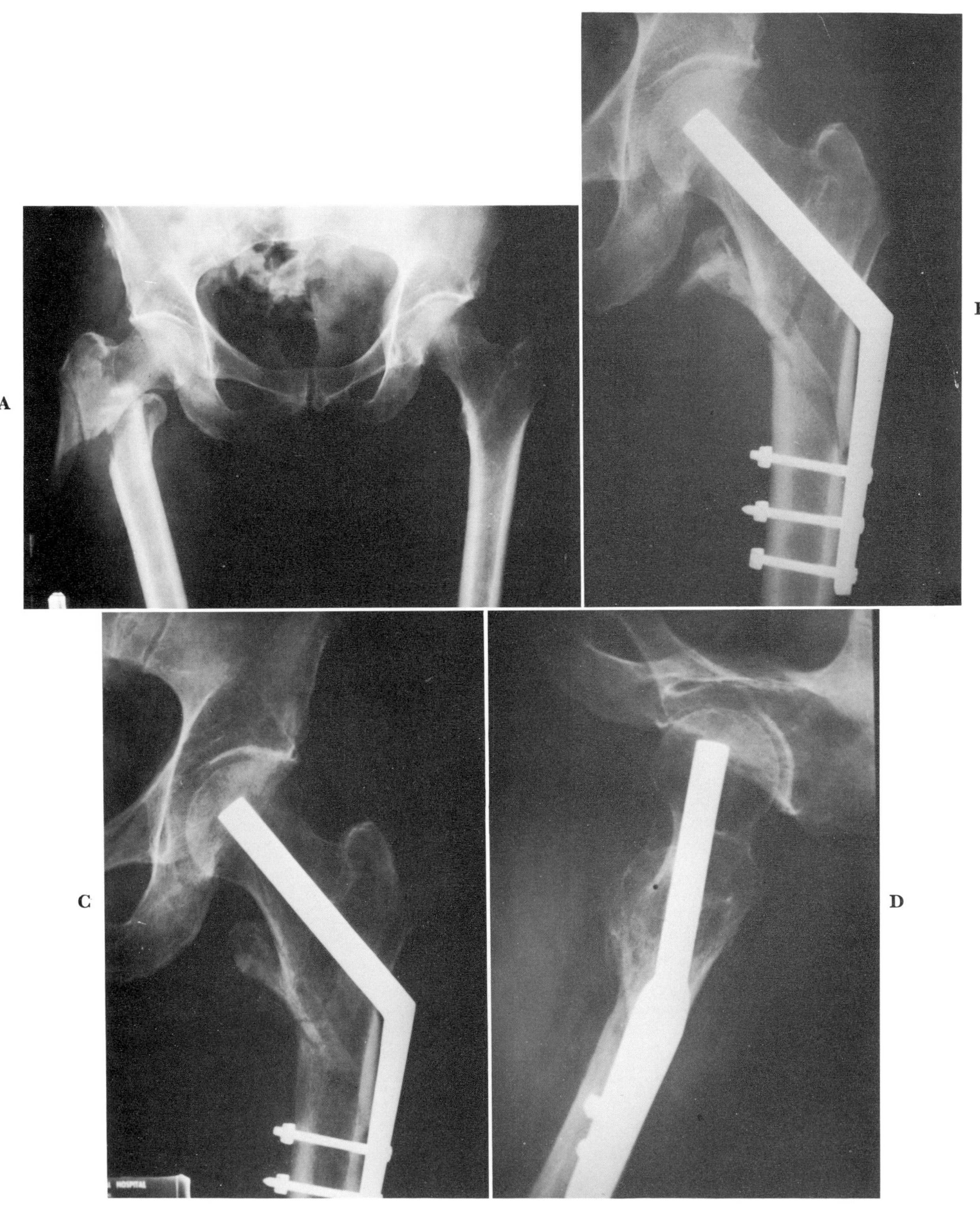

Fig. 8-26. See text.

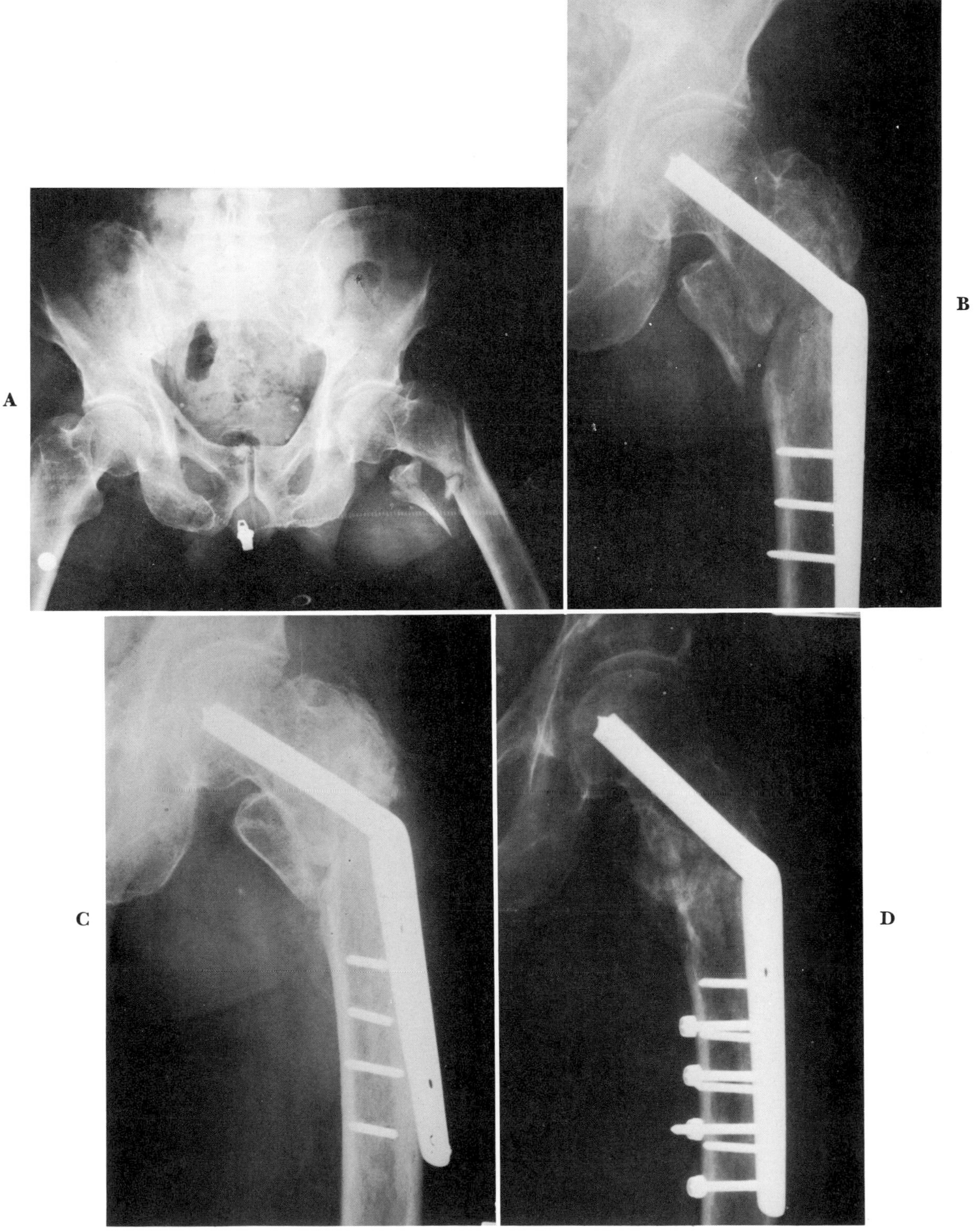

Fig. 8-27. See text. *Continued.*

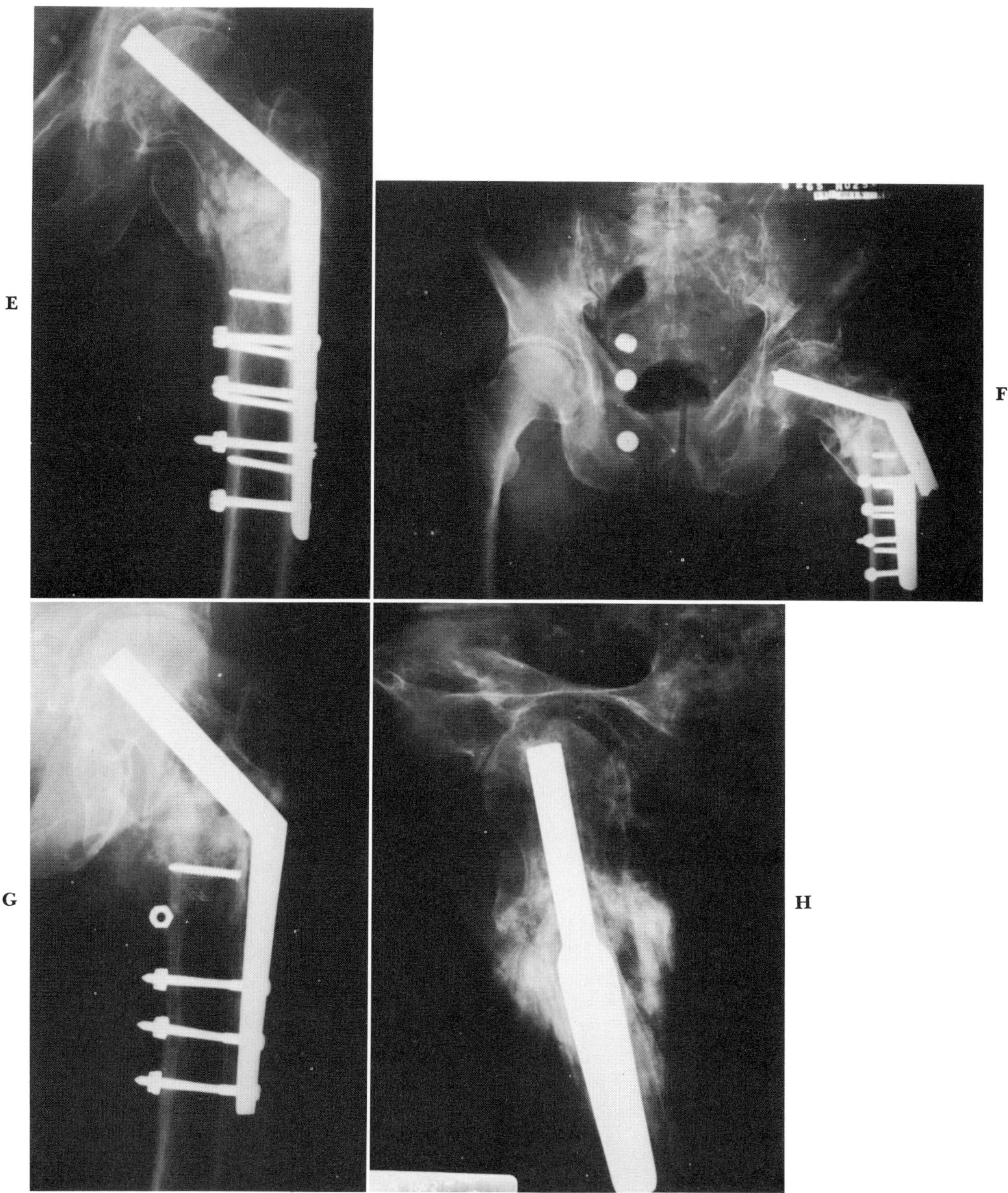

Fig. 8-27, cont'd. See text.

acetabulum were not counted as complications.

I cannot believe that Georgian hips are any different from Missouri hips, either in age at time of injury, osteoporosis, or percentage of those to be considered unstable. We are treating the same condition. I can only wish that Dr. Dimon would alternate his method for my method for a few years and see which group does the best, the primary shaft displacements with the short Jewett nail or the anatomic reductions fixed with a strong nail and early weight bearing.

REFERENCES

1. Dimon, J. H., III, and Hughston, J. C.: Unstable intertrochanteric fractures of the hip, J. Bone Joint Surg. **49A**:440, 1967.
2. Foster, J. C.: Trochanteric fractures of the femur treated by the vitallium McLaughlin nail and plate, J. Bone Joint Surg. **40B**:684, 1958.
3. Holt, E. P., Jr.: Hip fractures of the trochanteric region: treatment with a strong nail and early weight bearing, J. Bone Joint Surg. **45A**:687, 1963.
4. Hughston, J. C.: Unstable intertrochanteric fractures of the hip, J. Bone Joint Surg. **46A**:1145, 1964.
5. Johnson, L. L., Lottes, J. O., and Arnot, J. P.: The utilization of the Holt nail for proximal femoral fractures, J. Bone Joint Surg. **50A**:67, 1968.

Chapter 9

Troublesome fractures and dislocations of the hand

HERBERT H. STARK, M.D.
Los Angeles, California

Ideally, all fractures of the hand should be properly reduced and held immobile long enough to heal, but not so long that the finger joints stiffen. Proper reduction includes physiologic alignment with suitable bone contact and correct rotation. If fractures of small parallel bones such as metacarpals and phalanges are not aligned exactly and rotated correctly, the fingers will deviate or overlap when flexed. In adults, finger joints tend to stiffen when immobilized longer than 3 weeks; therefore, rigid splinting is mandatory until a fracture will not displace, but joint motion is encouraged as soon as it is safe to do so.

Most fractures of metacarpals and phalanges can and should be treated by closed reduction and external immobilization. Since several muscles that move the fingers have tendons that cross the wrist, immobilization of the wrist, usually in slight dorsiflexion, is essential to maintain reduction of a metacarpal or phalanx fracture. Unless there is some specific reason to do otherwise, metacarpophalangeal and proximal interphalangeal joints should be immobilized in semiflexion, not in extension or in acute flexion. One excellent method of external immobilization is illustrated (Fig. 9-1). After applying a short arm plaster cast to stabilize the wrist, a wire splint is anchored to the plaster and bent to hold a particular finger in semiflexion, which is the functional position. A sling of adhesive tape is affixed to the wire splint. This sling supports the injured finger, and, since it is contoured, it avoids flattening the soft tissues or compressing the flexor tendons against underlying bones, practices that encourage the adherence of flexor tendons to bone. After manipulation and reduction of the fracture, be it metacarpal, proximal, or middle phalanx, the finger is placed on the adhesive sling and taped to it with adhesive. Thus, the injured finger is immobilized, but all uninjured parts are allowed to move.

Several bone and joint injuries of the hand are peculiar and do not respond to closed methods of treatment. Many of these can be treated successfully by open reduction and internal fixation. For convenience, these troublesome problems will be discussed under three headings.

TROUBLESOME FRACTURES

Dorsal intra-articular fracture of a distal interphalangeal joint

A mallet finger deformity occurs after rupture of an extensor tendon near its insertion, or after avulsion of the tendon, often with a tiny bone fragment, from its insertion. A similar deformity is caused by an intra-articular fracture of the dorsal lip of a distal phalanx (Fig. 9-2). Ordinarily, this fracture fragment includes more than one third of the articular surface, it is tilted and often malrotated, and the base of the distal phalanx may slide volar to the condyles of the middle phalanx. Closed reduction of the fracture is seldom successful, and when it fails the fracture should be exposed through a dorsal skin incision. After dividing one collateral ligament, preferably the ulnar,

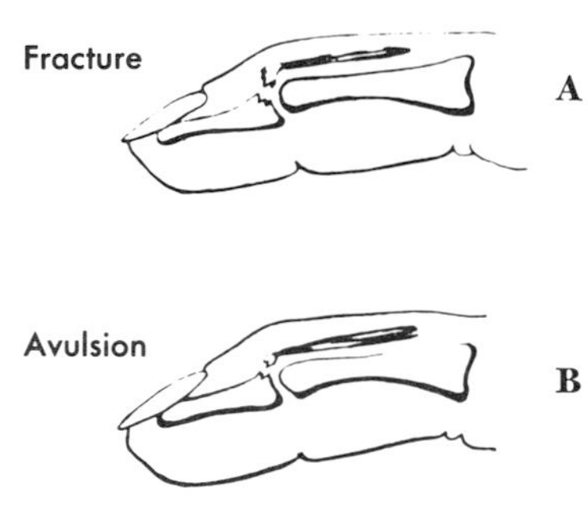

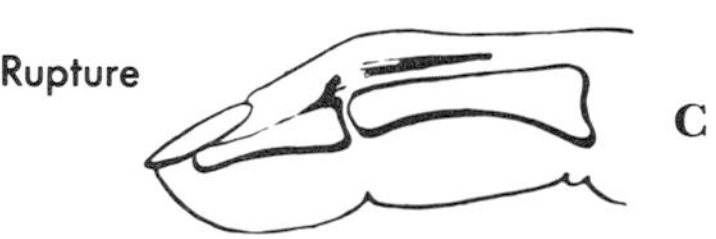

Fig. 9-2. Three causes of a mallet finger deformity are illustrated. **A** shows an intra-articular fracture. **B** shows a tiny bone fragment associated with a tendon avulsion. **C** shows tendon rupture without bone damage. Tendon avulsions and ruptures respond to routine mallet finger treatment; intra-articular fractures do not. The fracture should be reduced.

A

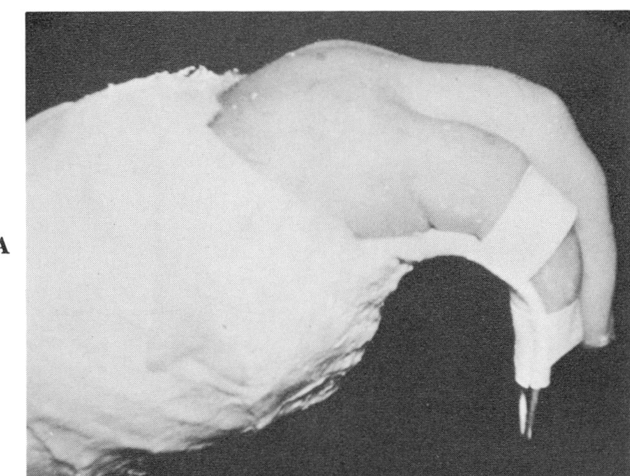

B

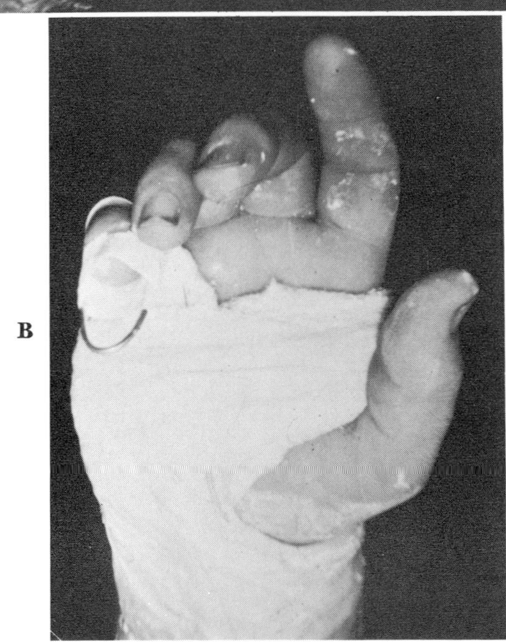

Fig. 9-1. A useful method of immobilizing fractures of metacarpals or phalanges after closed reduction. (In this instance, a fifth metacarpal neck fracture.) **A,** Adhesive tape strips, which conform to finger curvature, support the finger when affixed to a wire splint that is incorporated in a short arm plaster cast. The wire splint immobilizes the metacarpophalangeal and interphalangeal joints in semiflexion, but the plaster immobilizes the wrist in moderate dorsiflexion. **B,** Correct rotation is facilitated by directing the fingertip toward the thenar eminence and aligning the finger so that the plane of the fingernail corresponds with that of its counterpart on the opposite hand. Uninjured fingers are free to move, and the plaster does not block metacarpophalangeal flexion.

an exact reduction is obtained and the fracture is immobilized with one or two small Kirschner wires or with a pullout wire suture. The collateral ligament is repaired before skin closure.

Postoperatively, the finger is immobilized with plaster or with a metal splint that holds the proximal interphalangeal joint in moderate flexion, thus relaxing the extensor tendon apparatus and lessening stress on the replaced fracture fragment. The distal interphalangeal joint of the finger is immobilized in extension, but it is not hyperextended. After 3 weeks, splinting of the proximal interphalangeal joint is discontinued, but splinting of the terminal joint is continued until the fracture has healed, when the Kirschner wire is removed. Long-term follow-up examinations show that fingers treated by this method have regained almost normal motion, and the distal interphalangeal joint has remained healthy and free of degenerative arthritis (Fig. 9-3). By contrast, if the joint surface is not restored by accurate reduction, and if the fracture is allowed to unite in malposition, motion will be limited or painful, and probably both (Fig. 9-4).

Oblique intra-articular fracture of a proximal interphalangeal joint

This fracture is frequently overlooked by the patient, the first treating physician, or both. It is a

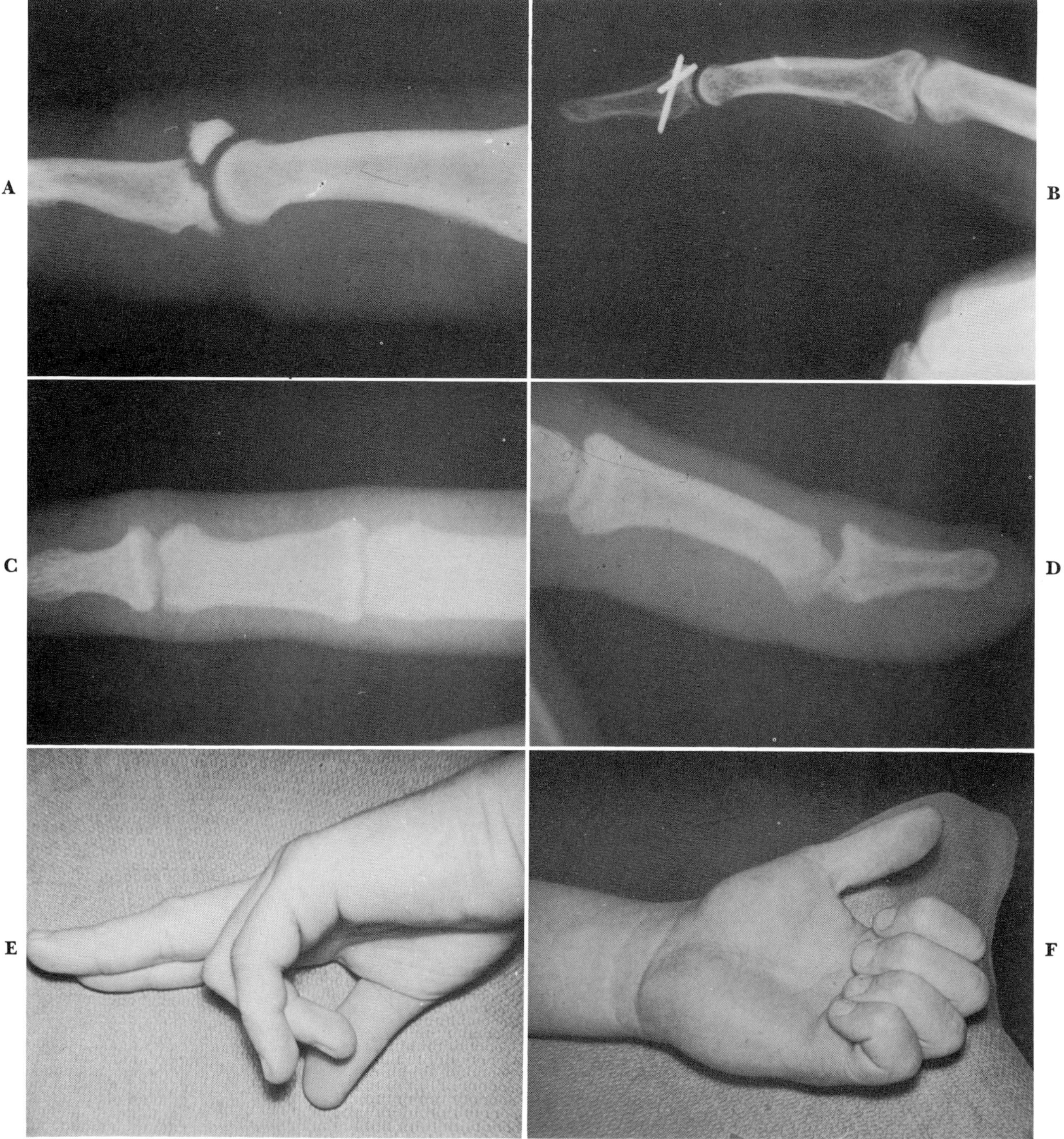

Fig. 9-3. A, Closed intra-articular fracture of the distal joint of a ring finger 3 days after injury. (From Stark, H. H., Boyes, J. H., and Wilson, J. N.: J. Bone Joint Surg. 44-A: 1061, 1962.) **B,** Five weeks after internal fixation. **C** and **D,** Appearance of joint 1 year after surgery. **E** and **F,** Motion of finger 1 year after surgery.

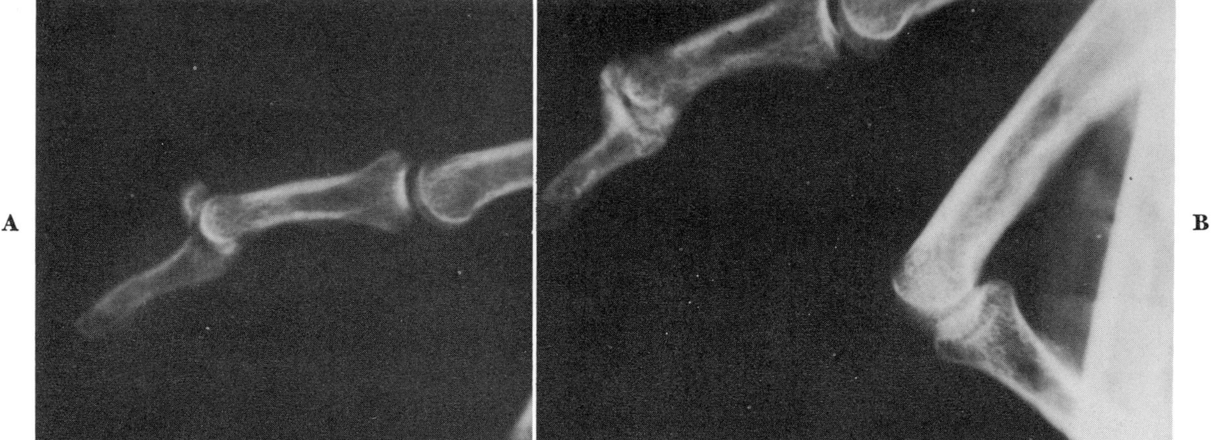

Fig. 9-4. A, A fracture similar to that in Fig. 9-3, which was treated for a "mallet finger" by splinting. **B,** An arthritic and deformed joint was present 1 year later. Fusion was necessary to relieve pain.

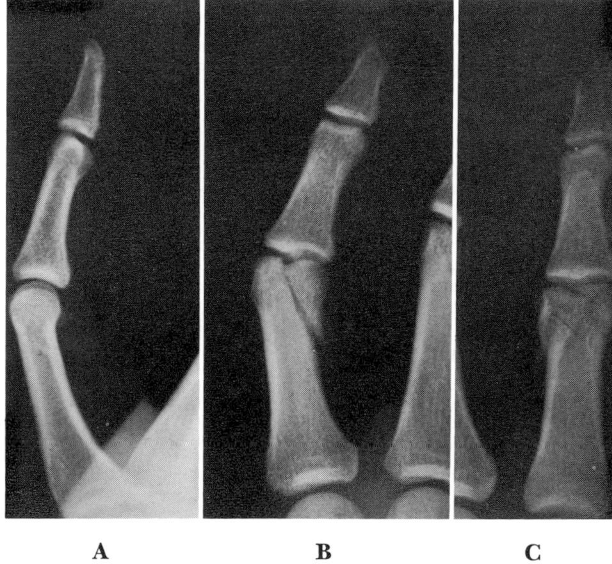

Fig. 9-5. Three views of an intra-articular proximal phalanx fracture. The fracture is not seen on the lateral roentgenogram, **A;** it appears slightly displaced on the anteroposterior roentgenogram, **C,** but on the oblique roentgenogram, **B,** the significant displacement is clearly shown. At least three roentgenographic views are needed to demonstrate bone injuries about finger joints.

common athletic injury, and because the finger can be moved immediately after injury, it is often treated as a sprain. Almost invariably, the fractured condyle slides proximally and the finger angulates and rotates through the proximal interphalangeal joint (Fig. 9-5). Even when the fracture is recognized, the need for an exact reduction may not be appreciated. The surest way to get a perfect reduction is to open the finger through a dorsal zigzag skin incision, and after a longitudinal incision between one lateral band and the central slip of the extensor tendon, the fracture and joint are exposed (Fig. 9-6). Blood supply to the fracture fragment is provided by the intact collateral ligament, which is not disturbed. Accurate reduction of the fracture can be accomplished, two small Kirschner wires ensure fixation, and before skin closure a removable running wire suture is used to approximate the extensor tendon apparatus. The Kirschner wires are cut off beneath the skin, and they should be inserted so that they do not damage articular cartilage or the joint. Occasional voluntary motion is allowed two weeks postoperatively, but the finger is protected with a shaped aluminum or plastic splint until the fracture has healed, when the Kirschner wires are removed.

Spiral fracture of proximal phalanx

Transverse fractures of proximal phalanges respond nicely to closed treatment, but spiral fractures do not. Several ingenious methods of skeletal traction have been devised for treating the spiral fracture, but all are cumbersome and give less predictable results than open reduction and internal fixation. This fracture is unstable, the finger will rotate and shorten, and radiographs are misleading because they fail to show the malrotation (Fig. 9-7). We can restore almost normal finger motion by surgical treatment, a method that also allows

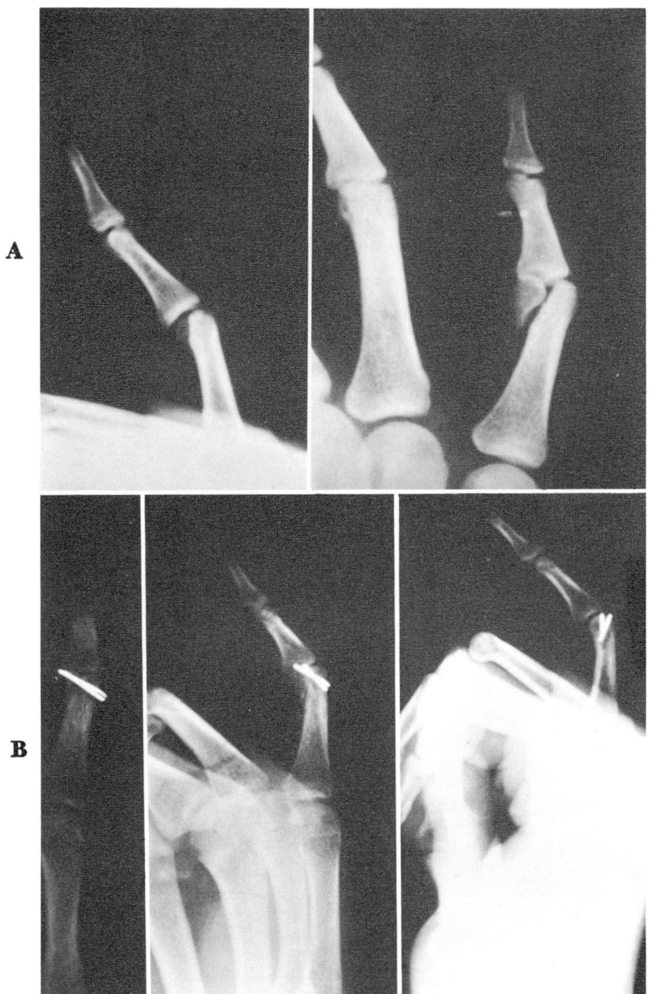

Fig. 9-6. A, An oblique intra-articular fracture of a proximal interphalangeal joint. The fracture fragment is rotated almost 180°; the malrotation is not shown on the lateral view but is evident on the oblique view. **B,** Anatomic reduction obtained by surgery. Two small Kirschner wires give excellent fixation; they do not cross the joint or violate the articular cartilage.

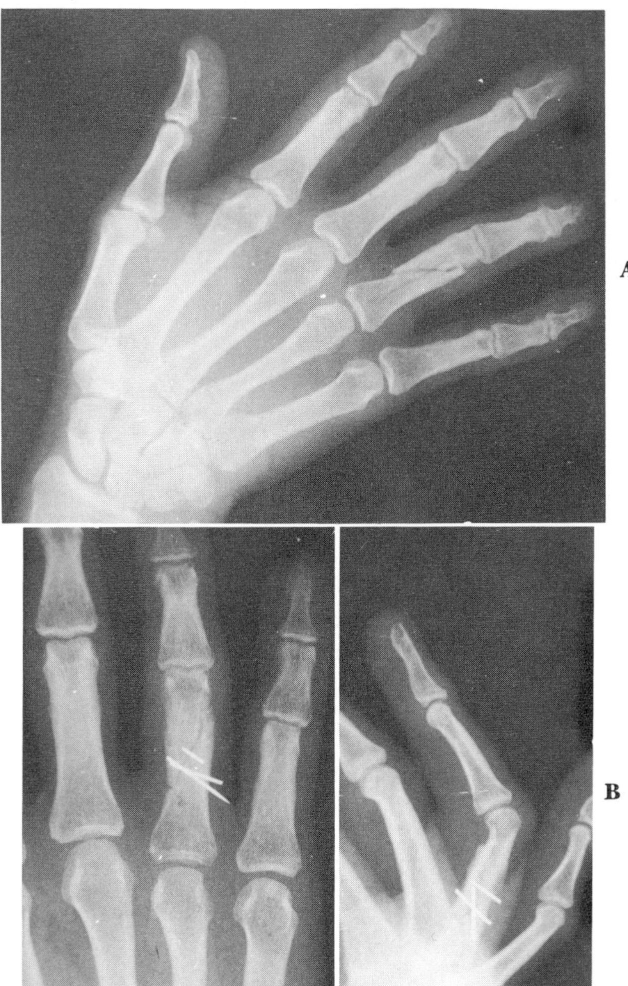

Fig. 9-7. A, A closed spiral fracture of the proximal phalanx causes a finger to shorten and rotate. **B,** Fracture has healed 9 weeks after operation. Normal finger length and correct rotation assured by internal fixation.

voluntary motion as soon as the skin has healed. Either a midlateral or extensor tendon splitting incision gives excellent exposure.

Intra-articular fracture of base of proximal phalanx

In this injury, it is possible to achieve a painless and mobile proximal interphalangeal joint, factors that guarantee a useful finger, by open reduction and internal fixation (Fig. 9-8). Even though badly comminuted, if we are patient and if we have the proper tools, the multiple fragments can be replaced accurately. Fragmentation and the amount of bone displacement are best shown by right and left oblique roentgenograms. A curved dorsal skin incision and longitudinal splitting of the extensor tendon afford excellent exposure. By direct vision, Kirschner wires are used to hold the fracture fragments in correct position; they need not cross the joint. Motion is started 3 weeks after surgery, and the Kirschner wires are removed under local anesthesia when the fracture has healed.

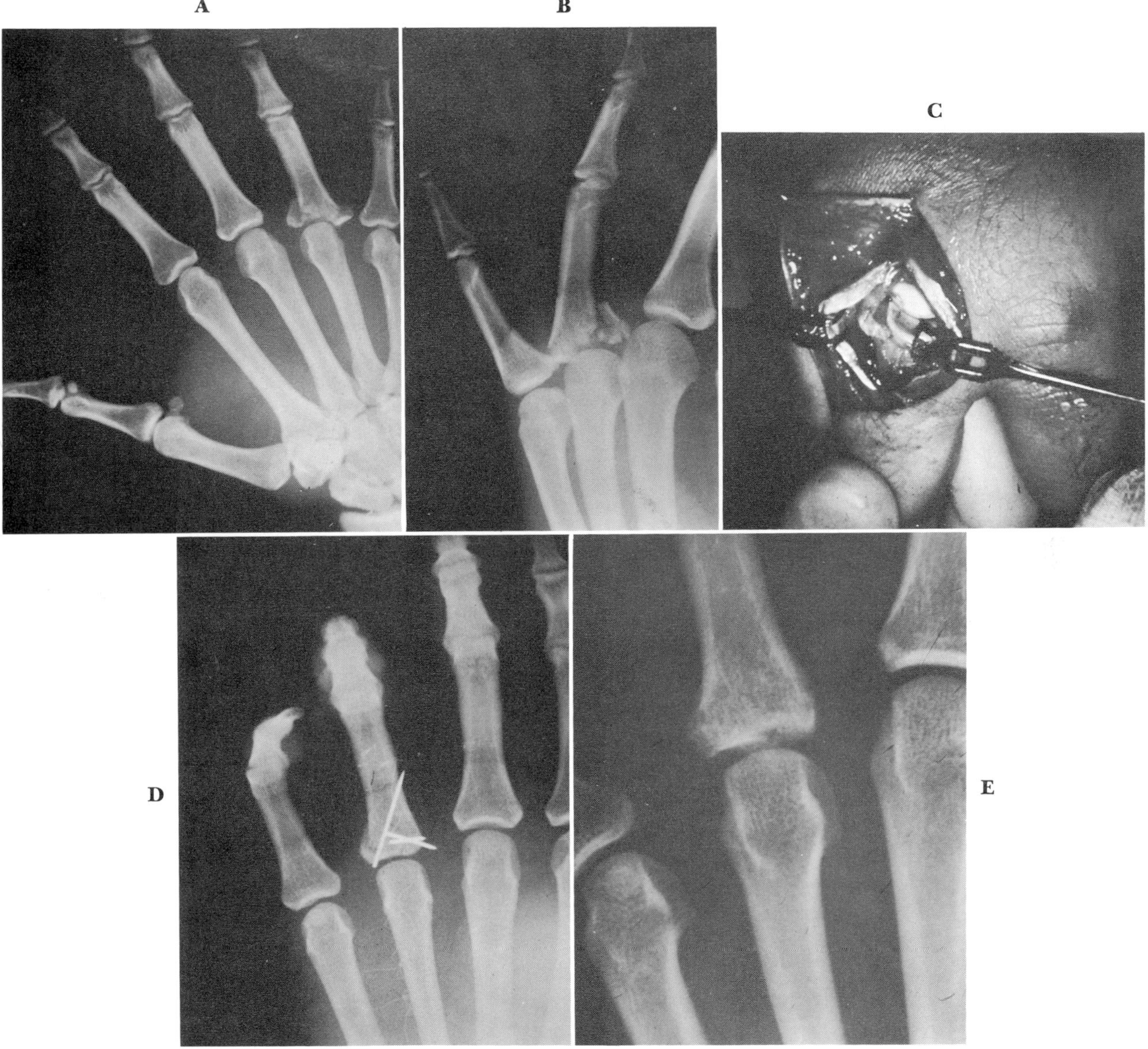

Fig. 9-8. Comminuted fracture of proximal phalanx involving metacarpophalangeal joint. **A** and **B,** Marked comminution and displacement of fracture fragments. **C,** The fracture and joint are exposed through an extensor tendon-splitting incision. **D,** Reduction of fracture and method of fixation. Extensor tendon was reapproximated with a removable stainless steel wire suture. **E,** Six months after surgery joint space is adequate, but there is some irregularity of the articular surface. Two years later, motions and grip were normal and painless.

Fracture of the metacarpal head

The result after treatment of this fracture is most unpredictable (Fig. 9-9). Fortunately, this fracture is rare, but it is easily overlooked because of minimal displacement. Since it occurs through soft cancellous bone, internal stabilization is precarious, and open reduction usually fails. Even when there is minimal displacement of the fracture and very little visible destruction of the articular surface of the metacarpal head, joint motion usually remains painful for many weeks. Some patients will regain painless motion after prolonged

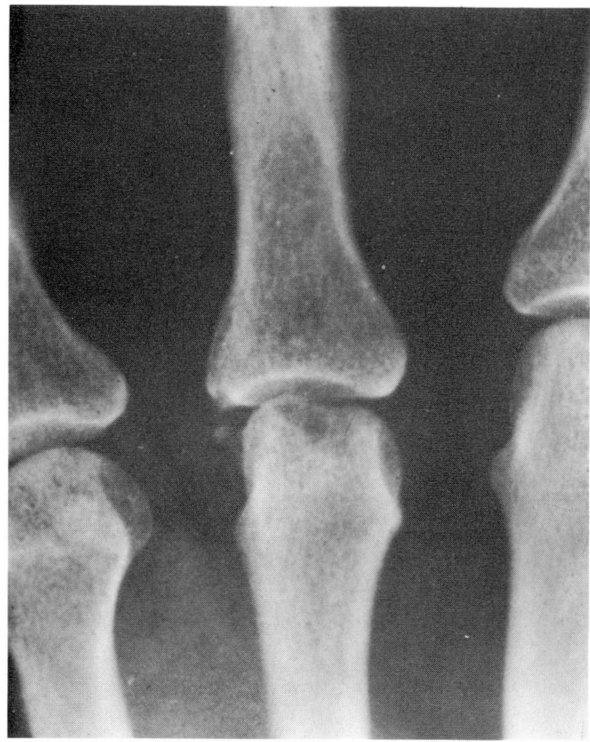

Fig. 9-9. Metacarpal head fracture with minimal displacement, 2 weeks after injury. In spite of prolonged conservative splinting, pain persisted. Arthroplasty was performed, but the joint was still painful. Fusion eliminated the pain.

splinting, but others will not. If pain continues after conservative treatment, arthroplasty or joint fusion are indicated.

Unstable metacarpal shaft fractures

Occasionally a metacarpal fracture cannot be reduced or maintained in an acceptable position by external splinting. A short oblique fracture through the midshaft of a fifth metacarpal is likely to angulate sharply and be unstable (Fig. 9-10). Such a fracture should be opened and fixed internally. This avoids deformity, prevents discomfort from prominence of the metacarpal head in the palm, and restores a near-normal grip. It is essential that metacarpal shaft fractures heal in correct rotation; hence, if malrotation persists after manipulation and external splinting, open reduction should be performed.

Ununited metacarpal neck fractures

Although extremely uncommon, sometimes metacarpal neck fractures do not heal, even though

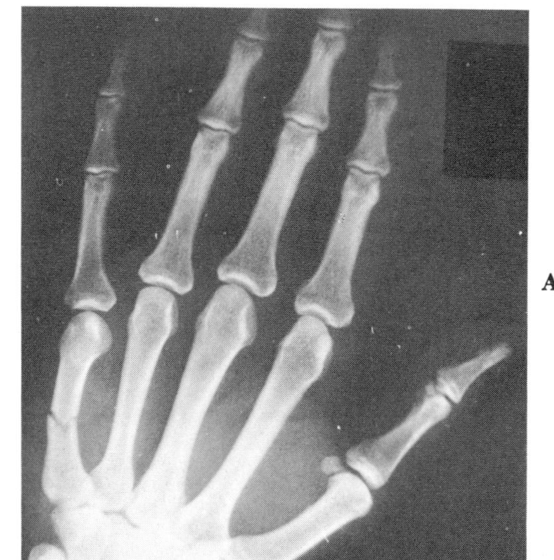

A

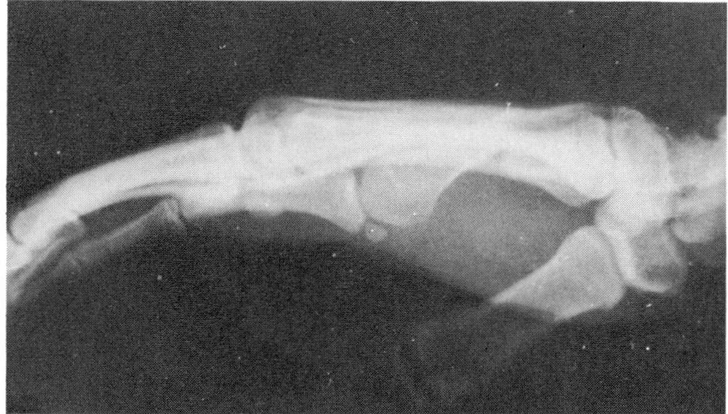

B

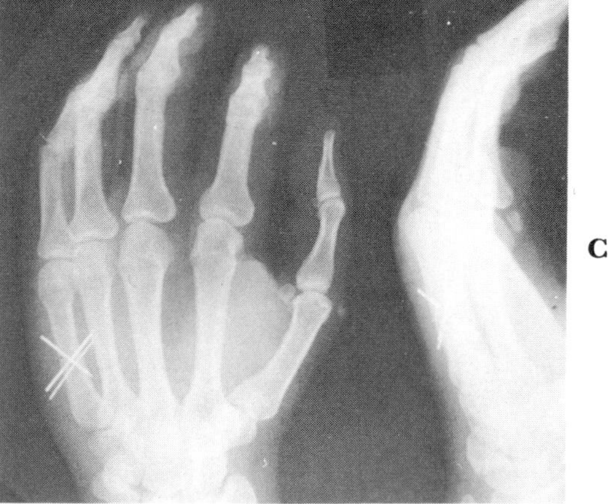

C

Fig. 9-10. A and **B,** Anteroposterior and lateral views of closed oblique fracture of the fifth metacarpal shaft. Reduction could not be maintained by external splinting. **C,** Fracture healed 8 weeks after open reduction and internal fixation.

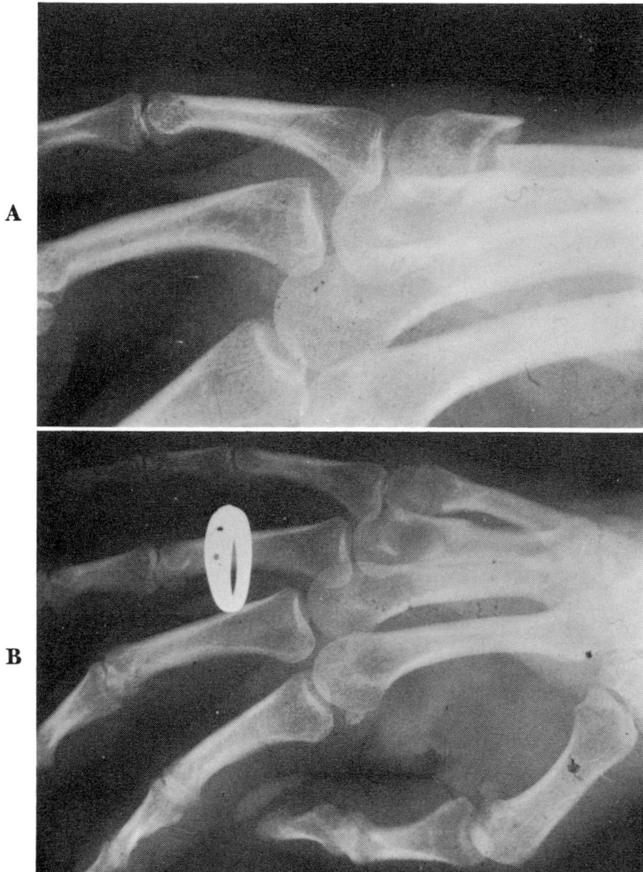

Fig. 9-11. A, Nonunion of metacarpal fracture 3 months after injury. Fracture was immobilized properly from day of injury. **B,** After removing the interposed soft tissue, the fracture was immobilized with two Kirschner wires. Appearance of the fifth metacarpal 4 months after surgery for the nonunion.

treated properly from the time of injury (Fig. 9-11). Interposition of soft tissue causes the nonunion. If the soft tissue is removed and the fracture immobilized by internal fixation, bone healing will occur. The solution is simple, but unless aware of the possibility of a nonunion, it will be overlooked. Then much useless effort will be spent in persistent and prolonged splinting.

TROUBLESOME DISLOCATIONS

Rupture of volar plate of proximal or distal interphalangeal joint

A dorsal dislocation of the proximal interphalangeal joint is a common injury. The middle phalanx shifts dorsalward and, in order for this to occur, the volar plate must disrupt. If the dislocation is reduced soon after injury and the finger is

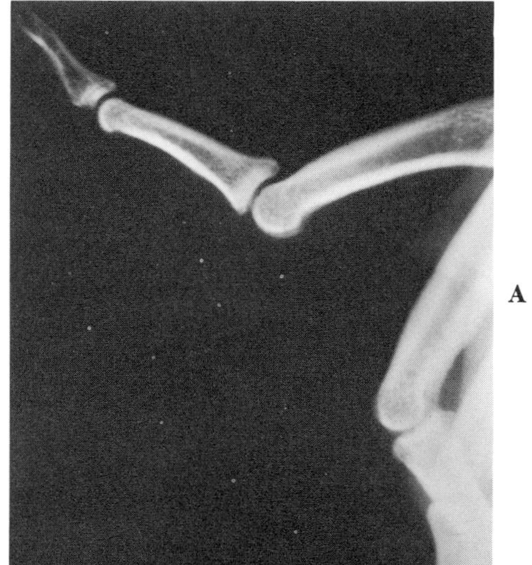

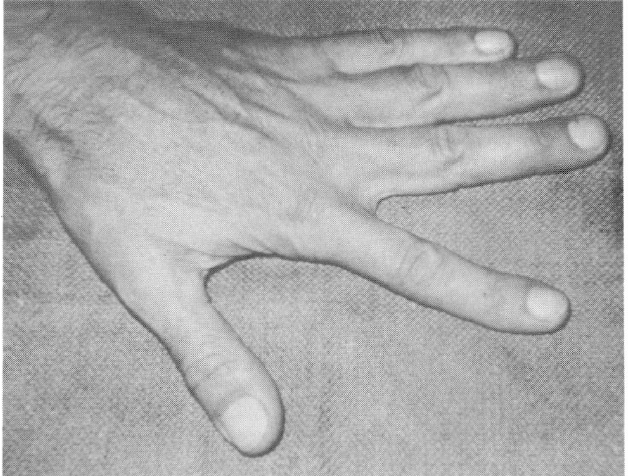

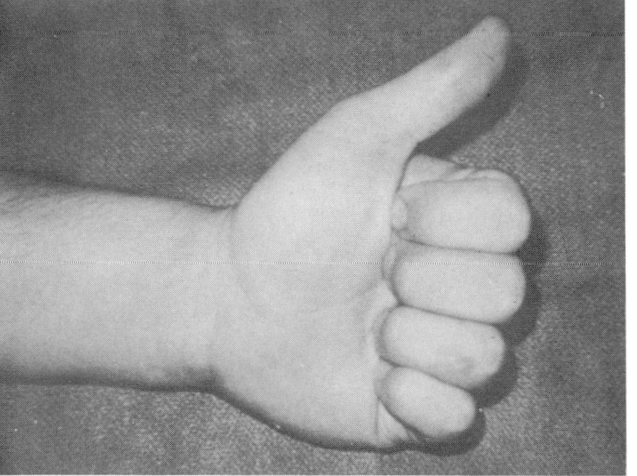

Fig. 9-12. A, Marked hyperextension of proximal interphalangeal joint of ring finger 2 years after injury. Volar plate has been avulsed at its distal attachment, but there is no fracture. **B** and **C,** Flexion and extension of ring finger 9 weeks after repair of volar plate.

immobilized in semiflexion for 2 or 3 weeks, the volar plate will heal, the joint will be stable, and satisfactory motion will return to the finger. If the finger is not splinted soon after injury, the volar plate will not heal, and a chronic hyperextension deformity may result. Since the middle phalanx catches in hyperextension, patients with this deformity find it difficult to initiate flexion of the proximal interphalangeal joint, and the finger is awkward to use. These complaints and the deformity can be eliminated by surgery (Fig. 9-12).

The finger is opened through a midlateral incision, the flexor tendons are retracted volarward, and the volar plate is identified. Usually, the plate has ruptured near its distal attachment, and a small flake of bone, which has pulled loose from the middle phalanx base, may be attached to the free end of the plate. The volar plate can be reattached to the middle phalanx with a pullout wire suture, and, as a precautionary measure, the proximal interphalangeal joint should be immobilized in about 45° of flexion with a small Kirschner wire for 2 or 3 weeks. Voluntary motion is allowed 3 weeks after repair, but complete extension of the proximal interphalangeal joint is prevented until 6 weeks after operation.

Disruption of the volar plate of a distal interphalangeal joint is much less common and more disabling. Because of joint instability, the fingertip sags into hyperextension with pinching, pushing, or percussive motions (Fig. 9-13). The plate should be reattached to the distal phalanx and the terminal joint immobilized with a transarticular Kirschner wire for 3 weeks. Immobilization of the proximal interphalangeal joint is unnecessary.

Volar dislocation of proximal interphalangeal joint

For a volar dislocation to occur, the middle slip of the extensor tendon must disrupt, but the volar plate remains intact. This dislocation can be reduced without surgery, and if the proximal interphalangeal joint is splinted in extension and the distal interphalangeal joint allowed to flex, when the middle slip heals there will be satisfactory balance between the intrinsic and extrinsic finger extensors (Fig. 9-14). Six weeks of splinting is usually sufficient, but during this time, splinting must be continuous and the patient must actively flex the distal interphalangeal joint over the end of the splint.

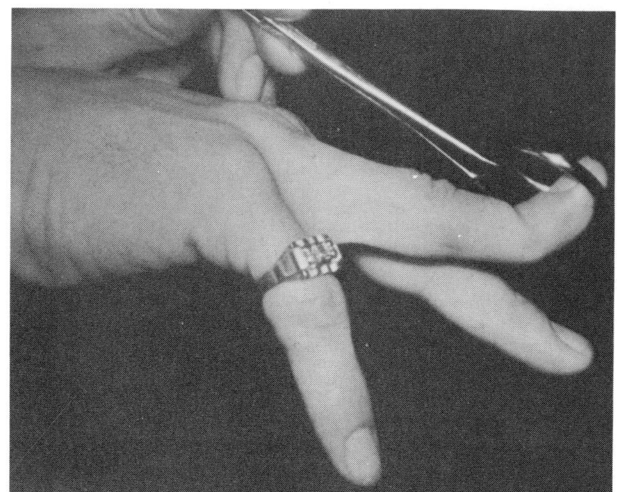
A

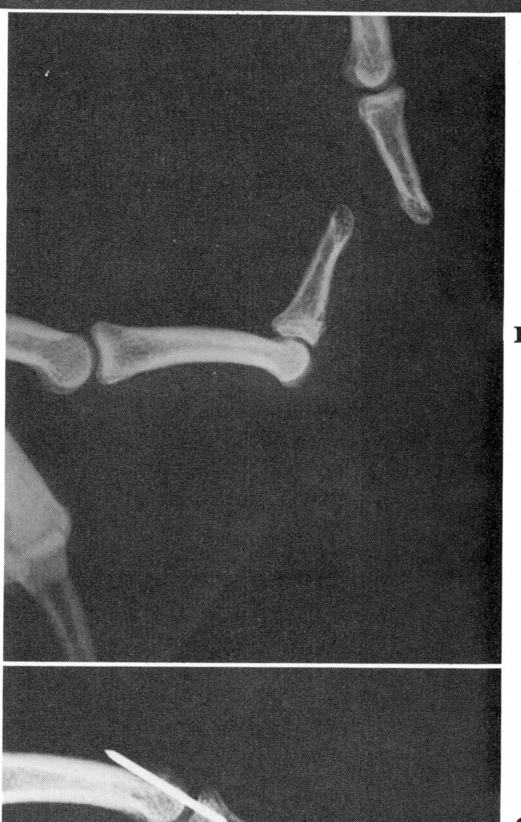
B

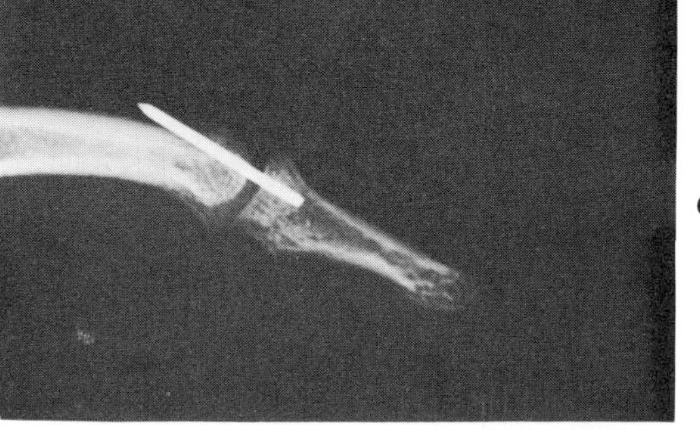
C

Fig. 9-13. A and **B,** Hyperextension of terminal joint and roentgenographic appearance 10 months after disruption of volar plate. **C,** Temporary immobilization of joint with Kirschner wire after repair of volar plate. This protects the repair until the plate heals to the bone.

A

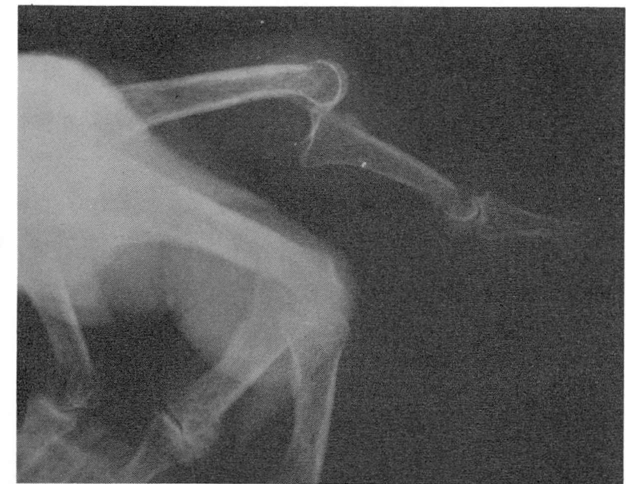

B

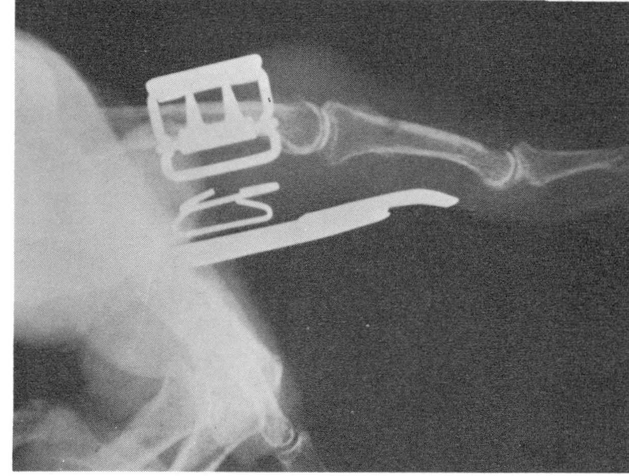

Fig. 9-14. A, Two-week-old volar dislocation of proximal interphalangeal joint in a 62-year-old patient. **B,** After reduction, finger immobilized with metal splint that holds the proximal interphalangeal joint in extension, but allows active flexion of the distal joint. The patient regained satisfactory motion and had a stable joint.

Dorsal dislocation of metacarpophalangeal joint

Ordinarily, this dislocation afflicts the index finger of children, but it can occur in adults, and it may, in rare instances, occur in other fingers (Figs. 9-15 and 9-16). It results from a fall on the outstretched hand, which causes the base of the proximal phalanx to slide dorsal to the metacarpal head. The proximal phalanx becomes locked in this position. The stance of the finger is characteristic; it is malrotated and overlaps the middle finger, flexion is limited, and the metacarpal head is prominent beneath the palmar skin. We need to know two things about this dislocation. First, it is seldom possible to reduce it by closed manipulation and, second, open reduction should be done through a palmar incision. Even if unfamiliar with the injury, the treating physician will soon discover that he cannot reduce the dislocation by manipulation. If he is unaware of the reason why, he is likely to operate on the finger through a dorsal or midlateral incision. Usually, a satisfactory reduction cannot be accomplished with such exposures.

In this dislocation, the volar plate ruptures at the metacarpal neck but remains attached to the base of the proximal phalanx. The volar plate and the transverse metacarpal ligament become wedged between the metacarpal head and the proximal phalanx, and this is the major obstacle to reduction. When the joint is exposed through a transverse palmar incision, the metacarpal head will be found immediately beneath the skin. The radial neurovascular bundle will be radial and *dorsal* to the metacarpal head, and the ulnar neurovascular bundle and flexor tendons will be in an abnormal location *dorsal* and ulnar to the metacarpal head. After visualizing and protecting these structures, the transverse metacarpal ligament is divided longitudinally on the ulnar side of the metacarpal and lifted from behind the metacarpal head. After removing this obstacle, reduction of the dislocation is easy. The finger is immobilized semiflexed for 3 weeks. Recovery of normal finger function is anticipated when reduction is achieved soon after injury.

When the dislocation has persisted for several weeks, reduction is more difficult and cannot be accomplished through a single palmar incision. The collateral ligament and soft tissue on the ulnar side of the metacarpophalangeal joint are contracted and adherent, and they prevent reduction even though the blocking soft tissue has been removed from within the joint. The transverse metacarpal ligament should be divided through a palmar incision, and the ulnar collateral ligament and associated scarred soft tissues are excised through a separate dorsal longitudinal incision. To ensure relocation, the joint is pinned with a transarticular Kirschner wire for 3 weeks. When reduction is delayed longer than 3 weeks, there will be some permanent loss of finger motion, but, even so, the dislocation should be corrected.

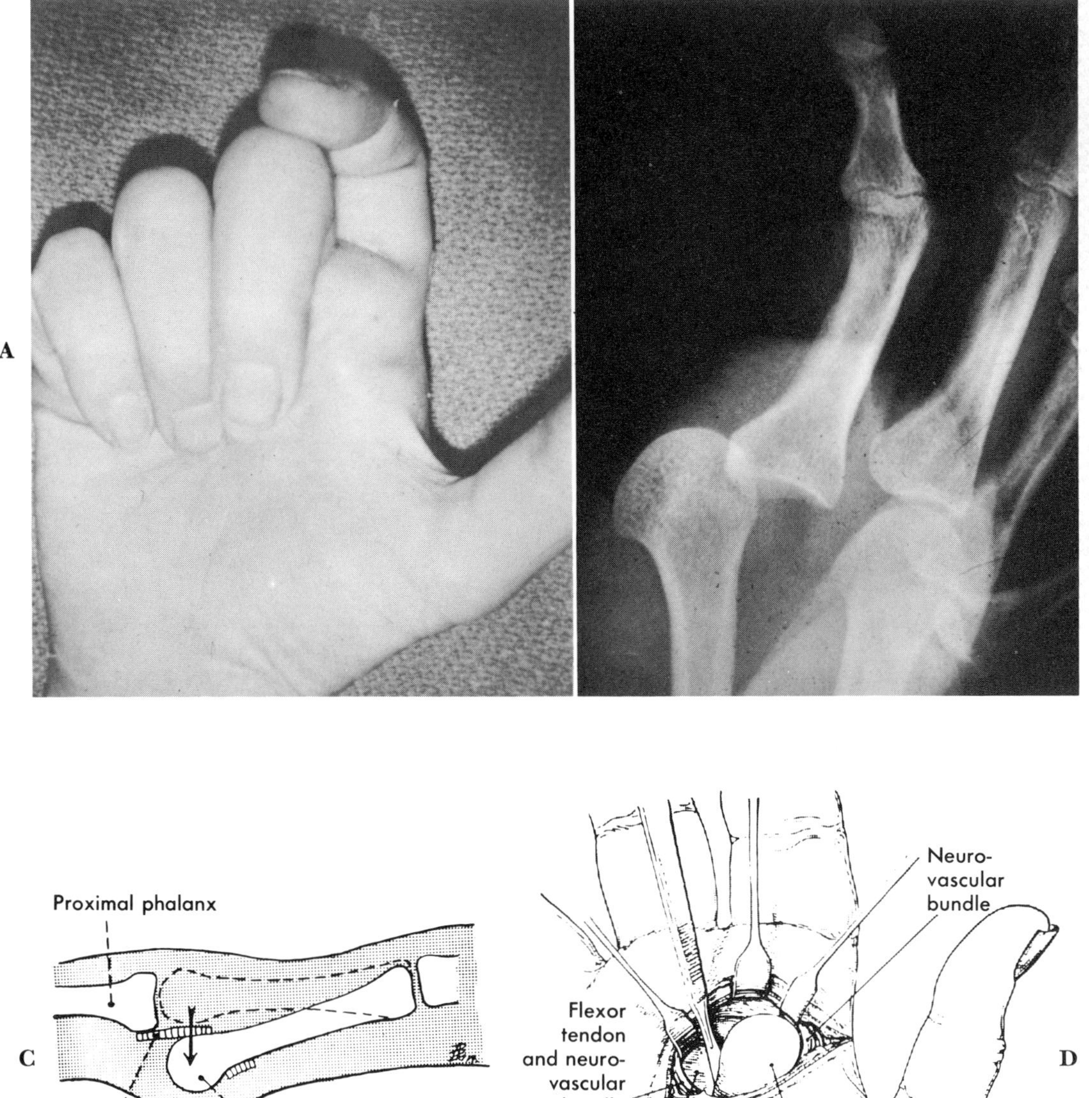

Fig. 9-15. Dorsal dislocation of metacarpophalangeal joint of index finger. **A,** Typical appearance of the hand. The metacarpal head is prominent in the palm, the finger is malrotated, and the distal two joints of the finger are semiflexed. **B,** In a typical dislocation, the proximal phalanx lies dorsal to the metacarpal head, and the space between the second and third metacarpal bones is increased. **C,** The major obstacle to reduction is the transverse metacarpal ligament, which becomes wedged between the metacarpal head and the proximal phalanx. **D,** Recent dislocations are exposed through a transverse palmar skin incision. After longitudinal division of the transverse metacarpal ligament, the interposed tissue is removed, and reduction is accomplished.

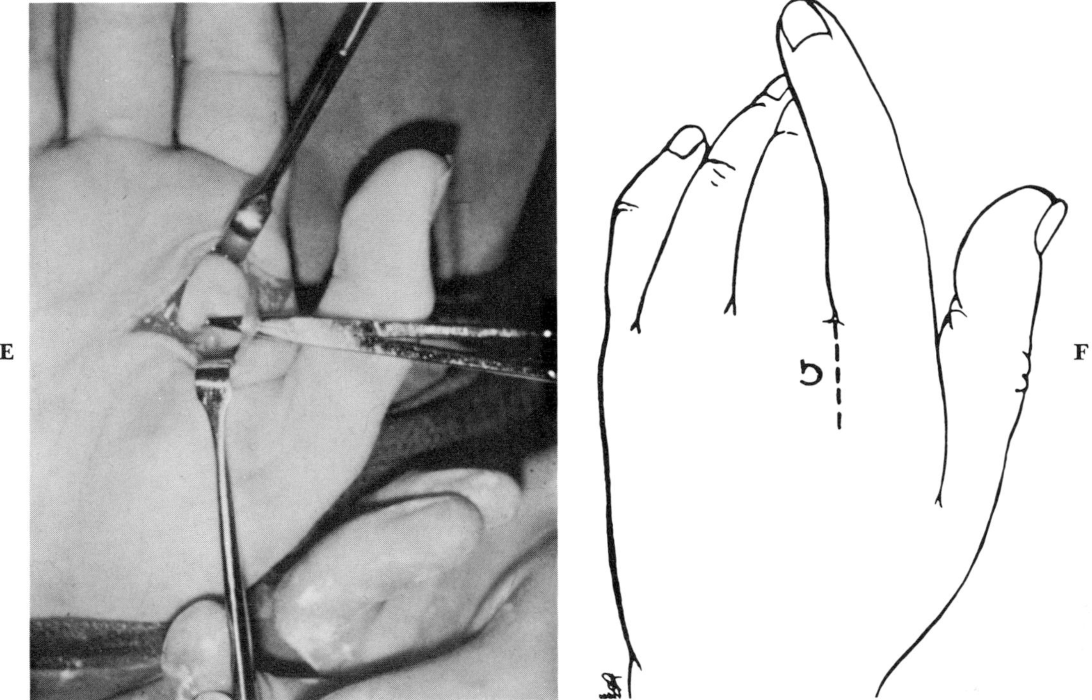

Fig. 9-15, cont'd. E, The metacarpal head is encountered just beneath the skin, and the neurovascular bundles, which are *dorsal* to the metacarpal head, should be isolated and protected. **F,** If reduction has been delayed longer than 3 weeks, the ulnar collateral ligament of the metacarpophalangeal joint must be excised through a special dorsal incision before reduction can be accomplished. (**A-D** and **F,** From Murphy, A. F., and Stark, H. H.: J. Bone Joint Surg. **49-A:**1579, 1967.)

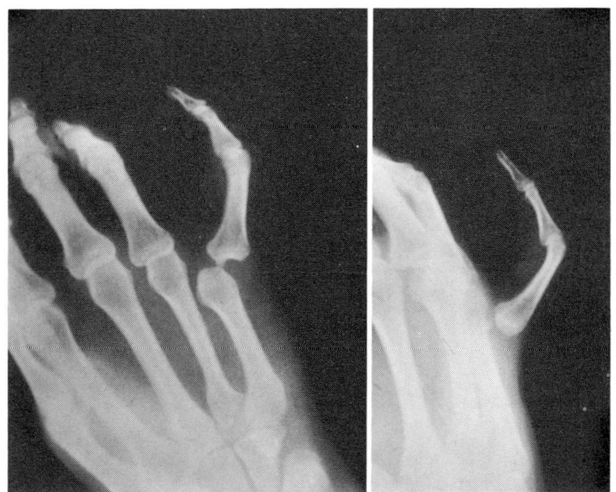

Fig. 9-16. A dorsal dislocation of the metacarpophalangeal joint of little finger, which is an unusual injury. Best treatment is open reduction through a palmar incision.

Carpometacarpal dislocations

Since this dislocation is often associated with extensive soft tissue damage, it may be unrecognized because of hasty primary treatment or failure to obtain adequate roentgenograms of the hand. Diagnosis can be made on the anteroposterior or oblique views, but a true lateral view or "prayer view" of both hands is best to demonstrate the dislocation (Fig. 9-17). Immediately after injury, closed reduction is easy, but the reduction may be unstable. If so, percutaneous pinning with Kirschner wires will maintain reduction until the torn joint capsules heal. The Kirschner wires are removed about 5 weeks after injury.

When the dislocation is either missed or left unreduced, the dorsal prominence on the hand is bothersome, the mechanics and muscle balance of the hand are upset, and the grip is weak. For these reasons, it is desirable to effect reduction even though it has been present for several weeks, or even months. Correction of the dorsal deformity and surgical fusion of the involved joints through

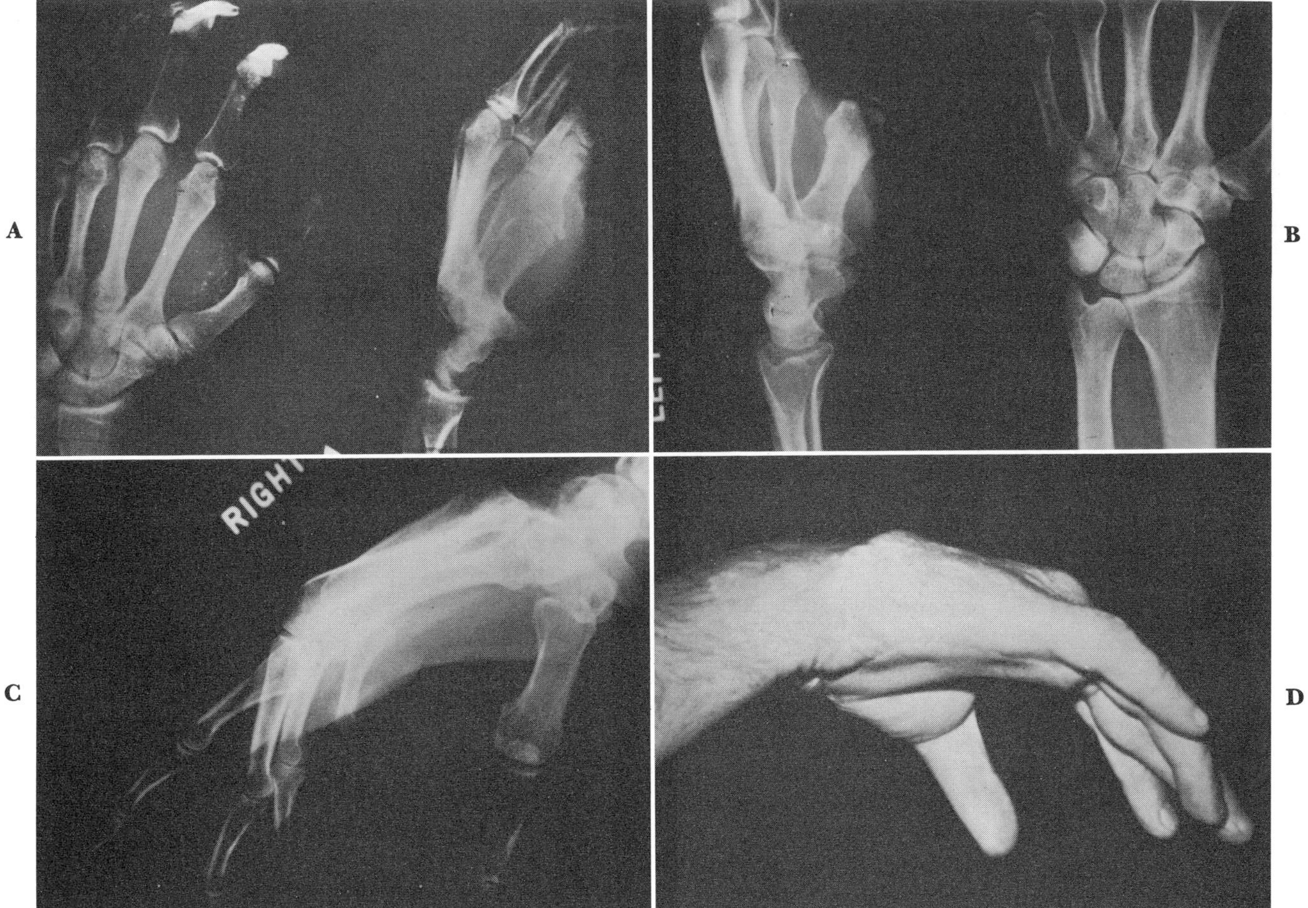

Fig. 9-17. A, Dorsal dislocation of the fourth and fifth metacarpal bones was overlooked in these roentgenograms. The hand was badly crushed, and there was extensive soft tissue injury. **B,** Comparative views of the uninjured hand show the normal joint space between the hamate and the fourth and fifth metacarpal bones on the anteroposterior view, and on the lateral view the head and base of each of the ulnar four metacarpals are in the same horizontal plane. These *normal* relationships are not present in **A. C,** A true lateral roentgenogram of the injured hand demonstrates the dislocation clearly. **D,** Bony prominence caused by the persistent dislocation 1 year after injury. Even in long-standing dislocations, open reduction of the joint dislocation and joint fusion improve the mechanics and function of the hand.

a dorsal skin incision restore strength and usefulness to the hand. Care must be taken to avoid injuring the motor branch of the ulnar nerve; it is close to the volar surface of the fourth metacarpal bone and must be protected.

Closed rupture of collateral ligaments of a metacarpophalangeal joint of the thumb

Patients with a closed rupture of either the ulnar or radial collateral ligament of this joint seldom seek treatment immediately after injury. If they do, and treatment is begun within 10 days of injury, plaster immobilization for 4 weeks may allow the ligament to heal and the joint to become stable. If this fails, or if initial treatment is delayed for more than 10 days, surgical repair of the torn ligament is indicated, although joint fusion is a simple and good solution for older patients. Disruption of the ulnar collateral ligament is somewhat more common than the radial, but the pathology encountered at surgery is similar in either instance. A characteristic abnormal and visible soft tissue prominence usually accompanies this ligament rupture. When doubtful about the diag-

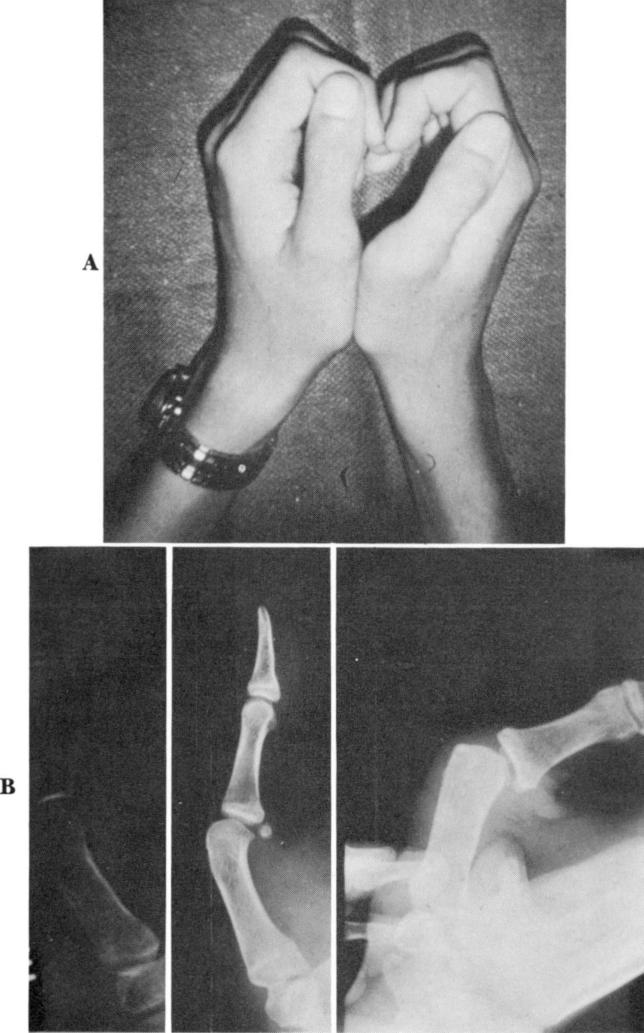

Fig. 9-18. A, Clinical deformity caused by old rupture of radial collateral ligament of metacarpophalangeal joint of thumb. **B,** A roentgenogram with the joint under stress aids in diagnosis.

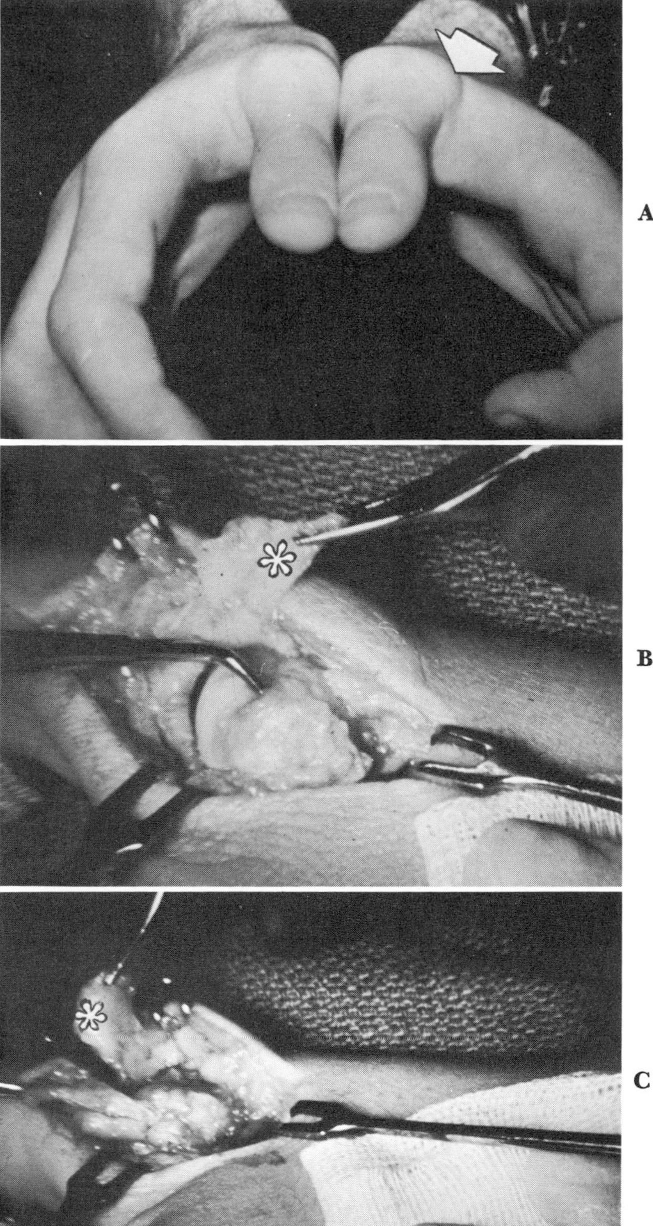

Fig. 9-19. A, Appearance of thumb 10 weeks after rupture of ulnar collateral ligament. The soft tissue prominence is caused by the disrupted collateral ligament folding proximalward, arrow. **B,** Usual finding at surgery. The hemostat is holding the reflected portion of the adductor aponeurosis, *, and the probe points to the folded collateral ligament, which has been avulsed from its distal attachment. **C,** The scar covering the torn ligament has been removed, the ligament has been unfolded, and its free margin is covering the joint and is ready for attachment to the proximal phalanx. Reflected part of adductor aponeurosis has been cut to expose the joint and torn ligament, *.

nosis, a stress roentgenogram should be obtained. This can be taken without anesthesia (Fig. 9-18).

A detailed description of the peculiar pathology of this lesion has been published by Stener.[12] This should be understood before attempting surgical repair of either collateral ligament.

Through a midlateral skin incision, the reflected portion of the adductor or abductor aponeurosis (depending upon whether the radial or ulnar side of the joint is exposed) is divided, thus exposing the joint and the torn ligament. Although the collateral ligament may rupture at any location, the usual rupture occurs at or near the phalangeal

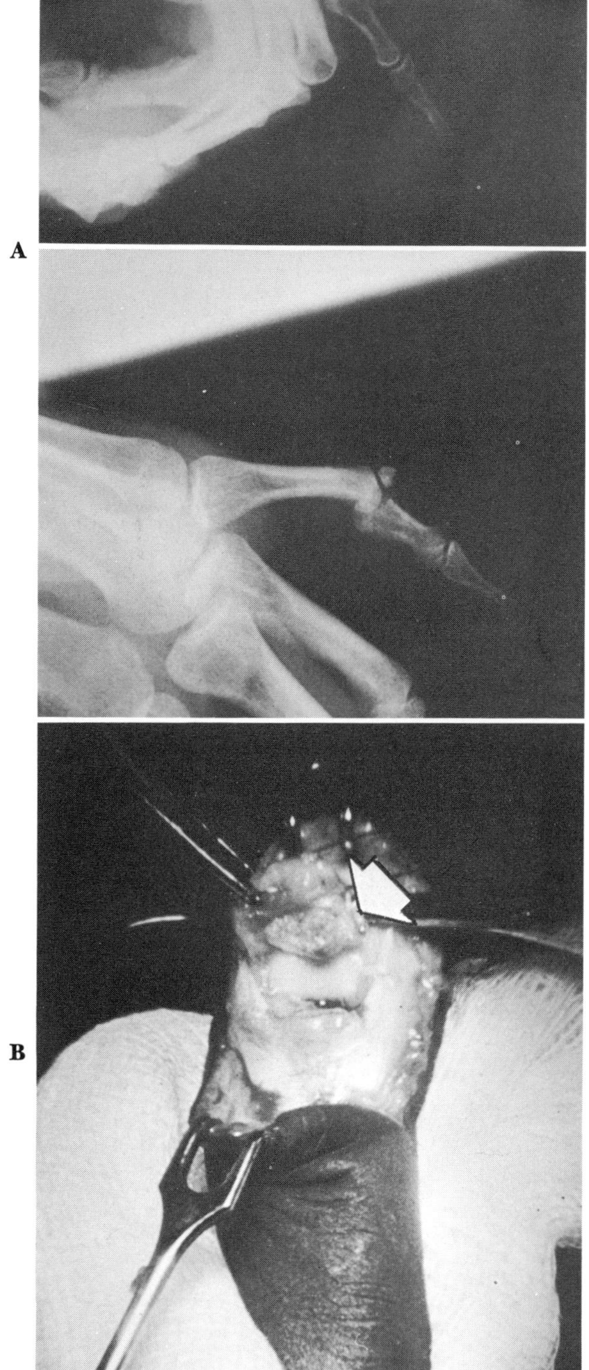

Fig. 9-20. A, A fracture of the dorsal lip of the middle phalanx allows the middle phalanx to dislocate volarward. **B,** The fracture fragment, arrow, which is attached to the middle slip of the extensor tendon, is ready for reattachment to the middle phalanx. Good fixation is accomplished with pullout wire suture.

insertion. The torn ligament, which is folded on itself and which may be partly obscured by scar tissue, is unfolded and reattached to the proximal phalanx with a pullout wire or with chromic sutures (Fig. 9-19). The divided aponeurosis is reapproximated, and, although not mandatory, it is usually wise to immobilize the joint with a small Kirschner wire for about 3 weeks. Plaster immobilization is continued for a total of 5 weeks after operation. If surgical repair cannot be accomplished, joint fusion usually gives a better functional result than attempted tendon grafting or ligamentous reconstruction with a free graft.

FRACTURE-DISLOCATIONS

Three fracture-dislocations are particularly troublesome; two of these involve the middle joint of a finger and one the base of the thumb.

Fracture of dorsal lip of middle phalanx

The central slip of the extensor tendon inserts into the dorsum of the middle phalanx; therefore, when the dorsal lip of this bone fractures, not only is a boutonniere deformity produced, but also the middle phalanx dislocates volarward. The fracture fragment should be repositioned through a curved dorsal incision and immobilized with a small Kirschner wire or with a pullout wire suture (Fig. 9-20). Postoperatively, the proximal interphalangeal joint is immobilized in extension, but gentle flexion should be started no later than the fourth week after surgery. After accurate reduction and secure fixation, the proximal interphalangeal joint should regain a good degree of motion.

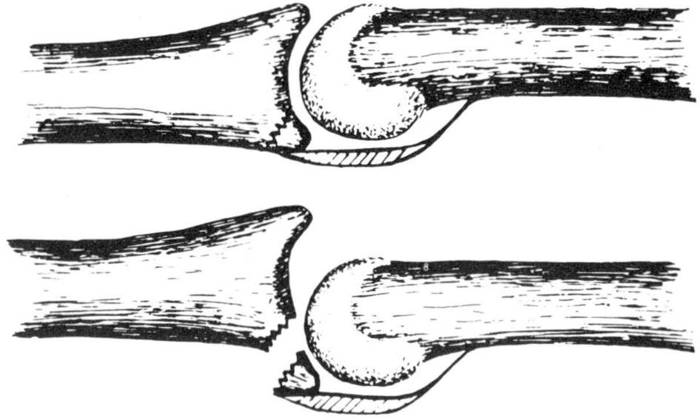

Fig. 9-21. When the volar lip of the middle phalanx fractures, loss of the buttressing effect of this bone fragment, which also affords attachment of the volar plate, permits the middle phalanx to dislocate dorsalward.

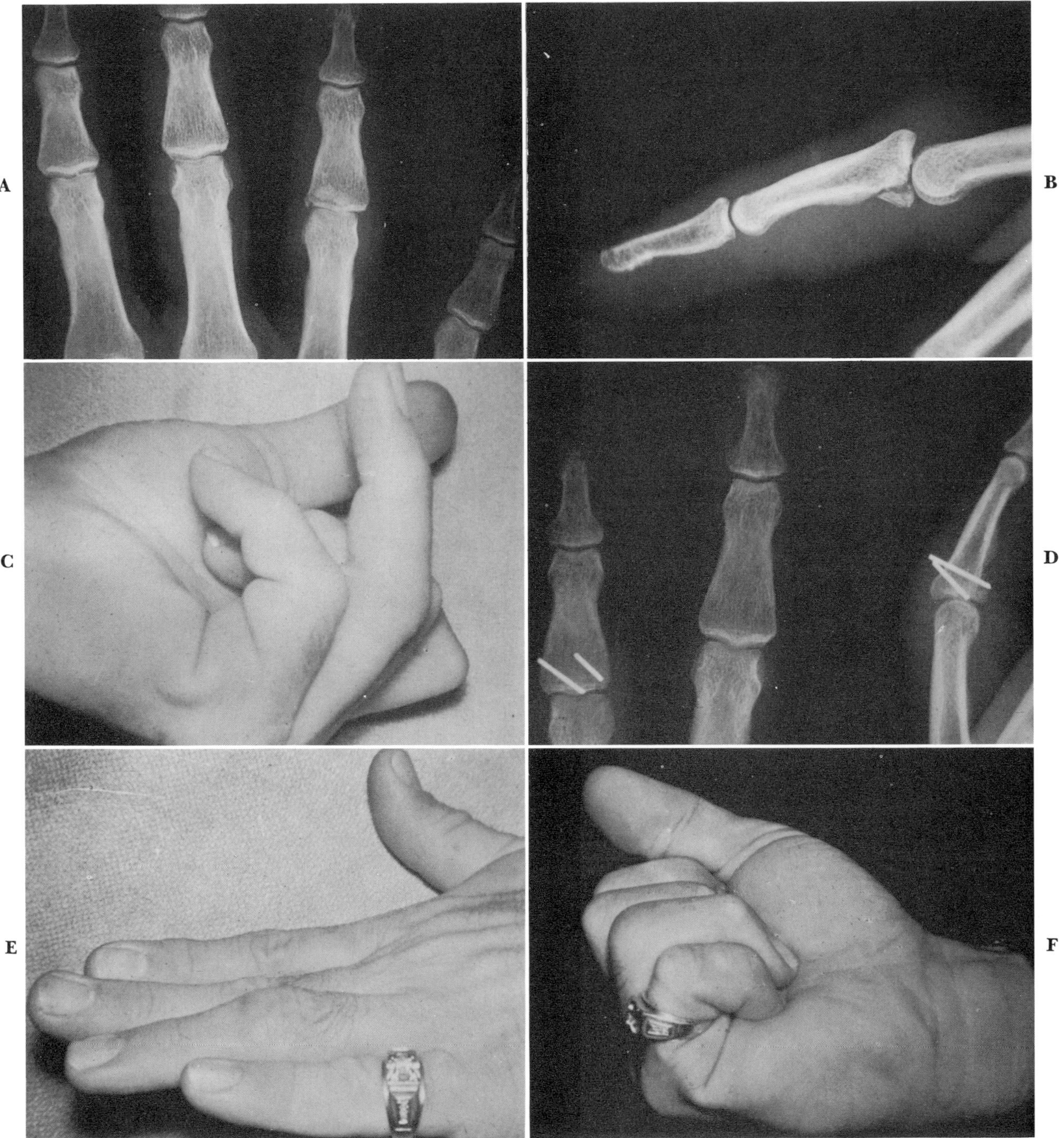

Fig. 9-22. A and **B,** Roentgenograms showing fracture dislocation of proximal interphalangeal joint 6 weeks after injury. Without a lateral view, the dislocation may be unrecognized. **C,** Preoperative limitation of finger motion is illustrated. Because of the dislocation, flexion of the injured ring finger is restricted, and this also limits flexion of the contiguous uninjured fingers. **D,** By surgery, this reduction was obtained; the fracture fragment was fixed with two Kirschner wires, which do not interfere with flexor tendon gliding. Usually the joint is immobilized for 3 weeks with another transarticular Kirschner wire; this prevents redislocation and facilitates replacement of the fracture fragment. **E** and **F,** Motion of finger 3 years after surgery.

Fracture of volar base of middle phalanx

A fracture of the volar base of the middle phalanx is deceptive. Roentgenograms immediately after injury often show an undisplaced or minimally displaced fracture. The volar plate inserts into the base of the middle phalanx, and when this portion of the bone fractures, all volar support of the joint is lost, and there is nothing to stop the middle phalanx from dislocating dorsalward (Fig. 9-21). If soon after injury the significance of this fracture is recognized, a good result can be obtained by splinting the proximal interphalangeal joint in semiflexion for 3 weeks. If the magnitude of this injury is unrecognized, or if the finger is splinted improperly, the fracture will displace and the joint will dislocate within a few days following injury. When this happens, fixed extension of the injured finger prevents complete flexion of adjacent uninjured fingers.

True lateral roentgenograms are essential to avoid missing this fracture. Once dislocation has occurred, the best treatment is reduction by surgery even if several weeks have elapsed since the injury (Fig. 9-22). If the dislocation and fracture are not reduced, the joint surfaces will remain incongruous, and surgical fusion will probably be needed unless the joint fuses spontaneously.

The proximal interphalangeal joint is exposed through a midlateral incision. One collateral ligament is divided, and the fracture fragment, which is still attached to the volar plate, is identified. The dislocation is reduced; it may be necessary to disrupt adhesions beneath the dorsal joint capsule with a probe, or to divide the dorsal fibers of the opposite collateral ligament before reduction is possible. The proximal interphalangeal joint should be placed in 45° of flexion, and it is advisable to transfix the joint in this position with one small Kirschner wire. The fracture fragment is then replaced and immobilized with one or two small Kirschner wires or, occasionally, with a pullout wire suture.

When there is much comminution and crushing of the subchondral bone, a free bone graft obtained from the distal radius should be packed beneath the replaced fracture fragment. This graft adds stability to the fracture fragment and forms a prop to restore the proper curvature to the base of the phalanx. If the fracture has united in malposition, it is separated from the middle phalanx shaft, replaced, and immobilized with a small Kirschner wire and supported with a bone graft. By using an electric drill, magnification, and precise and gentle technique, a reasonably smooth joint surface can be fashioned. The divided collateral ligament is repaired before skin closure. The Kirschner wire crossing the joint is removed at 3 weeks, and gentle but limited voluntary finger motion is started shortly thereafter. If a pullout wire suture is used, it is also removed at 3 weeks, but if the fracture has been immobilized with a second Kirschner wire, which is a better method, that wire is removed when the fracture has healed, which is usually 5 or 6 weeks after surgery. Fingers treated by this method have usually regained useful and painless joint motion even when reduction has been delayed for as long as 4 months after injury.

Bennett's fracture-dislocation

Many types of treatment have been advocated for this fracture. We should remember that this is an intra-articular fracture of a very mobile joint that is moved innumerable times each day (Fig. 9-23). Accurate restoration of the articular surface affords the best likelihood of the joint remaining

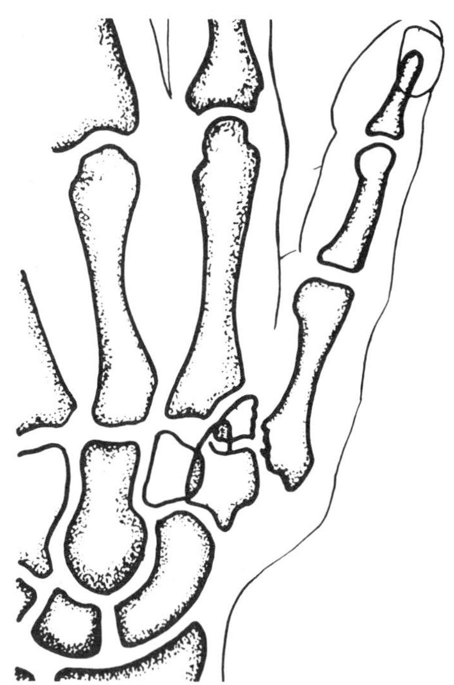

Fig. 9-23. Bennett's fracture is an intra-articular fracture. The base of the thumb dislocates, but the small fracture fragment remains in its normal position.

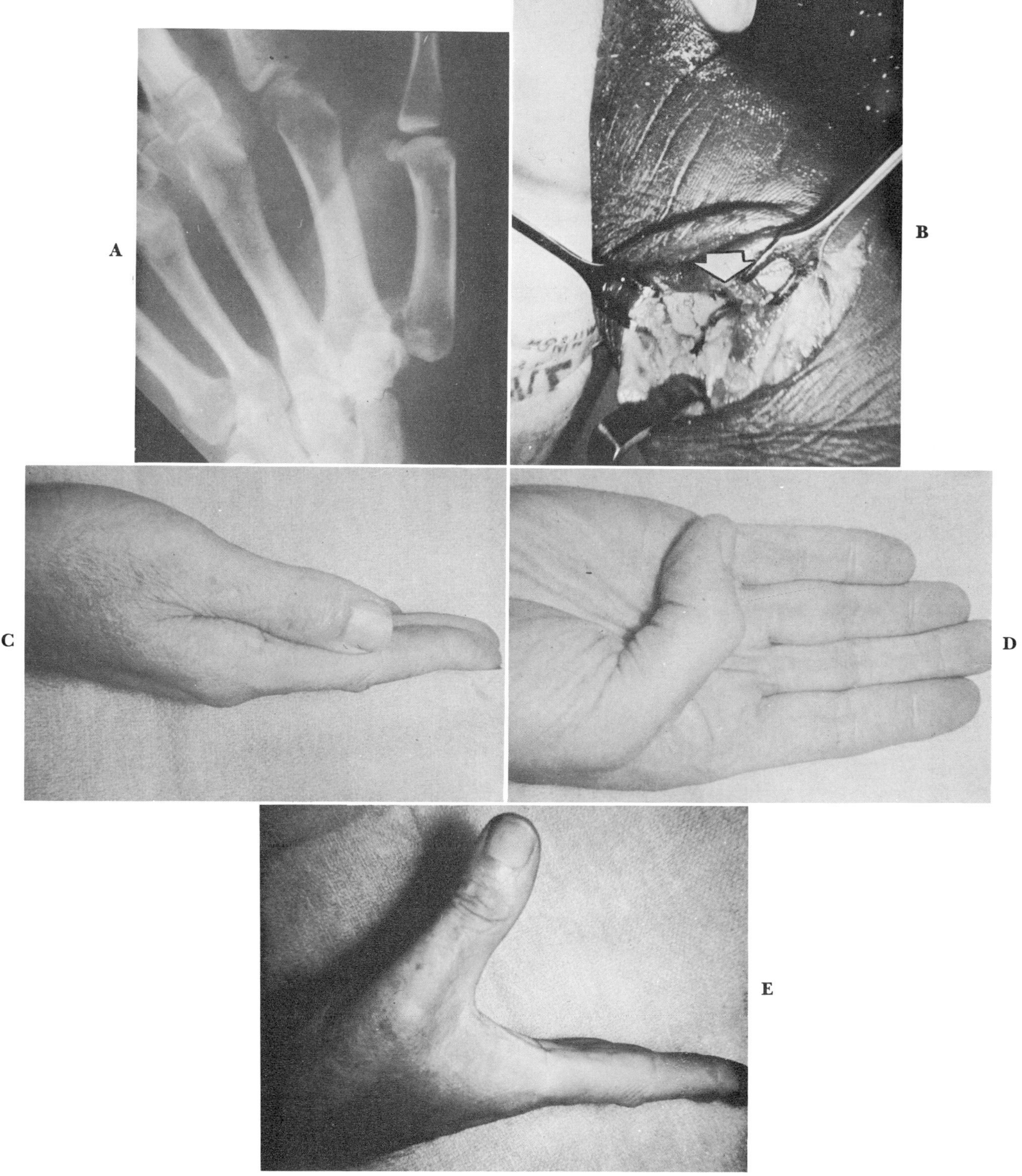

Fig. 9-24. A, Fracture-dislocation of the Bennett type 2 weeks after injury. **B,** Exposure through a volar skin incision. The fracture has been reduced and transfixed with one small Kirschner wire, arrow. **C-E,** Motion of thumb 4 years after surgery. Adduction, abduction, and flexion-adduction, which depend on metacarpal-carpal motion, are complete and painless.

healthy for many years after injury. Any closed method of treatment, including percutaneous pinning, makes us dependent on bone shadows for evaluation of the accuracy of reduction. Since roentgenograms can be misleading, particularly if taken through plaster, and assuming that a more anatomic reduction can be obtained by direct vision of the fracture, open reduction and internal fixation is a logical method of treating this injury.

A volar skin incision provides excellent exposure of the fracture and joint. The thumb metacarpal is replaced on the saddle of the greater multangular bone and brought to the fracture fragment, which is relatively immobile because of its intact ligamentous attachments. The fracture fragment is fixed to the metacarpal shaft with one or two small Kirschner wires, and it is best to transfix the first metacarpal–greater multangular joint for 1 month with a separate Kirschner wire. The remaining wires are removed when the fracture has healed (Fig. 9-24). Postoperatively, plaster immobilization is continued until bone healing is complete.

Patients treated for this fracture-dislocation should be evaluated at least 2 years and preferably 5 years after injury and treatment. Even with poor reduction and an incongruous joint, thumb motion may remain relatively painless for many months, but if a smooth articular surface is not restored, the joint surface will usually deteriorate and patients will seek further care several years later. Billing and Gedda[1] described a special roentgenographic view that shows the true lateral displacement of the metacarpal dislocation, and Lasserre, Pausat, and Derrennes[7] illustrated a technique of obtaining a roentgenogram showing the contour of the first metacarpal–greater multangular joint (Fig. 9-25). This latter view, as well as conventional views, should be taken routinely for suspected injuries about the base of the thumb.

In this presentation, various fractures, dislocations, and fracture-dislocations of the metacarpals and phalanges have been described. It is hoped that the aids in diagnosis, the methods of treatment, and the specific details of surgical technique that have been discussed will be helpful to other surgeons who treat such injuries.

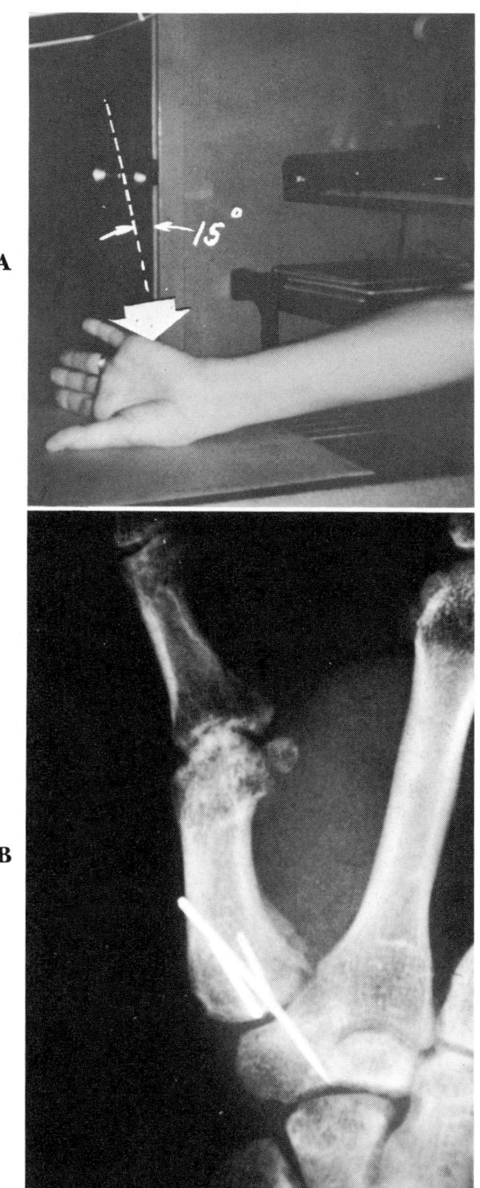

Fig. 9-25. A, Technique of obtaining a special roentgenographic view of the first metacarpal-greater multangular joint. The roentgenogram tube is tilted 15° toward the head, and the thumb is positioned with the forearm in pronation and the shoulder internally rotated. **B,** Roentgenographic view of the base of the thumb obtained by this method. The fracture has healed, and reduction was assured by a temporary transarticular Kirschner wire. Placing a small Kirschner wire across this joint is not harmful.

REFERENCES

1. Billing, Lars, and Gedda, K. O.: Roentgen examination of Bennett's fracture, Acta Radiol. **38**:471, 1952.

2. Boyes, J. H.: Bunnell's surgery of the hand, ed. 4, Philadelphia, 1964, J. B. Lippincott Co.
3. Gedda, K. O., and Moberg, E.: Open reduction and osteosynthesis of the so-called Bennett's fracture in the carpo-metacarpal joint of the thumb, Acta Orthop. Scand. **22**:249, 1953.
4. Hazlett, J. W.: Carpometacarpal dislocations other than the thumb: a report of 11 cases, Canad. J. Surg. **11**:315, 1968.
5. Howard, L. D., Jr., Niebauer, J. J., Pratt, D. R., and Brown, R. L.: Fractures of the small bones of the hand. (Instructional course booklet.)
6. Kaplan, E. B.: Dorsal dislocation of the metacarpophalangeal joint of the index finger, J. Bone Joint Surg. **39A**:1081, 1957.
7. Lasserre, C., Pausat, D., and Derrennes, R.: Osteoarthritis of the trapeziometacarpal joint, J. Bone Joint Surg. **31B**:534, 1949.
8. Murphy, A. F., and Stark, H. H.: Closed dislocation of the metacarpophalangeal joint of the index finger, J. Bone Joint Surg. **49A**:1579, 1967.
9. Pratt, D. R.: Exposing fractures of the proximal phalanx of the finger longitudinally through the dorsal extensor apparatus, Clin. Orthop., no. 15, pp. 22-26, 1959.
10. Stark, H. H., Boyes, J. H., and Wilson, J. N.: Mallet finger, J. Bone Joint Surg. **44A**:1061, 1962.
11. Stener, B.: Displacement of the ruptured ulnar collateral ligament of the metacarpo-phalangeal joint of the thumb, J. Bone Joint Surg. **44B**:869, 1962.
12. Stener, B.: Hyperextension injuries to the metacarpophalangeal joint of the thumb—rupture of ligaments, fracture of sesamoid bones, rupture of flexor pollicis brevis, Acta Chir. Scand. **125**:275, 1963.
13. Wilson, J. N., and Rowland, S. A.: Fracture-dislocation of the proximal interphalangeal joint of the finger, J. Bone Joint Surg. **48A**:493, 1966.

Chapter 10

Fractures in children

Part I

PAUL P. GRIFFIN, M.D.
Washington, D. C.

FRACTURES OF THE CLAVICLE

A fracture of the clavicle is one of the most common skeletal injuries in children. The fracture is usually sustained by a force directed medially along its longitudinal axis from either a direct fall on the shoulder or from a fall on the elbow with the shoulder abducted. In children under 7 to 8 years of age, most fractures of the clavicle are of the greenstick type. Complete fractures with displacement occur with greater frequency than do greenstick fractures in older children. In children below 8 to 9 years of age, all fractures can be treated by immobilization of the clavicle with a figure-of-eight bandage, as shown in Fig. 10-1. This bandage is made with sheet wadding covered by stockinette and will stretch after several days. It needs to be tightened every 3 or 4 days to keep the bandage snug enough to maintain abduction of the scapulae.

Greenstick fractures with angulation of 15° or less do not need to be reduced, but those with angulation in excess of 15° should be reduced by gentle, firm pressure applied to the apex of the angulation. A displaced fracture of the clavicle can usually be reduced adequately by adducting the scapula. As the scapula is adducted, the clavicle is lengthened and aligned. In children 9 years of age and younger, a bayonet position, as shown in Fig. 10-2 is adequate, but in older children this position may leave an obvious residual prominence at the fracture line. Most displaced fractures in older children can be reduced by manipulation under local anesthesia, and the reduction can be maintained by keeping the scapulae adducted with a figure-of-eight plaster bandage. When a plaster figure-of-eight bandage is used, one must be certain that the bandage is rolled beneath the axilla so that no sharp edges exist and that the bandage is molded adequately around the anterior portion of the shoulder to keep the shoulders back yet not compromise circulation.

Open reduction should never be needed to reduce and immobilize the fracture of the clavicle in a child. Nonunion and infection are complications that occur all too frequently with open reduction and never with closed treatment.

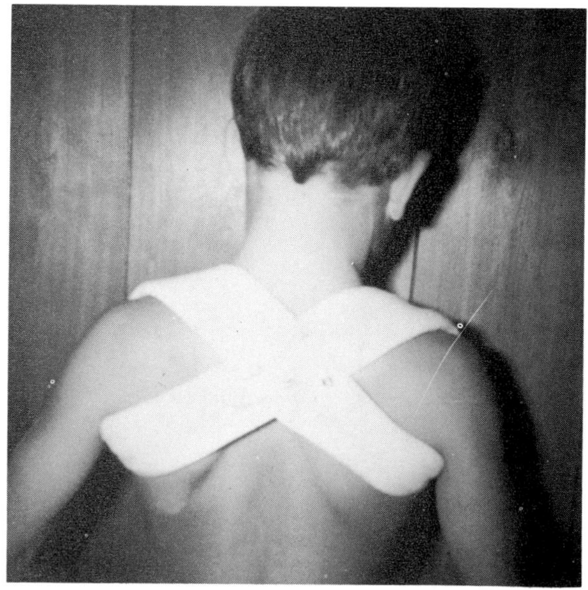

Fig. 10-1. Figure-of-eight bandage.

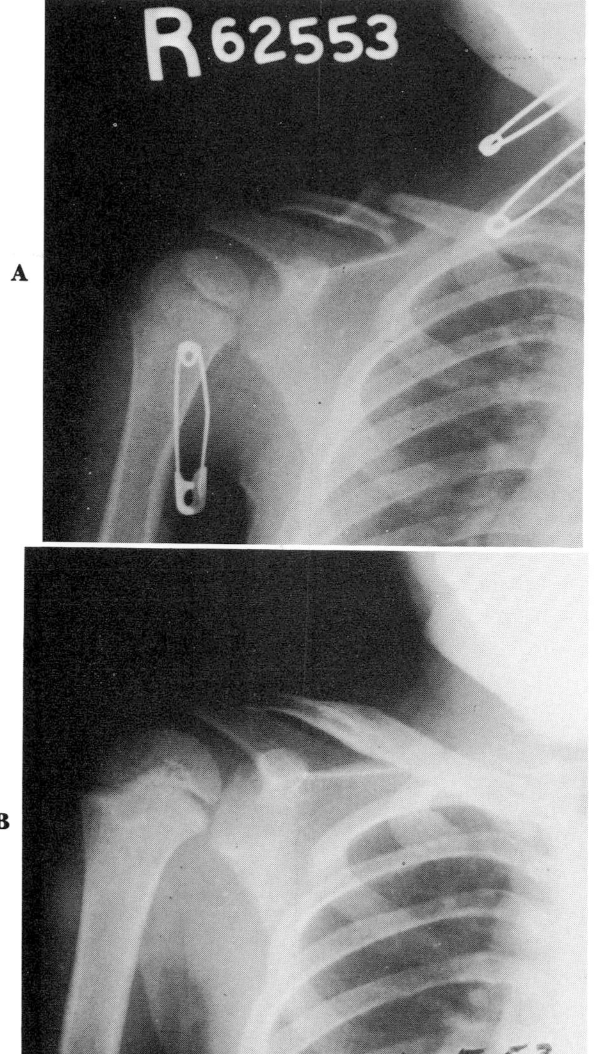

Fig. 10-2. A, Fracture of the clavicle with complete displacement in a 7-year-old child. The fragment position was accepted. **B,** The fracture healed without deformity and is seen here 4½ months after the injury.

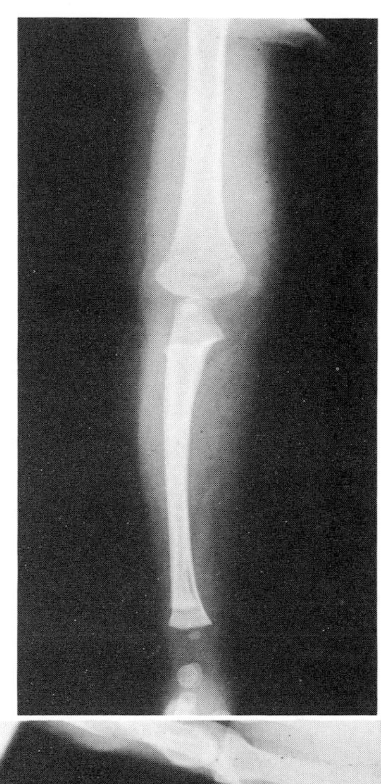

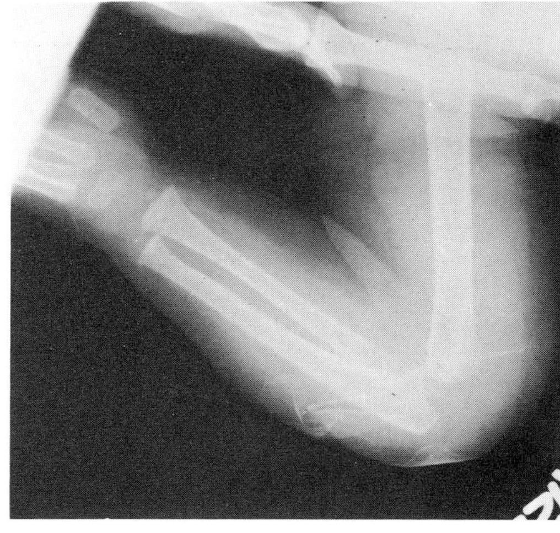

Fig. 10-3. Undisplaced supracondylar fracture of the humerus in an 18-month-old child.

SUPRACONDYLAR FRACTURES OF THE HUMERUS

Whereas the fracture of the clavicle is one of the most common fractures in children, the supracondylar fracture of the elbow is the most serious fracture occurring in children. Management of a supracondylar fracture can be difficult and the complications crippling. No fracture occurring in children deserves more careful attention to every detail than the supracondylar fracture. Even those fractures that are undisplaced and seem to be relatively minor may be followed by serious complications.

The usual supracondylar fracture of the elbow is one in which the distal fragment is either angulated or displaced posteriorly. This fracture is produced by falling on the hand with the elbow in extension. The less common supracondylar fracture in which the distal fragment is displaced anteriorly is sustained by direct fall on the elbow.

The treatment of the supracondylar fracture depends upon the severity of the displacement, the

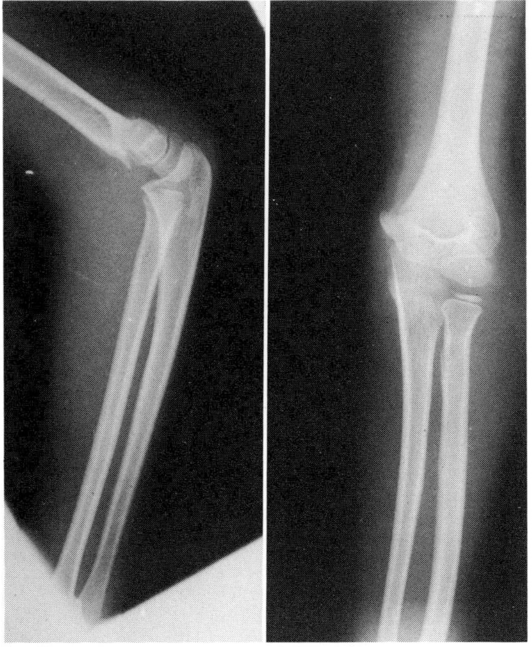

Fig. 10-4. Supracondylar fracture of the humerus with posterior angulation.

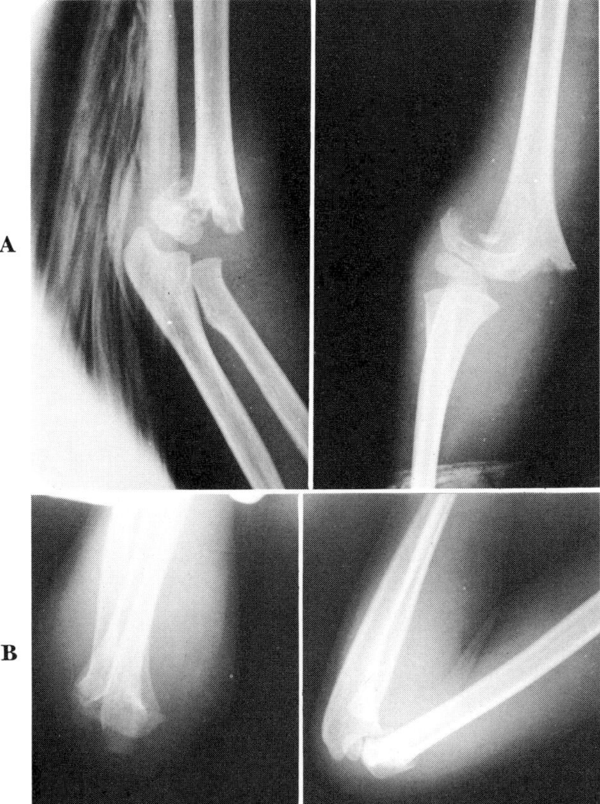

Fig. 10-5. A, Supracondylar fracture with posterolateral displacement of the distal fragment. **B,** After reduction.

length of time between fracture and treatment, and the presence or absence of vascular or nerve impairment.

A simple undisplaced supracondylar fracture, such as the one in Fig. 10-3, can be treated by immobilization of the elbow in flexion with a posterior plaster splint and a sling. The undisplaced supracondylar fracture must not be treated lightly, for with excessive swelling following the fracture vascular difficulties can occur. If the elbow is not immobilized beyond 90°, the undisplaced fracture can lose position and develop an angulation deformity. If swelling is so excessive that the elbow cannot be flexed to 90° without decreasing the radial pulse, the fracture should be treated in Dunlop's traction. In those patients in whom the elbow can be flexed to 90° but not above, this position of the elbow can be accepted, but the degree of flexion should be increased daily as the swelling subsides.

Supracondylar fractures that angulated posteriorly (Fig. 10-4) but are not displaced can be realigned by flexing the elbow and at the same time applying gentle pressure to the distal fragment. A fracture such as this should be in acute flexion for about 3 weeks, after which active flexion extension exercises should be started and the arm protected with a sling for another week. A completely displaced supracondylar fracture as in Fig. 10-5 must be reduced either by traction or manipulation. The technique of reducing a supracondylar fracture by manipulation varies between individuals, but the success of the reduction is directly related to the length of time between injury and treatment. If the patient with such a fracture is seen before excessive swelling has occurred, a satisfactory closed reduction can usually be obtained. The technique of reducing a supracondylar fracture that we use is to apply gentle traction on the forearm for several minutes with the elbow in extension. Traction will usually align the distal fragment from its previous medial or lateral displacement. If the lateral or medial displacement is not corrected by gentle traction, pressure on the distal fragment in the appropriate direction applied while the traction is maintained will usually complete the alignment in this plane. The posterior displacement is partially corrected by traction in extension and is completed by flexing the elbow while the traction is maintained on the forearm.

As the elbow is flexed, pressure with the thumb

is applied to the distal fragment to complete the reduction. The posterior periosteum and triceps act as a hinge, which helps reduce the posteriorly displaced distal fragment. It is important that the lateral or medial displacement be corrected before the elbow is flexed. After the elbow is flexed, medial or lateral displacement cannot be corrected because the posterior hinge of the periosteum and triceps locks the fragments, preventing the distal fragment from moving medially or laterally. The reduction is maintained by the acute flexed position of the elbow. The lower portion of Fig. 10-5 shows this fracture reduced. The internal or external rotation of the distal fragment must also be corrected by appropriate pronation and supination of the forearm while the elbow is in extension. Just

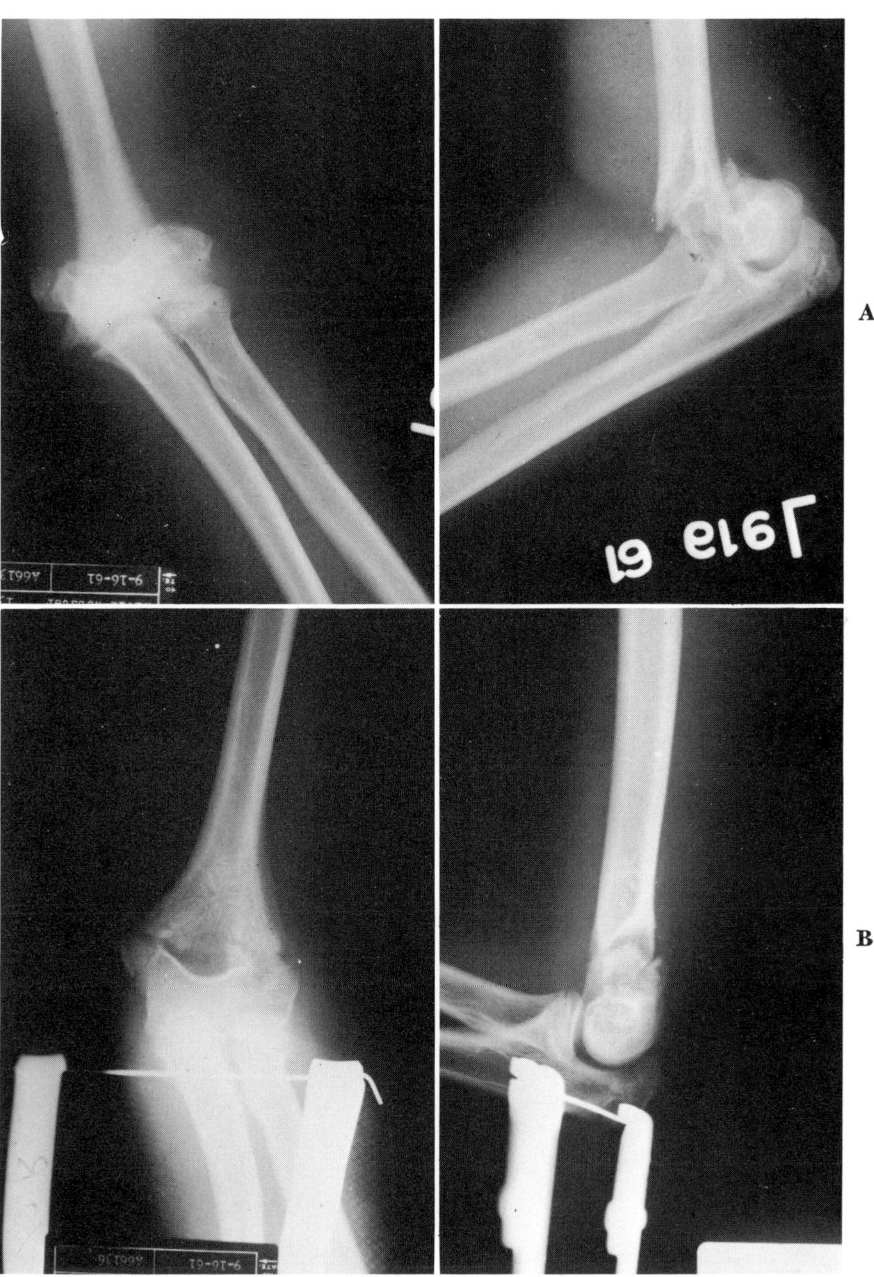

Fig. 10-6. A, Supracondylar fracture with posterior displacement. **B,** Supracondylar fracture after Kirschner wire was placed in olecranon and fracture was reduced by traction.

as the medial or lateral displacement cannot be corrected once the elbow is flexed, the rotation cannot be corrected with the elbow in the flexed position. It may be difficult to be certain by roentgenographic examination that rotation has been completely corrected. Clinically one can usually tell whether the fracture is reduced in all its elements by comparing the condyles and olecranon prominences of the fractured elbow with the prominences of the opposite elbow. When the rotation is not corrected, a triangle formed by the medial and lateral condyles and the olecranon will not be equal on the two sides.

The elbow should be immobilized by a posterior splint with the splint held in place by an Ace bandage and reinforced by tape going from the forearm up to the arm. No bandage should be placed in the antecubital fossa, and a circular plaster cast should not be used to immobilize supracondylar fractures of the elbow.

If there is significant vascular or neural impairment following the supracondylar fracture of the elbow or if there is swelling about the elbow that prevents adequate flexion without the radial pulse being obliterated, the fracture should be treated with traction. Fig. 10-6, *A* is a radiograph of a 12-year-old boy admitted 3 hours after injury. His radial pulse was absent, and he had severe pain in his hand with hypesthesia of his fingers. The fracture was reduced by traction, and as the traction was applied, the radial pulse returned. However, when the elbow was flexed beyond 90°, the pulse disappeared. For this reason the fracture was reduced, and reduction was maintained by skeletal traction with the Kirschner wire in the olecranon, as shown in Fig. 10-6, *B*. A Bradford frame is

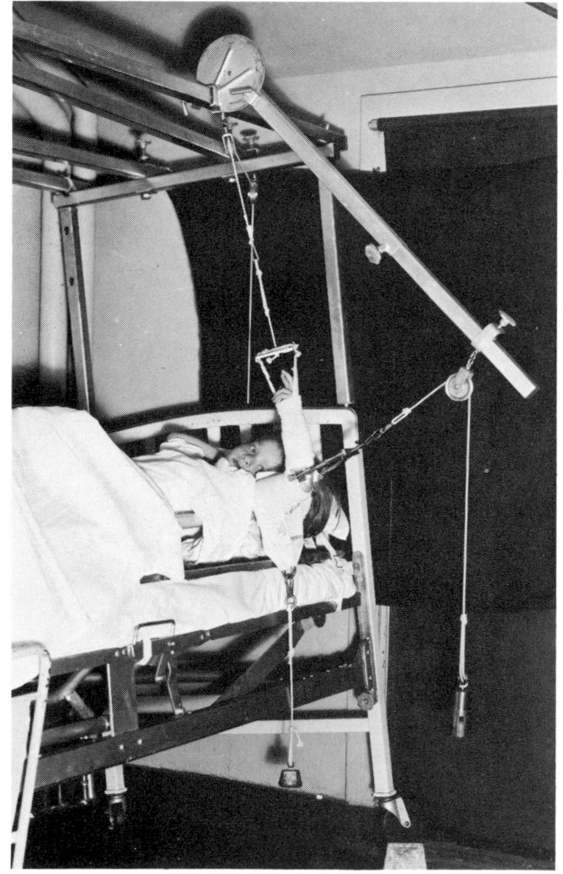

Fig. 10-7. Child in skeletal traction for treatment of a supracondylar fracture of the humerus. (Used on the Orthopedic service of Children's Hospital Medical Center in Boston, Mass.)

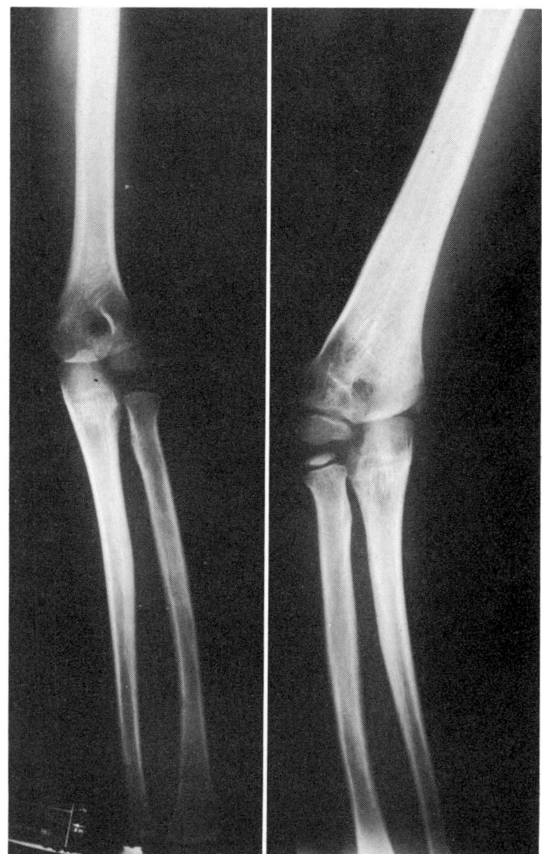

Fig. 10-8. Cubitus varus of right arm following supracondylar fracture.

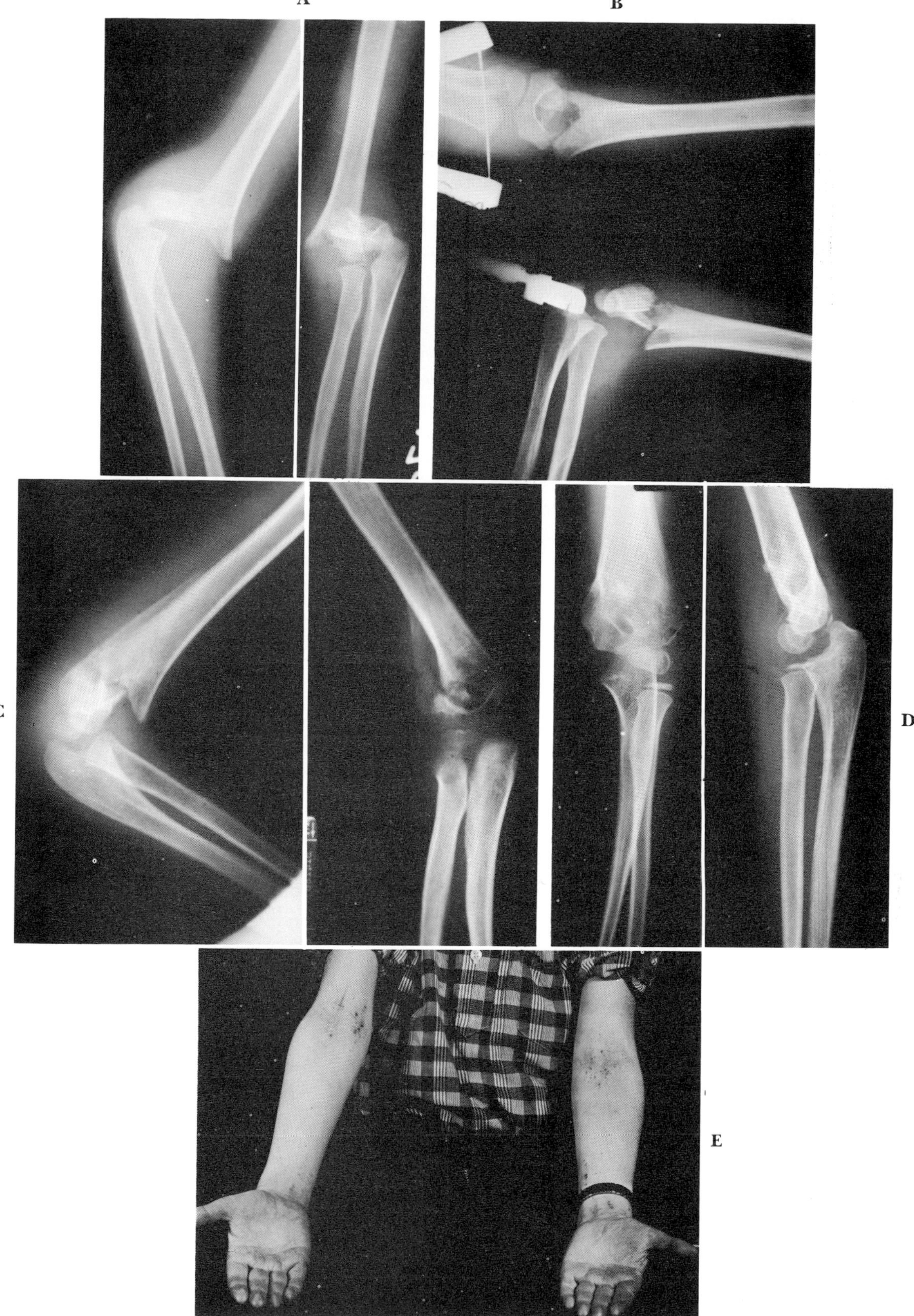

Fig. 10-9. A, Supracondylar fracture with posteromedial displacement. **B,** Supracondylar fracture in **A** after skeletal traction by means of a Kirschner wire in the olecranon. Rotation not corrected. **C,** Four months after the injury. **D,** Fourteen months after the injury. **E,** Carrying angle of both arms is about equal.

beneficial in controlling the body position in small children who are treated with traction (Fig. 10-7).

The most common complication following a supracondylar fracture is a varus deformity of the elbow. As a rule the varus is minimal, but frequently it is severe enough to produce a so-called Gunstock deformity as seen in Fig. 10-8 on the right. The patient whose radiograph is shown in Fig. 10-8 is a 7-year-old boy who had a closed reduction of a supracondylar fracture with immobilization of the elbow at a right angle, with a circular cast. The varus deformity is a result of angulation of the distal fragment in relation to the proximal fragment, but angulation does not occur easily except when rotation has not been corrected. If the distal fragment is rotated internally on the proximal fragment, muscle pull will easily angulate the distal fragment, producing a varus deformity. If traction is maintained in proper alignment with the proximal fragment, angulation does not occur to any significant degree even though rotation is not corrected. In Fig. 10-9, *A* and *B,* a fracture is shown that was treated by skeletal traction in which the rotation was not corrected. The radiograph in Fig. 10-9, *C* shows the persisting rotation deformity in the healing fracture. The anterior beak on the proximal fragment in the lateral projection is the radiographic sign of rotation of the distal fragment. As can be seen in Fig. 10-9, *D* and *E,* this child did not have a significant alteration of his carrying angle.

Although the varus deformity is the most common complication following supracondylar fractures, the most serious complication is Volkmann's ischemic contracture. The typical deformity in Volkmann's ischemic contracture is one in which the wrist is flexed and the fingers extended at the MP joint and flexed at the IP joints. Active extension of the wrist and interphalangeal joints is limited because of myostatic contracture and paresis of the flexors of the wrist and fingers and of the intrinsic muscles of the hand. This complication can usually be prevented by use of traction to reduce and immobilize the fracture and by early surgical intervention with decompression of the forearm if the ischemia persists in spite of traction. In general, a relative state of ischemia is usually obvious by the presence of poor capillary return, pain, pallor, and paralysis of the muscles of the hand. However, the development of a Volkmann's ischemic contracture may be so gradual that it is difficult to recognize until there is loss of sensation and paralysis of a severe degree. A good clinical sign of impending Volkmann's contracture is pain in the forearm on attempting to extend the fingers passively, and if there is a progressive loss of passive extension of the fingers, it should be indicative of increasing ischemia.

When vascular impairment is present on admission following a supracondylar fracture and does not immediately improve with traction on the forearm and reduction of the fracture, the antecubital fossa should be explored and the forearm decompressed by opening all fascial compartments of the forearm down through the transverse carpal ligament. The brachial artery may be caught on the proximal fragment. Almost always the brachial artery at the level of the fracture will be constricted with severe arterial spasm. Pulsations will be seen to come down to the level of the constriction and stop. The spasm of the artery may be treated by soaking the artery in an anesthetic agent, by sympathetic block, by mechanically expanding the constricted area with an intra-arterial injection of saline at the point of constriction with clamps above and below the constricted area. If more of these procedures improve the circulation of the forearm and fingers, resection of the constricted area will usually be followed by dilatation of the collateral circulation about the elbow and immediate improvement in circulation of the hand.

If a Volkmann's ischemic contracture is seen several weeks following the initial injury, improvement, and in many patients complete recovery, of function can be obtained by resecting the fascia about the muscles in the anterior compartment of the forearm.

FRACTURES OF DISTAL THIRD OF RADIUS AND ULNA

The distal third of the forearm is usually fractured by a fall on the hand with the wrist in extension. With this type of injury the distal fragment is either angulated with the apex of the angulation anteriorly, or the distal fragment is displaced posteriorly frequently with either lateral or medial displacement, as seen in Fig. 10-10, *A.* As in all fractures, the reduction of a distal forearm fracture is easier if the reduction is attempted immediately after injury. Several days delay in the reduction, increases the difficulty with which an anatomic reduction is obtained, and, in fact, the end-on-end

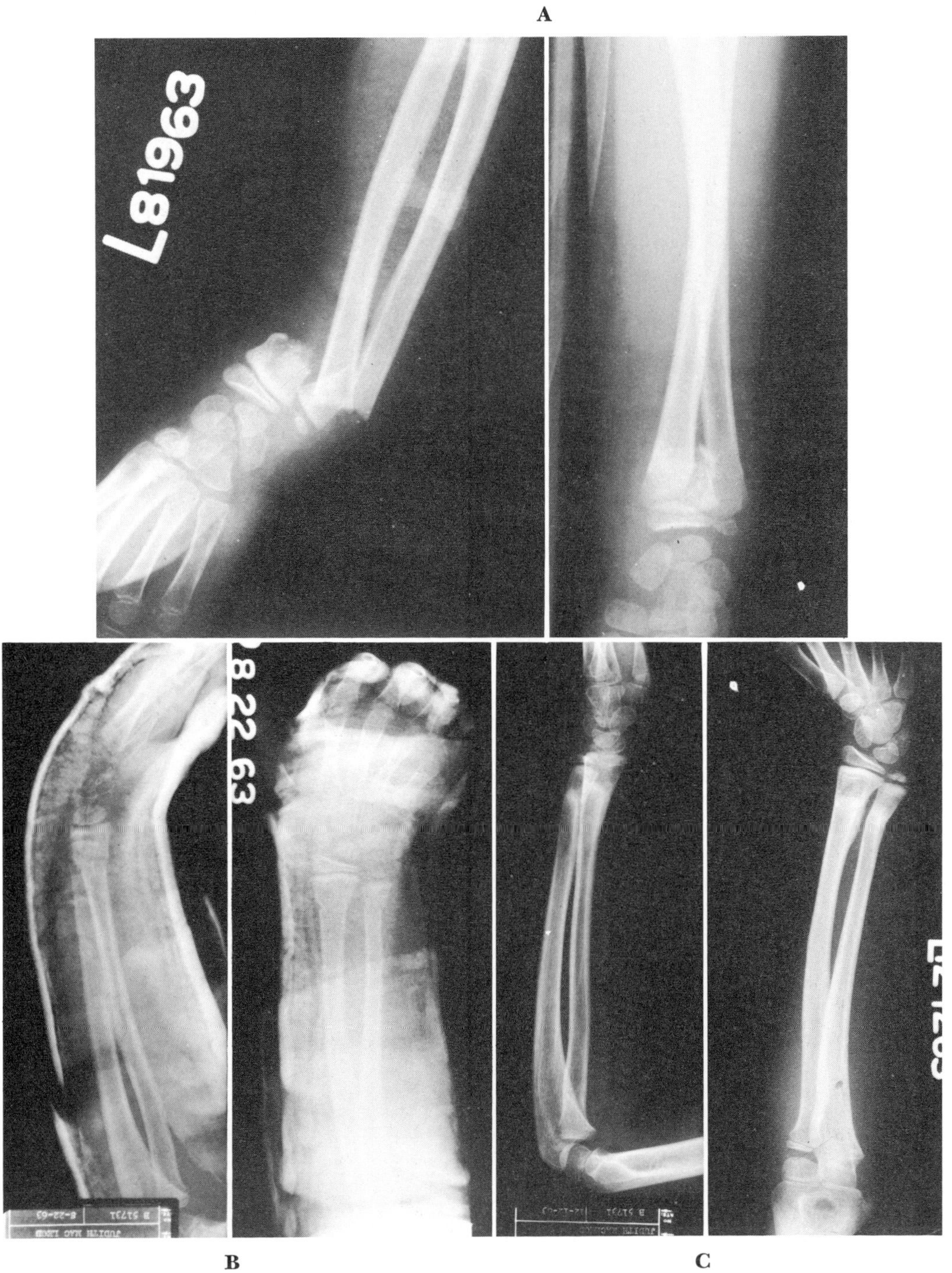

Fig. 10-10. A, Distal radius and ulna fracture in an 8-year-old girl with posterior displacement of the distal fragment. **B,** Three days after reduction with good position. **C,** Four months after reduction the fracture is well healed.

reduction may be impossible after several days. Good anesthesia with relaxation of the muscles is an important factor in obtaining the reduction.

The technique of reduction should include traction applied slowly for several minutes on the hand with countertraction above the elbow. As the muscles relax the length of the radius and ulna is restored. While the traction is maintained, direct pressure is applied on the distal fragment, forcing it forward in apposition with the proximal fragment. If the distal fragment does not go into its proper position easily, the degree of pronation or supination should be changed while traction and direct pressure on the distal fragment are continued. With the proper degree of supination and pronation, the fracture will usually reduce. Al-

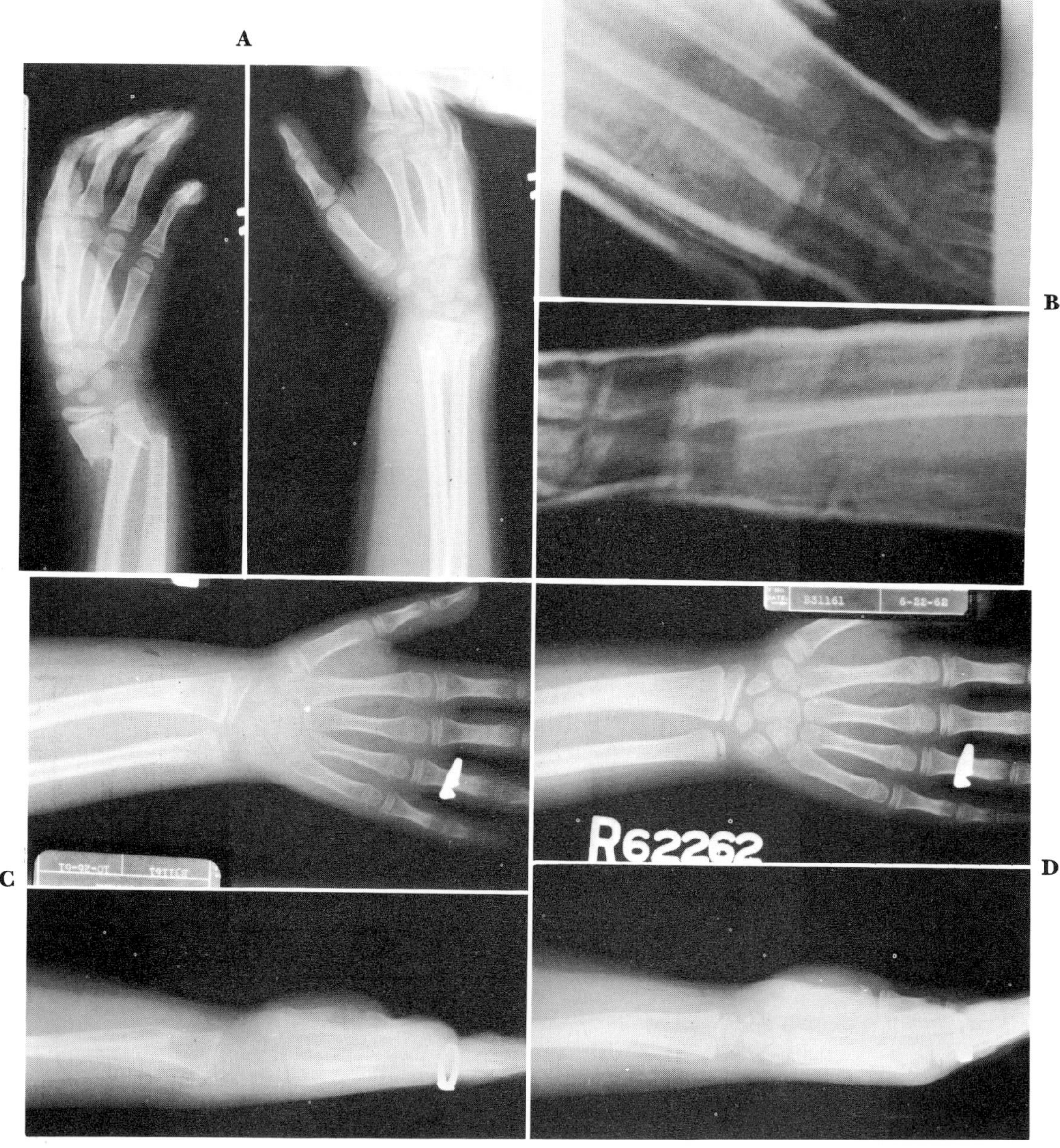

Fig. 10-11. A, Fracture of the distal radius and ulna in an 8-year-old girl. **B,** The bayonet position was accepted. Alignment is excellent. **C,** Two and one-half months after injury the fracture is remodeling very well. **D,** Ten months later no deformity of significance is present.

though pronation is a classical position used in reducing fractures of the distal third of the forearm, it is not always necessary and in certain instances the fracture is more easily reduced if the distal fragment is supinated. Such a fracture is shown in Fig. 10-10, *B*.

An anatomic reduction of a two-bone forearm fracture of the distal third in a child is not necessary. With the fragments left in side-by-side position, an excellent result can be expected, providing the alignment is good. The fracture in Fig. 10-11, *A* could not be reduced by manipulation. A bayonet position was accepted, as in Fig. 10-11, *B*. The remodeling is very rapid, as shown in Fig. 10-11, *C*. When a bayonet position is accepted, excessive overriding may occur. If the overriding becomes a problem, traction applied to the metacarpal with a Kirschner wire will correct and prevent overriding. Open reduction should not be necessary.

FRACTURES OF MID SHAFT OF FEMUR

Fractures of the mid shaft of the femur are the most frequent fractures that occur in the lower extremities in children less than 5 or 6 years of age. The frequency of fractures of the femur becomes much less after the age of 9 to 10 years. With the fracture reduced in the bayonet position, healing is rapid and is thought by many to be the position of choice. The callus produced in the healing of the fracture comes from both the periosteum and the endosteum, with the osteocytes at the ends contributing nothing to healing. Side-by-side apposition gives more periosteal elevation, and a more massive callus is produced. The massive callus gives greater surface contact between the callus and the fractured fragments. In our experience the bayonet position did not shorten the period of immobilization. The average period of immobilization is not significantly different between those fractures that were allowed to override and those that were reduced end to end.

Fractures of the femoral shaft usually stimulate the rate of growth of the femur. In a series of seventy-three fractures followed for a period of 1 year following the fracture, 81% of children over 2 years of age showed 3 mm. or more of stimulation of growth (Fig. 10-12). The median effect of this group of patients was 8 mm. of stimulation. The maximum stimulation occurs within the first year following the fracture but can continue for several years. Stimulation of growth in the femur was less in children under 2 years of age and in those over 10 years of age. Inhibition of growth following fracture in the teen-ager and in the child less than 2 may occur without radiographic evidence of epiphyseal damage.

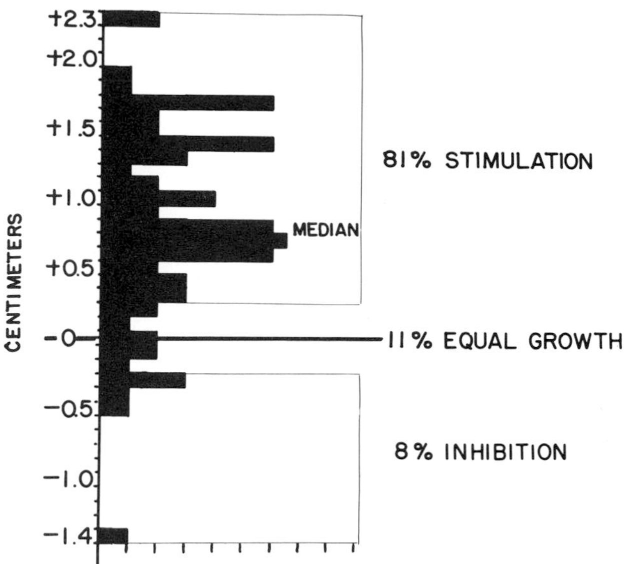

Fig. 10-12. The effect of a fracture of the femur on femoral growth, seventy-three children, 2 to 12 years after fracture.

The degree of displacement of the fractured fragment is another factor that influences the degree of stimulation of growth following a fractured femur. Repeated manipulation of a fracture probably increases the degree of stimulation following a fracture. In children between 2 and 8 years of age, the statistical chance of having equal leg lengths is probably greater if the fragments are allowed to override 1 cm., providing there is no angulation. Angulation of the fractured fragments effectively shortens the length of the bone and must be considered in the over-all measurement of the factor in the degree of overriding that one accepts. In children less than 2 years of age and in those over 10, overriding of the fragments should be minimal if at all.

Part II

CHARLES M. HAMILTON, M.D.
Nashville, Tennessee

TRANSVERSE FRACTURE OF HUMERUS

Transverse fractures of the humerus result from a direct blow or a fall. A spiral fracture of the humerus, like all spiral fractures, occurs as a result of a torsion injury. One of the more frequent ways of producing this fracture is by throwing a heavy object such as a rock or a baseball. Both these fractures can be treated with consistently good results using a light hanging cast or a posterior splint (Fig. 10-13). If an infant should receive such a fracture, then lateral traction would probably be the treatment of choice. With the infant lying on his back, the forearm would be suspended perpendicularly, and horizontal traction would be applied to the upper arm. This would prevent malrotation until the fracture stuck sufficiently to use a Velpeau or sling and swathe bandage.

Case 1. This 11-year-old boy sustained a spiral fracture of the shaft of his humerus when he threw a rock (Fig. 10-14, *A*). It is interesting that he had a unicameral bone cyst of the proximal humerus, but he did not fracture through the cyst as one might have expected. Although no direct trauma

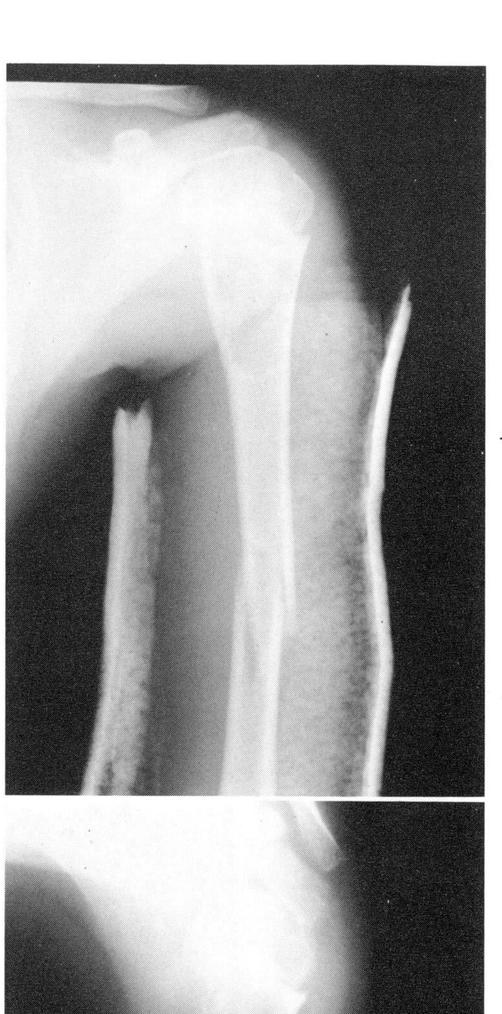

Fig. 10-14. A, Spiral fracture of the humerus. **B,** Five months postfracture.

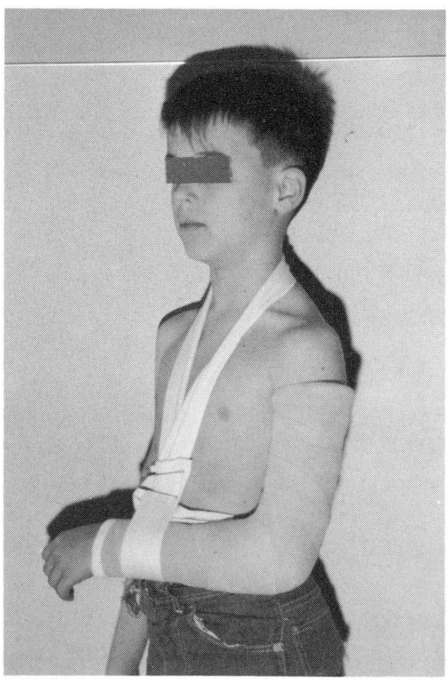

Fig. 10-13. A light hanging cast.

was involved, he also had a radial nerve palsy that gradually subsided over the ensuing 3 or 4 months. Fig. 10-14, *B* shows the last radiograph, 5 months postinjury, with the fracture solidly united.

DISLOCATION OF ELBOW

Dislocation of the elbow is a common injury in children.[1] It constitutes 6% of the elbow injuries in children who seek medical treatment. Fractures are associated with more than half of the dislocations. When seen within the first few hours following injury, closed reduction is usually very easy and can be accomplished with narcotic sedation alone, without requiring anesthesia. If treatment is delayed a week or two, open reduction may be necessary. If several months have elapsed, it is better to leave them dislocated rather than run the risk of serious impairment of motion that would probably follow any operative reduction and fixation at that time. Occasionally, one will see a dislocation of the radial head that has been untreated and unrecognized and that does not interfere with normal use of the elbow. A fresh dislocation should be immobilized in a plaster splint for 3 weeks.

Case 2. This is a posterior dislocation, without fracture, which was easily reduced and which regained full motion (Fig. 10-15).

Case 3. This is a more usual situation in which the medial epicondyle is fractured (Fig. 10-16, *A*). Fig. 10-16, *B* shows the postreduction film. The medial epicondyle has slipped back in good position. She regained normal use of her arm.

Case 4. This is a doctor's son who dislocated his left elbow in a football game when he was 17 years of age (Fig. 10-17, *A*). His father reduced the elbow

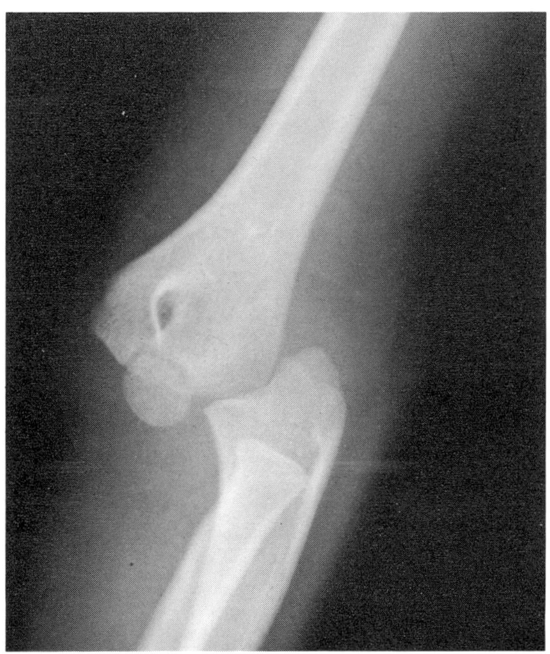

Fig. 10-15. Posterior dislocation of elbow without fracture.

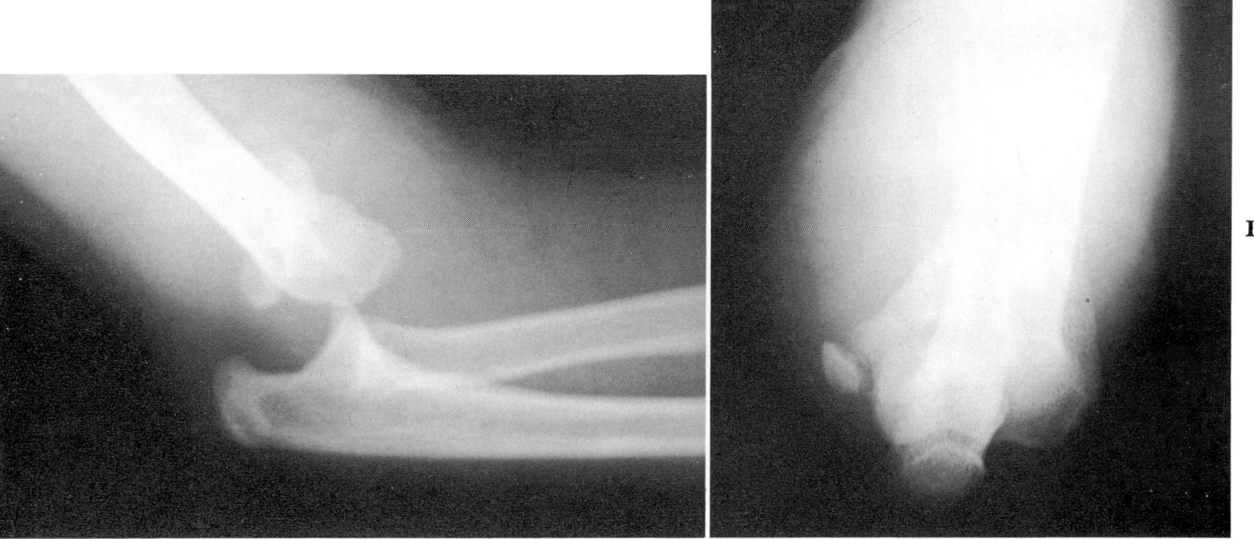

Fig. 10-16. A, Posterior dislocation of elbow with fracture of medial epicondyle. **B,** Postreduction.

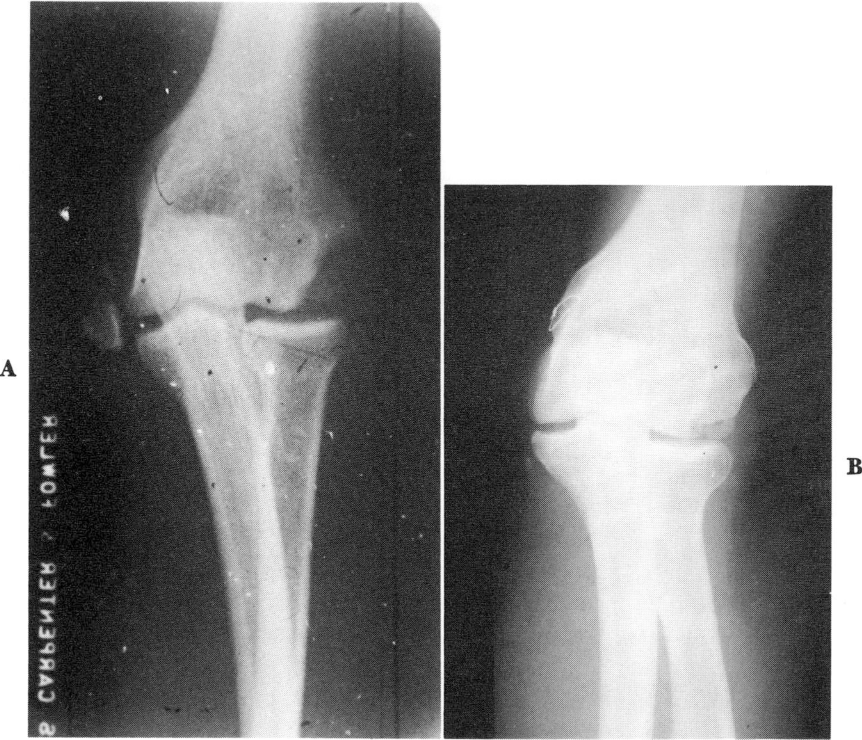

Fig. 10-17. A, Recurrent dislocating elbow showing deterioration of capitellum. **B,** Thirteen-year follow-up after capsulorrhaphy.

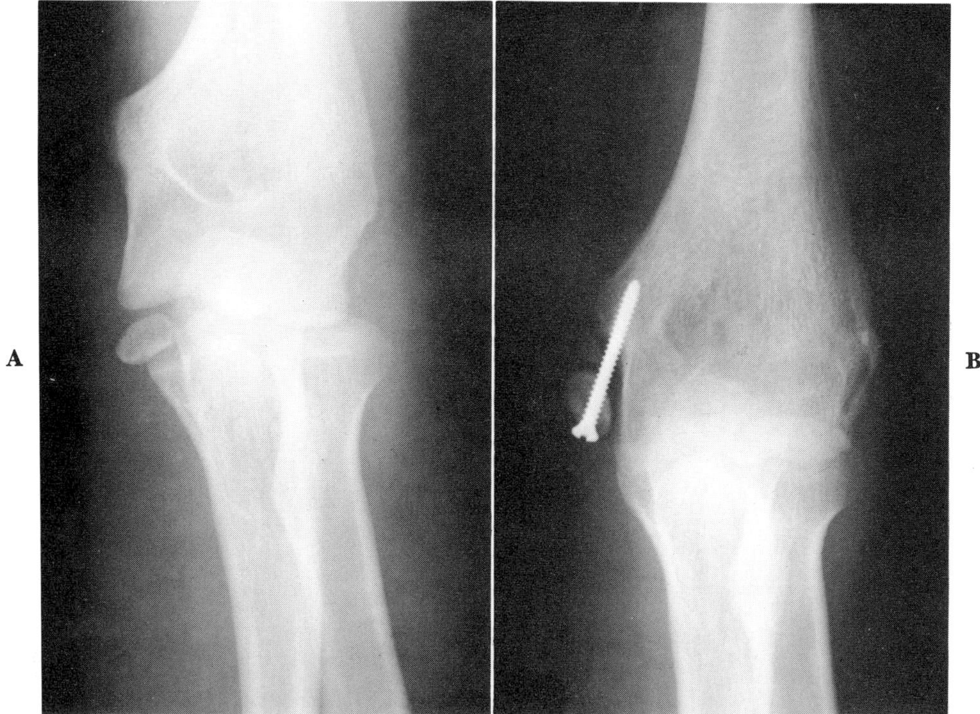

Fig. 10-18. A, Elbow subluxation with entrapment of medial epicondyle. **B,** Inadequate reduction and fixation of epicondyle resulted in loss of extension.

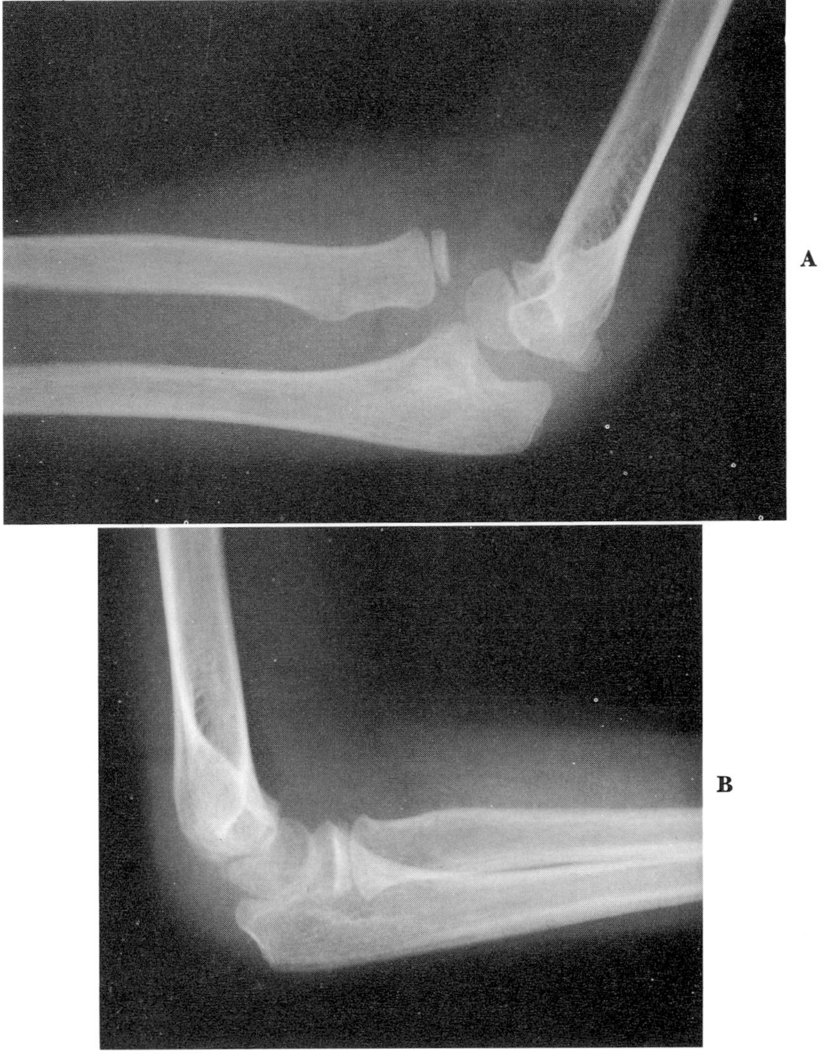

Fig. 10-19. A, Anterior dislocation of radial head. **B,** Six-month follow-up.

on the playing field but did not use any immobilization. He had recurrent dislocations, and 1 year later capsulorrhaphy with excision of the ununited fracture of the medial epicondyle was performed. Notice the deterioration of the capitellum. He obtained an excellent result from surgery. Fig. 10-17, *B* is a 13-year follow-up radiograph.

Case 5. This 16-year-old boy had a subluxation of his elbow with the medial epicondyle caught in the joint (Fig. 10-18, *A*). These undoubtedly represent dislocations that spontaneously reduced trapping the epicondyle fragment in the joint. Open reduction and fixation with a screw was done. Unfortunately, the epicondyle was not replaced accurately (Fig. 10-18, *B*) and resulted in limited extension of his elbow. He regained full motion after the epicondyle was excised.

Case 6. Rarely is it necessary to do a primary open reduction in an elbow dislocation, but here is an anterior dislocation of the radial head where this became necessary (Fig. 10-19, *A*). After two attempts at closed reduction had proved unsuccessful, the joint was entered and the radial head found to be lying over the orbicular ligament, which prevented its reduction. Follow-up radiographs taken 6 months later show her to have a normal elbow (Fig. 10-19, *B*).

FRACTURE OF NECK OF RADIUS

In fractures of the neck of the radius there is a divergence of opinions as to the degree of displacement acceptable without resorting to open reduction. Watson-Jones[7] believed that accurate restora-

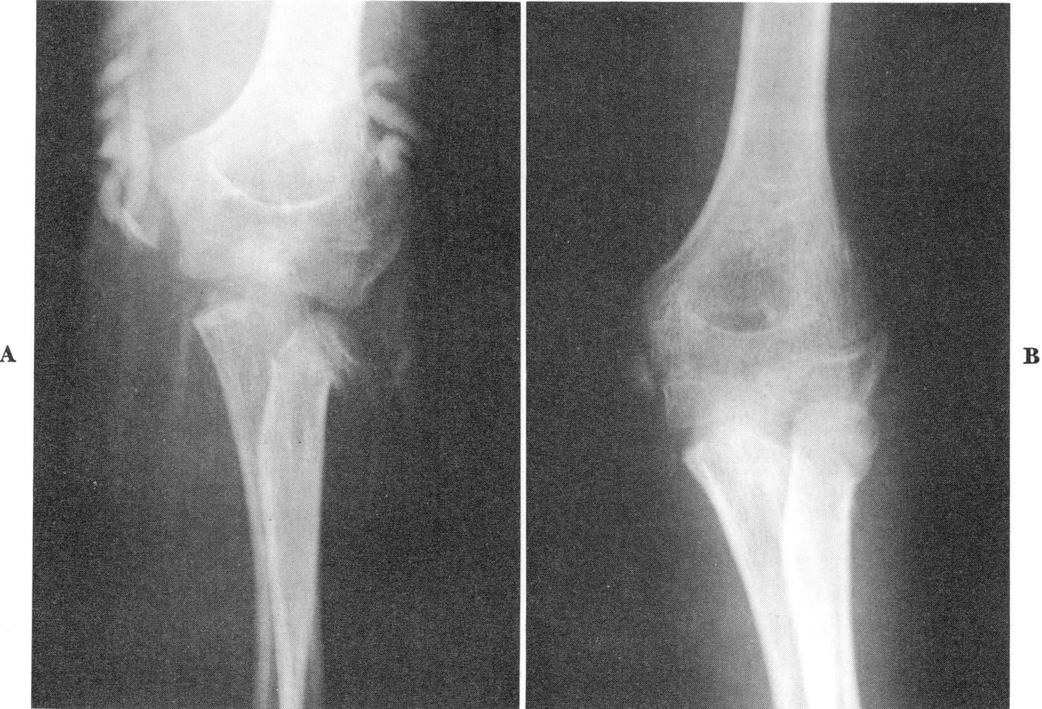

Fig. 10-20. A, Fracture of neck of radius with 50° to 60° tilting of head. **B,** Closed reduction.

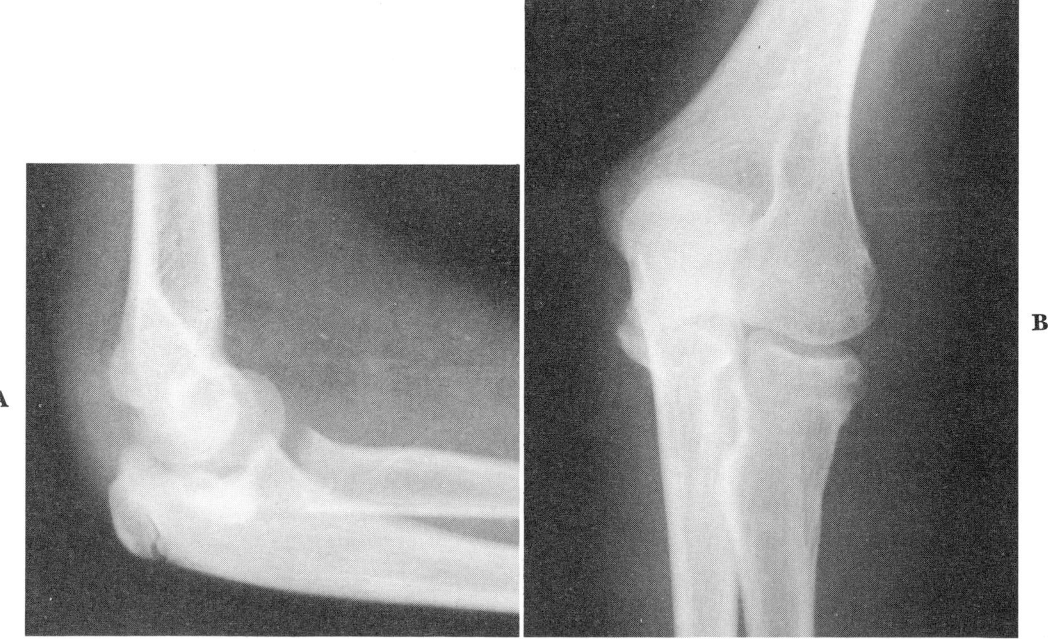

Fig. 10-21. A, Fracture of neck of radius with posterior dislocation of head. **B,** Sixteen-month follow-up.

tion of the joint surfaces between the capitellum and the head of the radius is necessary, and he would perform an open reduction on all such fractures that he was unable to reduce anatomically. However, Blount[1] and other writers on this subject[5] believed that an angle from 30° to 45° is acceptable and is compatible with good results. It is generally believed that displacement of more than 30° to 45° requires open reduction.

Case 7. Here is a fracture with 50° to 60° of angulation. We were fortunate in accomplishing almost anatomic reduction (Fig. 10-20).

Case 8. Here is a fracture of the neck of the radius with dislocation of the radial head posteriorly (Fig. 10-21, *A*). It required open reduction but was found to be very unstable, requiring insertion of a Kirschner wire. Ordinarily it is not necessary to use internal fixation as was done here. The Kirschner wire was removed at the end of 3 weeks,

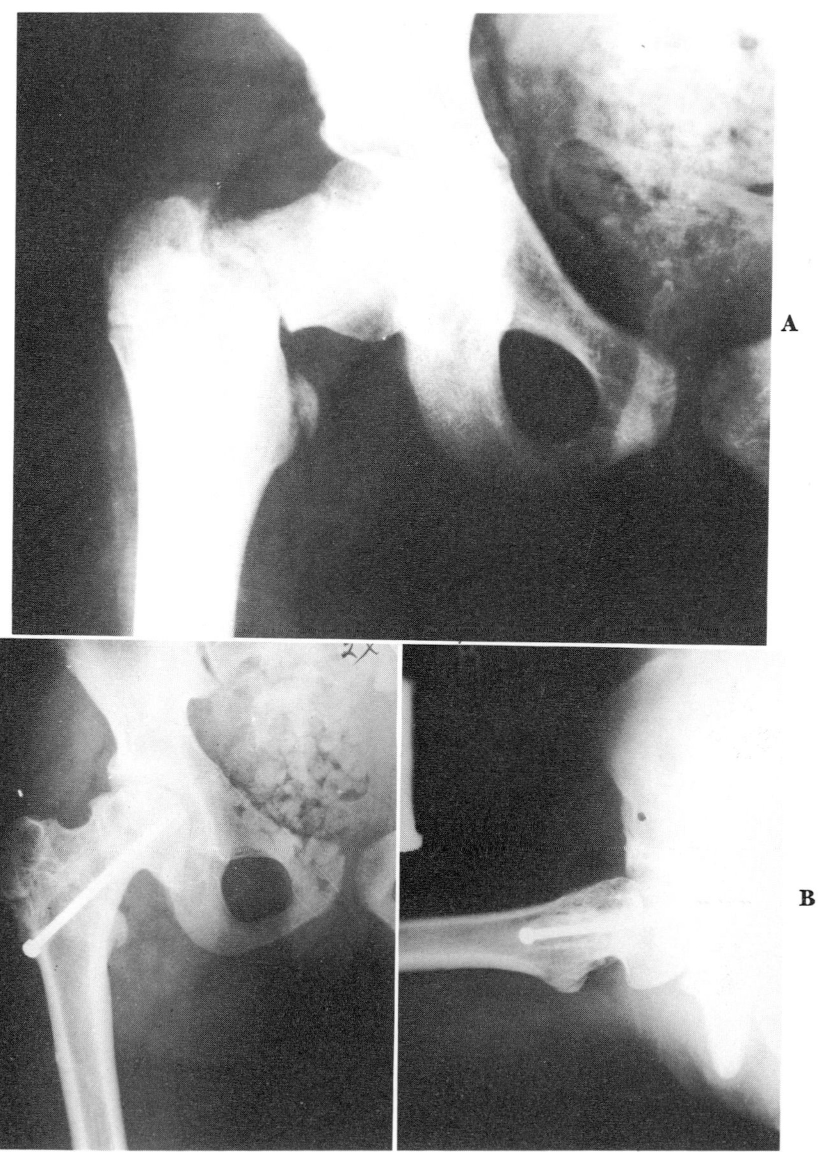

Fig. 10-22. A, Fracture of neck of femur near base of neck. **B,** Four-year follow-up after insertion of tibial graft and Knowles pins.

and the cast was removed at the end of 6 weeks. Here is the follow-up radiograph 16 months post-fracture (Fig. 10-21, *B*). She is now 13 years of age, and all the epiphyses at the elbow have closed. She has full flexion and full extension. Pronation is restricted to 40° and supination to 60°. There is no valgus or varus deformity. Incidentally, if there is any limitation of motion following fractures of the neck of the radius, it is usually rotation rather than flexion and extension that is restricted. She had a temporary radial nerve palsy, which recovered completely. One must never remove the radial head in a growing child. It results in gross deformity with radial deviation of the hand, shortening of the forearm, increase in the carrying angle, and weakness.

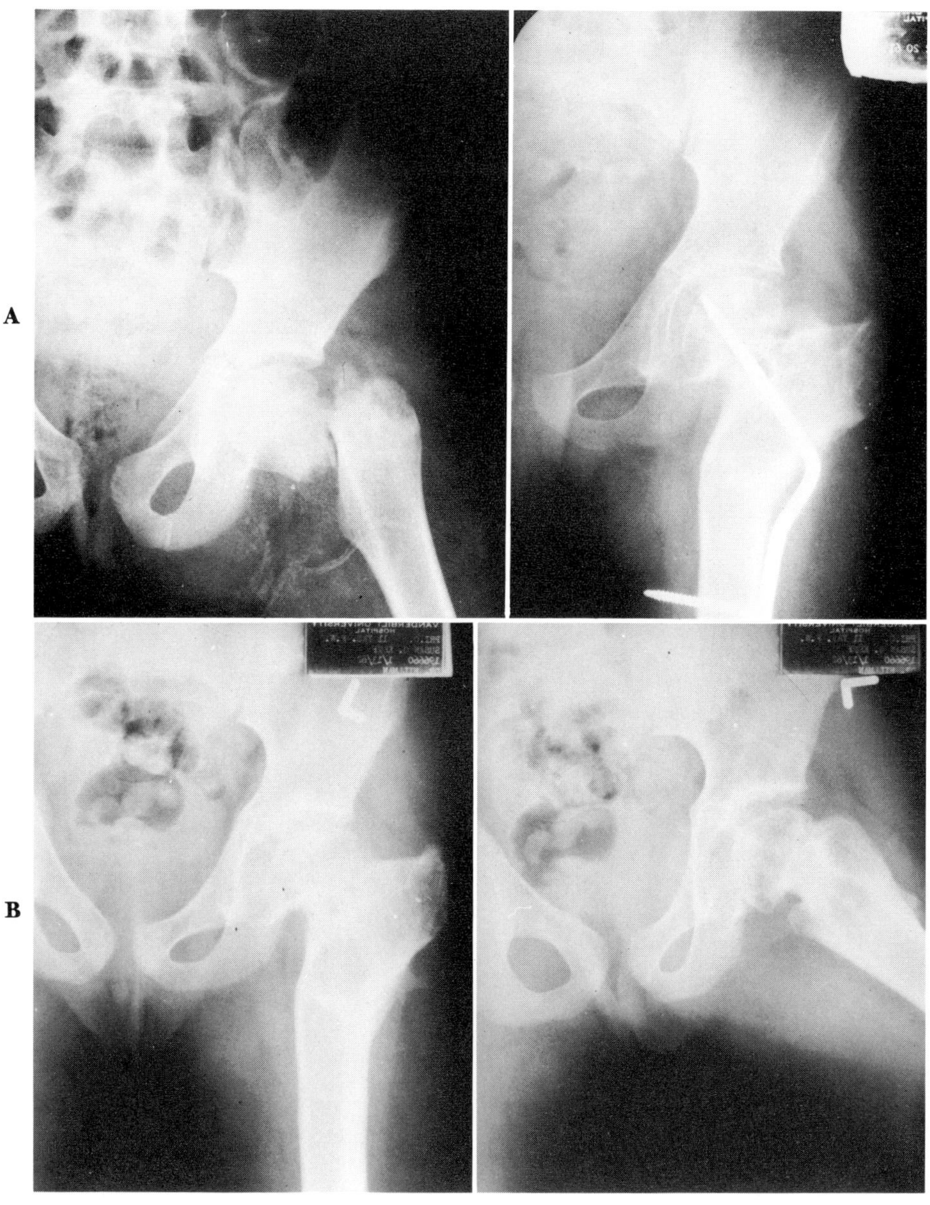

Fig. 10-23. A, Badly displaced fracture of femoral neck requiring osteotomy and bone grafting done 14 months after fracture. **B,** Fourteen months postosteotomy shows solid union but premature closure of epiphysis.

FRACTURE OF NECK OF FEMUR

Fractures of the neck of the femur in children are relatively infrequent injuries. However, careful treatment of this injury is important, for absolute immobilization of the fragments is imperative for union. It is nearly always a result of severe trauma. As you will see, the results are notoriously poor and fraught with many complications.

Ingram and Bachynski[2] reported fifteen cervical fractures with only eight good or fair cases and seven poor cases. McDougall[3] published twenty-one cervical fractures, of which seven were good, four were fair, and ten were poor. Ratliff[4] came up with an amazing series of seventy-one cases that he divided into undisplaced and displaced fractures. The undisplaced ones were fair or good with reasonable consistency and could be treated by

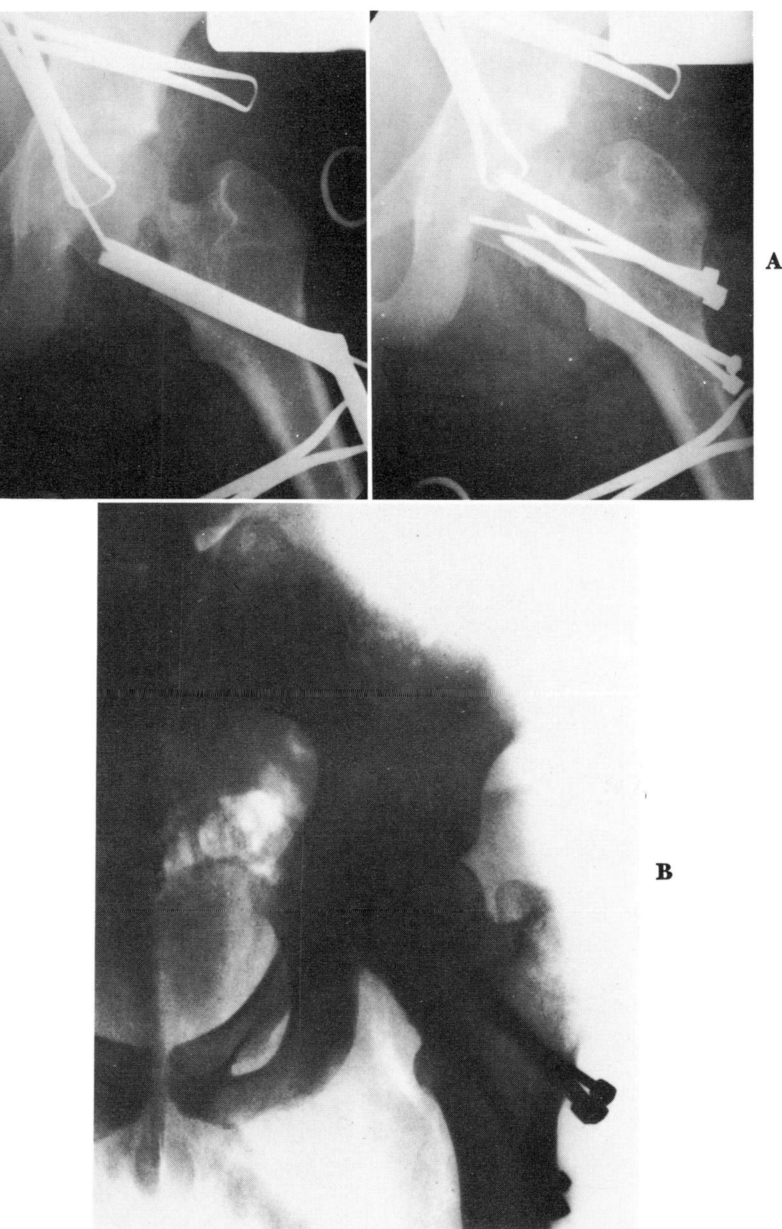

Fig. 10-24. A, A near catastrophe salvaged with Knowles pins. **B,** One-year follow-up.

simple plaster immobilization. Of his fifty displaced fractures, only twenty-two were good, fourteen were fair, and fourteen were poor. Combining these three series, there were 107 fractures with avascular necrosis in 45%, coxa vara in 24%, and nonunion in 12%, with many cases having more than one of these complications.

In order to understand the cause of this group of catastrophes, it is necessary to know the circulatory features of the head and neck of the femur in a growing child.[6] In the newborn infant the head has not yet ossified. There are vessels from the lateral epiphyseal group and from the metaphysis that cross, more or less at right angles to each other in a network through the cartilage of the head. The foveolar artery supplies a small area about the round ligament insertion. From 4 months to 3 years of age the ossification center appears in the head. The foveolar artery becomes less significant, as do the metaphyseal arteries. The lateral epiphyseal vessels increase in number and take over the principal role of the blood supply to the ossification center.

From 4 to 7 years of age, the epiphyseal plate becomes an effective barrier to vessels crossing from the metaphysis, and the foveolar artery has not yet developed to a significant degree. There is only one source of blood supply to the head during this period, which makes the risk of avascular necrosis extremely high in this age group. From

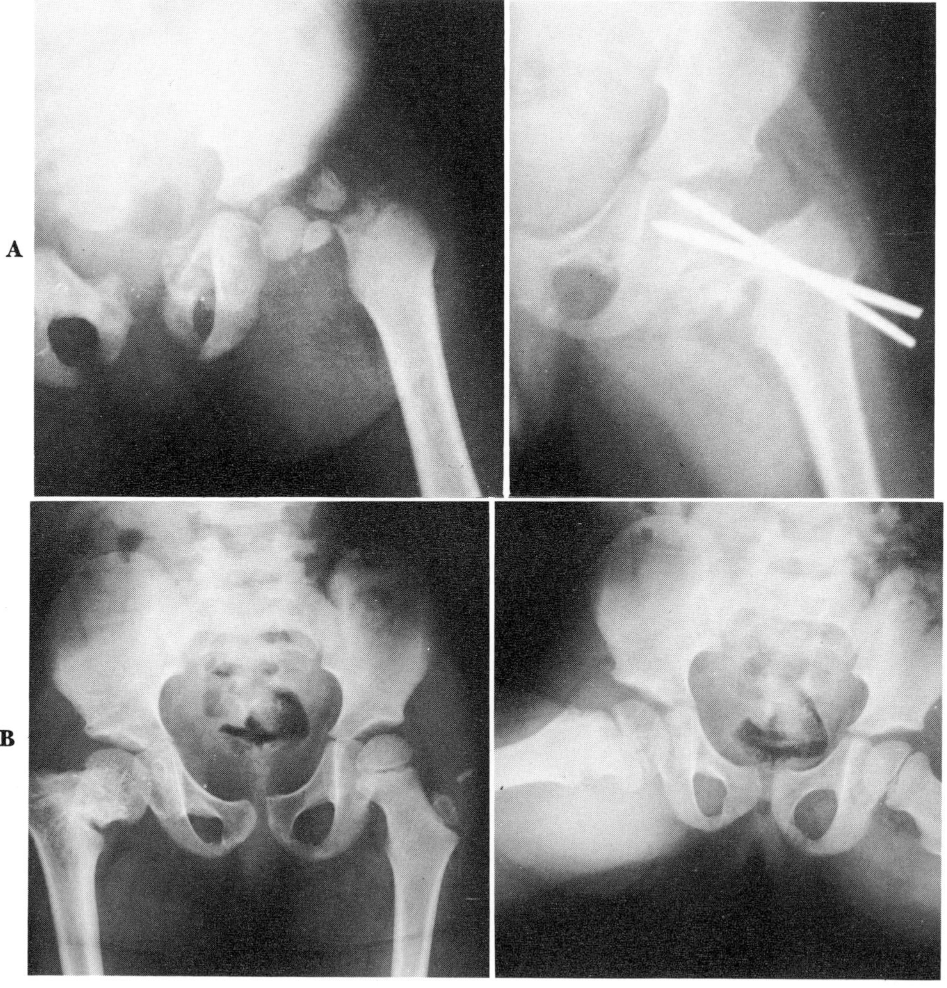

Fig. 10-25. A, Three-year-old girl with 1 month history of limp. **B,** Twenty-month follow-up.

7 to 14 years of age the foveolar artery finally reaches the ossification center and anastomoses with the lateral epiphyseal vessels. The metaphyseal vessels are still blocked by the epiphyseal plate. When the epiphyseal plate disappears in adolescence, the metaphyseal vessels once again combine with the other two sources of blood supply, and the free anastomosis that exists from now on through adulthood establishes itself. Impairment of blood supply results in delayed union, which enhances the possibility of coxa vara and nonunion.

Case 9. This 9-year-old girl was struck by a car while riding a bicycle (Fig. 10-22, *A*). A satisfactory reduction was accomplished by manipulation, and she was held in a plaster spica for 2 months. However, the fracture slipped, and she began to show early signs of avascular necrosis in the femoral head. A tibial bone graft and a Knowles pin were inserted. The follow up radiograph, 4 years later (Fig. 10-22, *B*) showed her to have degenerative changes in the joint with a cyst in the superior portion of the femoral head. She had 1 cm. shortening in this leg. In spite of these changes, she had no pain and had excellent motion.

Case 10. A 9-year-old girl sustained this badly displaced fracture of the femoral neck when she was struck by a car in Key West, Florida (Fig. 10-23, *A*). She was placed in a skintight plaster spica and transported to Nashville, Tennessee 5 days later. She had so much skin damage from the skintight plaster spica that surgery had to be postponed for 13 days. Open reduction and internal fixation with two Steinmann pins was done. Four months later the pins loosened and protruded through the skin, producing a pin tract infection. Fourteen months after injury, a second open reduction with subtrochanteric osteotomy and internal fixation with bone grafting was done (Fig. 10-23, *B*). This radiograph made 14 months postosteotomy shows solid union but premature closure of the epiphysis. She has a good range of motion and a good gait, but she has one-half inch shortening on this side.

Case 11. A 16-year-old boy fell when a park swing broke, sustaining a displaced fracture of his left femoral neck (Fig. 10-24, *A*). This shows clearly the disadvantage in using a triflanged nail. If one finds that the nature of the fracture requires the use of the Jewett nail, it can be accomplished by drilling into the head of the femur a preliminary hole that is almost as large as the flanges of the

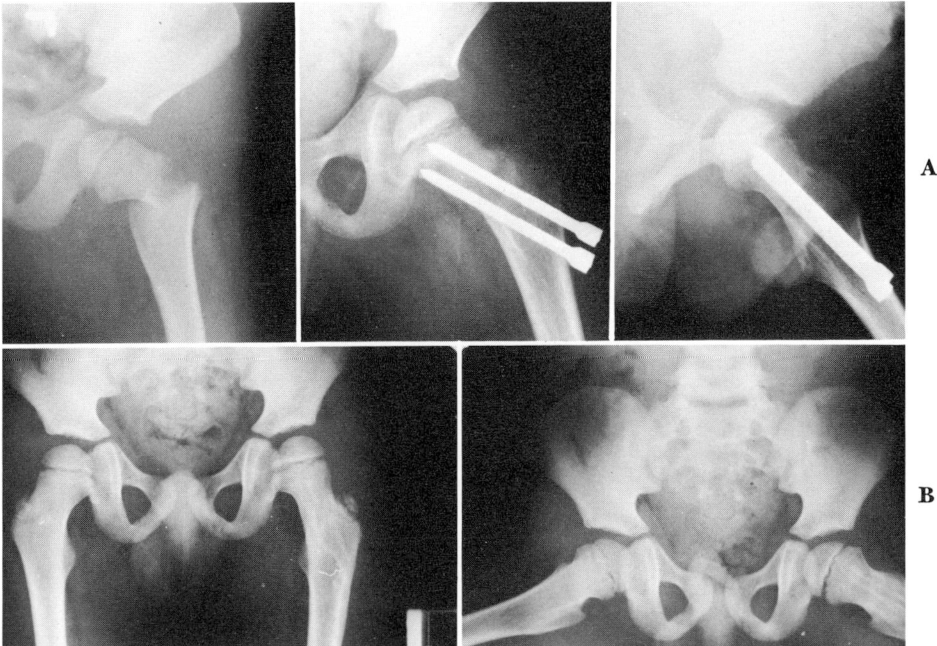

Fig. 10-26. A, A 4-year-old boy fixed with small Knowles pins. **B,** Twelve-month follow-up shows elongation of femoral neck.

nail. This boy is shown 1 year later in Fig. 10-24, *B* when he was serving in the Air Force and having no trouble with his hip.

Case 12. A 3-year-old girl was brought to our local Crippled Children's Service with this fracture of the left femoral neck and pelvis (Fig. 10-25, *A*). The parents had noticed a limp for 1 month but denied any injury to their knowledge. We suspect that this is another example of the battered child syndrome. Eleven months following injury, open reduction and internal fixation with two threaded Kirschner wires was done (Fig. 10-25, *B*). This follow-up film, made 20 months following open reduction, shows a persistent coxa vara with slight enlargement of the femoral head. There is some doubt, even yet, as to the state of healing.

Case 13. This 4-year-old boy fractured his left femoral neck and right clavicle when he was struck by a car. Fig. 10-26, *A* shows the method of treatment recommended, namely, closed or open reduction with internal fixation using Knowles pins. We prefer to use three pins but could get only two into this small femoral neck. Follow up radiographs (Fig. 10-26, *B*) at 12 months show a normal hip joint except for increased lengthening of the femoral neck.

COMPOUND FRACTURES

In the automobile age, compound fractures in children's bones occur not infrequently. When the child is brought to the Emergency Room the first thing the physician must do is to control shock and look for signs of other injuries such as fractured ribs or ruptured viscera. One must be careful not to be overly concerned with the fracture at the expense of overlooking other more vital injuries. Once the doctor is certain that the patient's general condition is satisfactory, he can assess the damage to the wound locally by inspection and determine whether there is any circulatory embarrassment or nerve damage. The wound is then covered with a temporary sterile dressing while a splint is applied to the extremity before making radiographs. Prophylactic antibiotics and tetanus immunization booster is then given. When these steps are completed, the child should be taken promptly to surgery for thorough cleansing and debridement of the wound.

The injured part is thoroughly scrubbed with surgical soap and copious quantities of sterile water. In preparing the skin with an antiseptic solution, care should taken not to allow the solution to flow into the open wound. The skin laceration must be extended sufficiently to allow meticulous examination of the entire depth of the wound for removal of particles of dirt, gravel, clothing, and other foreign material. If dirt is embedded into the bone fragment, this portion of the bone must be rongeured carefully to ensure removal of all particles of dirt. The wound should be irrigated with sterile saline, which facilitates the debridement of obviously necrotic fat, fascia, and muscle that must be trimmed away.

One must remember that it is not necessary to remove as much skin or tissue in a child as one would in an adult because of the excellent ability of children's soft tissue and blood vessels to survive trauma. Once the surgeon is satisfied that no gross contamination is still present, the fracture is reduced. It is neither necessary nor desirable to restore full length to the long bones as overgrowth can be anticipated. This acceleration in growth is exaggerated if the wound should become infected. Any significant bleeders are tied with absorbable suture material, leaving as little suture in the wound as possible. The skin is loosely closed with interrupted sutures, leaving small gaps to allow drainage to escape.

It is important not to leave the bone exposed. Where necessary, a relaxing incision can be made over the muscle to allow a flap of skin to be moved over the bone. The exposed muscle can be covered with a split-thickness skin graft, either immediately or at a later date. The wound is then covered with appropriate sterile dressings and a plaster cast. If the fracture should be totally unstable, one might elect to insert a skeletal pin distal to the fracture for traction purposes, but this pin should be incorporated in the plaster cast to prevent loosening of the pin in the bone and possible pin tract infection. A child can easily bridge a defect in the bone that would be unacceptable in an adult.

Radiographs at frequent intervals during the early postoperative period should be made to ensure proper position of the fracture. Wedging of the cast is done when necessary to improve alignment.

REFERENCES

1. Blount, W. P.: Fractures in children, Baltimore, 1955, The Williams & Wilkins Co.

2. Ingram, A. J., and Bachynski, B.: Fractures of hip in children, J. Bone Joint Surg. **35A**:867, 1953.
3. McDougall, A.: Fracture of the neck of femur in children, J. Bone Joint Surg. **43B**:16, 1961.
4. Ratliff, A. H. C.: Fractures of the neck of the femur in children, J. Bone Joint Surg. **44B**:528, 1962.
5. Reidy, J. A., and Van Gorder, G. W.: Treatment of displacement of the proximal radial epiphysis, J. Bone Joint Surg. **45A**:1355, 1963.
6. Trueta, J.: Normal vascular anatomy of human femoral head during growth, J. Bone Joint Surg. **39B**:358, 1957.
7. Watson-Jones, Reginald: Fractures and joint injuries, ed. 4, Baltimore, 1955, The Williams & Wilkins Co.

Chapter 11

Analysis and treatment of ankle injuries produced by rotatory, abduction, and adduction forces

THOMAS B. QUIGLEY, M.D.
Boston, Massachusetts

This presentation is concerned with the effects of stresses on the ankle, resulting from the moving body against the fixed foot. These fall into definite patterns in which, as forces increase, injury becomes more severe. The chaotic trauma produced by great kinetic energy, such as automobile accidents or falls from a height, constitute a small proportion of all ankle injuries, require individual analysis and treatment, and will not be discussed in this chapter.

Much of the data presented here are derived from observation and study of athletes wearing cleated shoes in contact sport, but apply, of course, to those injured elsewhere than on the playing field.

MECHANISM

As Lauge-Hansen,[1] of Denmark, showed in his basic studies on the cadaver, confirmed by clinical observation, three bones, three ligaments, and three forces are fundamentally involved in four patterns of injury.

The bones are the tibia, the fibula, and the talus-calcaneus as a unit. The ligaments are the deltoid, the fibular collateral, and the tibiofibular. Rarely are the three forces, rotatory, lateral, and supination-pronation applied singly.

Each of the four patterns of injury, as energy increases, progress from ligament sprain to combinations of fracture and ligament rupture or avulsion. They are as follows (Fig. 11-1):

1. Supination—external rotation
2. Supination—adduction
3. Pronation—external rotation
4. Pronation—abduction

DIAGNOSIS

Basically diagnosis must define ligament sprain or rupture, and fracture. Radiographs in at least two planes are absolutely essential for any but the most trivial ankle injury.

Sprain can be defined as a partial rupture of a ligament, which may or may not accompany fracture. In the presence of intact bone the degree of sprain can be graded in severity from one to four. *One* is the least degree of ligament stretch one can consider a sprain. *Two* is the most common. *Three* is severe, but the ligament is still in continuity. *Four* is complete rupture or avulsion. Grading is much more accurate if done a day after injury than immediately. It is of prognostic importance, particularly in athletes. What may appear as a trivial sprain immediately after injury, with minimal pain, tenderness, and edema, may have become severe and disabling when examined after 24 hours. Occasionally an apparently severe sprain will, after a day of treatment, be found to be of only moderate or minor degree. The most com-

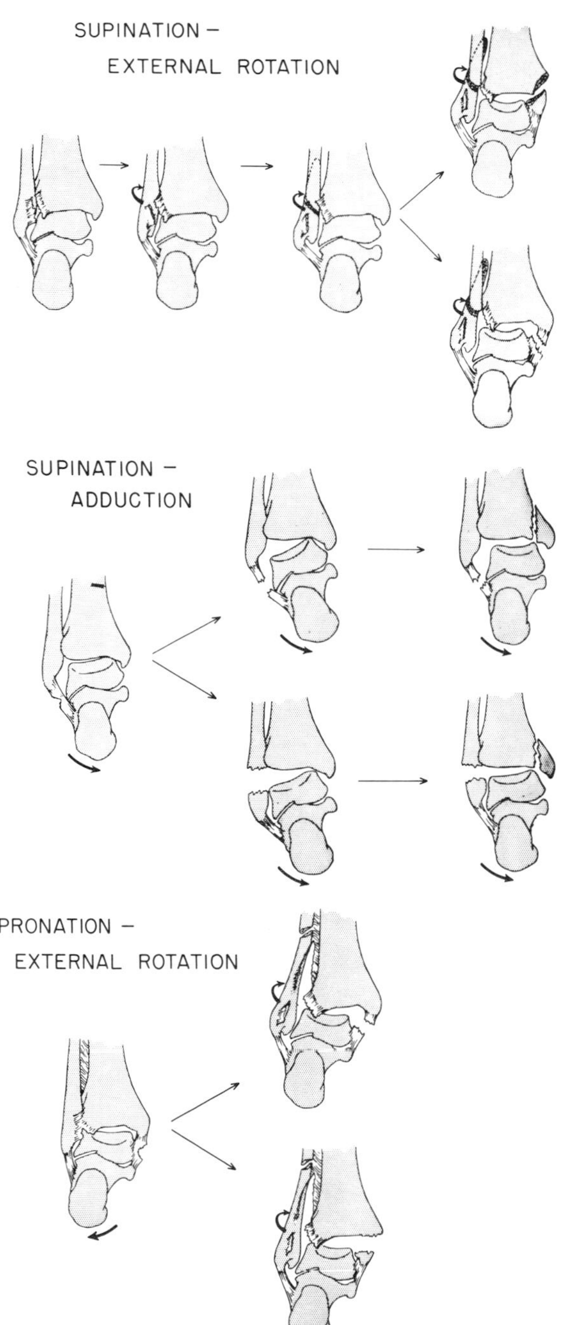

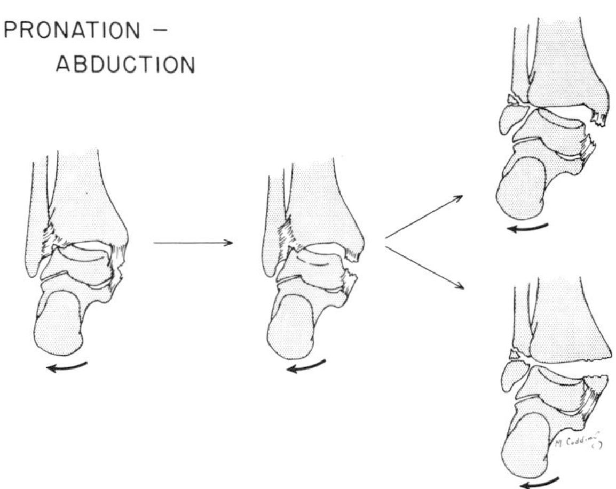

Fig. 11-1. Four patterns of increasing rotatory, coronal, and supination-pronation force. (From Quigley, T. B.: J.A.M.A. **169:**1431, 1959.)

mon ankle injury, a grade 2 sprain of the anterior tibiofibular and fibulotalar ligaments, if seen immediately after injury and treated as will be described, should be restored to full athletic activity 8 to 10 days after injury.

A golden opportunity for definitive diagnosis of ligament *rupture* or *avulsion* is present for about a half hour after injury. Gentle diagnostic manipu-

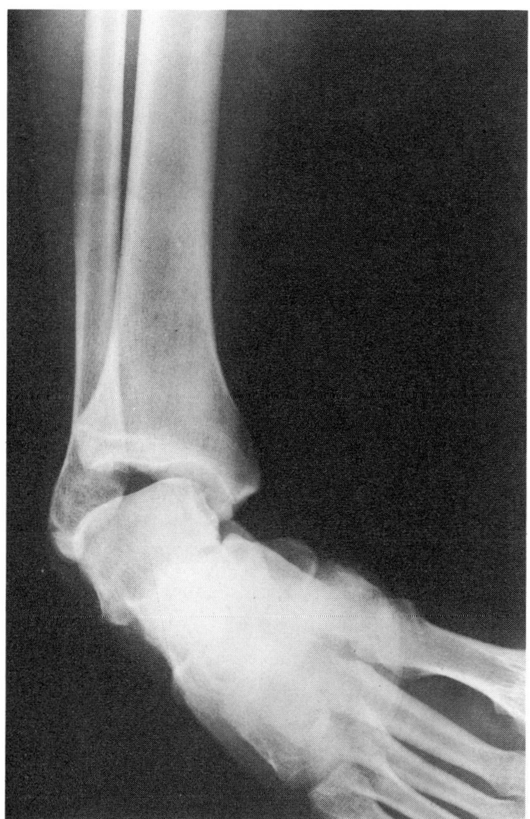

Fig. 11-2. Rupture or avulsion of the fibular collateral ligament is demonstrated by diagnostic supination. (From Quigley, T. B.: Instructional Course Lectures of the American Academy of Orthopaedic Surgeons, St. Louis, 1959, The C. V. Mosby Co., vol. 16, pp. 35-44.)

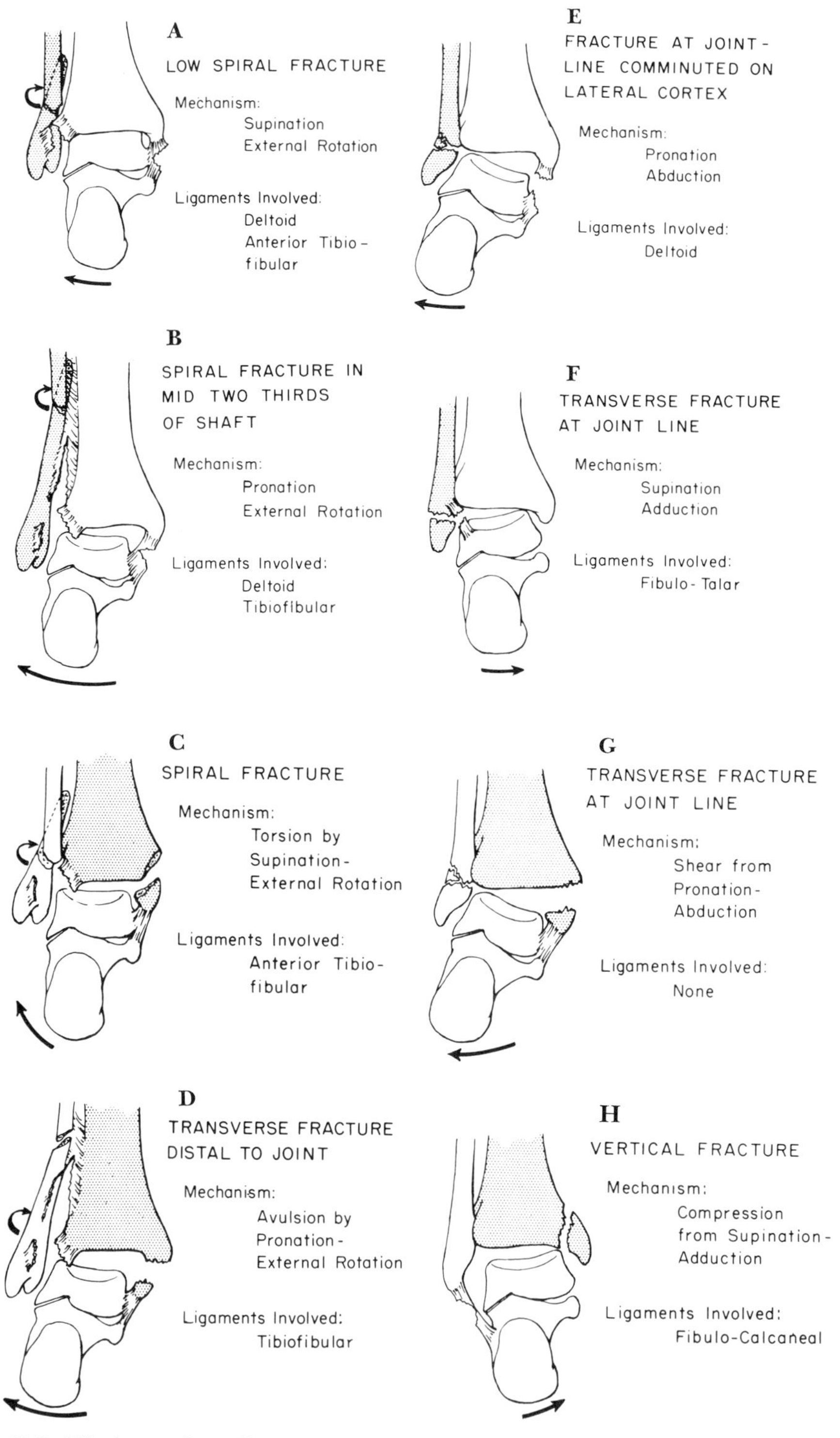

Fig. 11-3. Fibular and medial malleolar "keys" to the possibility of ligament rupture accompanying fracture. (From Quigley, T. B.: J.A.M.A. **169:**1431, 1959.)

lation, reproducing the mechanism of injury during this period, before edema and spasm have developed, is not uncomfortable. If the talus is seen to tilt in the joint mortise more than 15° in comparison to the opposite uninjured ankle in anteroposterior radiographs when such diagnostic stress in supination is applied, complete loss of continuity of the lateral ligament system can be considered to have occurred either as a result of the immediate injury or from some previous injury (Fig. 11-2). Such rupture or avulsion of the *fibular collateral ligament,* recent or old, is frequently unrecognized. A history of repeated sprain on the lateral side of the ankle with decreasing provocation is very suggestive of old rupture.

Rupture or avulsion of the *deltoid ligament* in the absence of fracture is very rare. Indeed it may not be possible without concomitant fracture of the lateral aspect of the joint.

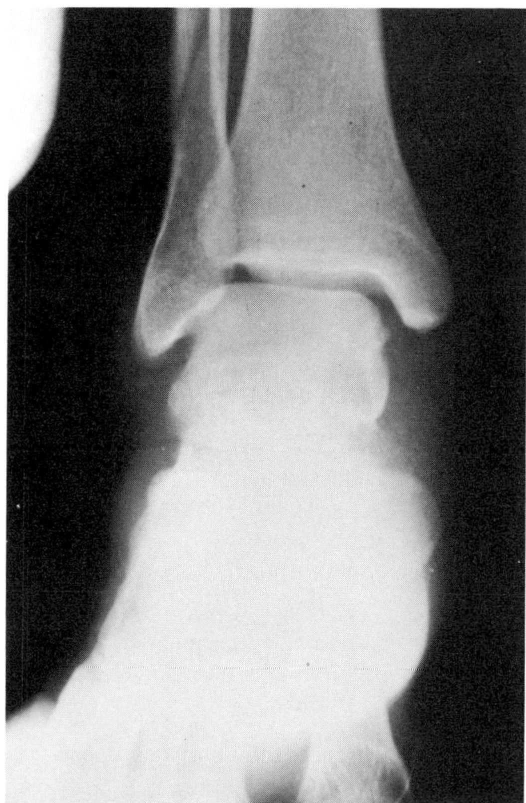

Fig. 11-4. A well-aligned supination-external rotation fracture of the distal fibula first seen 24 hours after injury on a ski slope. There is tenderness and edema on the medial aspect of the joint. Diagnostic manipulation without anesthesia is impossible. (From Quigley, T. B.: Instructional Course Lectures of the American Academy of Orthopaedic Surgeons, St. Louis, 1959, The C. V. Mosby Co., vol. 16, pp. 35-44.)

Rupture or avulsion of the *anterior tibiofibulotalar ligament* probably occurs more often than is realized, but definitive diagnosis is academic since surgical repair is almost never indicated.

When *fracture* has occurred, radiographs, with remarkable consistency, fall into the four patterns of stress that have been mentioned. The mechanism of injury and the possibility of *concomitant ligament rupture* can be deduced from study of anteroposterior radiographic views. Fig. 11-3 shows oversimplified but pragmatically useful "keys" showing the common patterns of ligament injury accompanying fracture of the fibula and of the medial malleolus.[3,4]

At the extreme of these torsional stresses or plantar flexion in older adults, the posterior lip of the tibia, the so-called third malleolus, may fracture, but this is uncommon in youth.

When the golden period of 20 to 30 minutes after injury has passed and diagnostic manipulation is no longer possible without anesthesia, arthrography may define the presence or absence of ligament rupture. Fig. 11-4 shows a well-aligned supination–external rotation fracture of the distal fibula first seen 24 hours after injury on a ski slope. Tenderness and edema are marked on the medial aspect of the joint. Diagnostic manipulation without an anesthetic is impossible. Is the deltoid ligament intact? Arthrography under local anesthesia answers the question (Fig. 11-5).

TREATMENT

The doctor, like the general in war, can initiate action only after assembling all the information available and making an appropriate diagnosis.

The principles of treatment of ligament sprain in the absence of fracture are cold, compression, rest, and elevation for the first 24 hours.[6]

Cold constricts the arteriolar bed and reduces hemorrhage at the site of injury. *Compression* disseminates edema and hematoma, facilitating its subsequent absorption. *Rest* is obvious. Activity beyond the threshold of pain is unnatural and only aggravates the injury.

Elevation enhances venous and lymphatic drainage.

Cold is applied over a compression dressing in the form of an ice pack for at least an hour and, if practically possible, overnight.

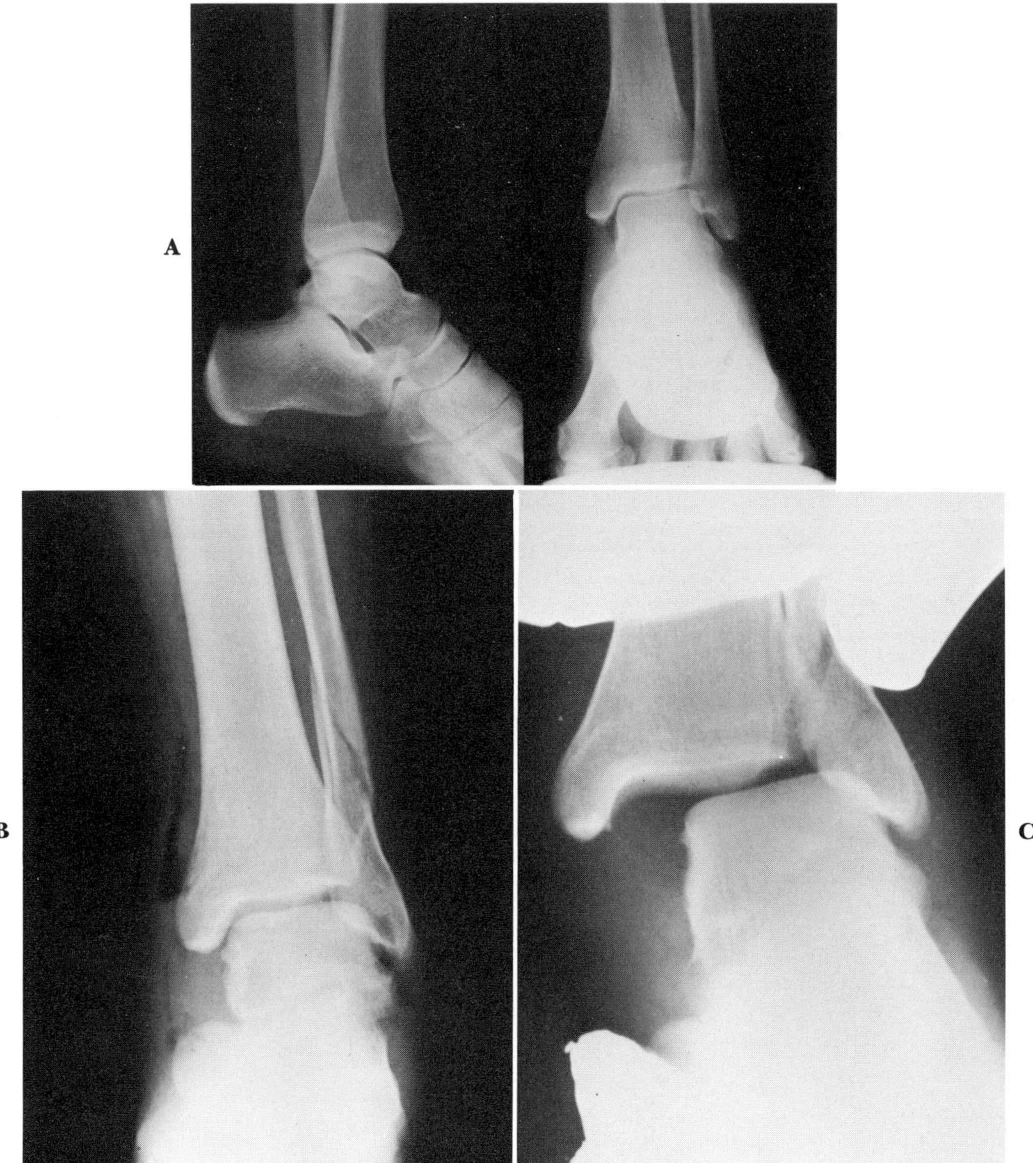

Fig. 11-5. A, Twenty cubic centimeters of air outlines a normal ankle. **B,** Twenty cubic centimeters of air injected into the ankle show a break in a capsule and air between the medial malleolus and the skin. **C,** Under spinal anesthesia, diagnostic manipulation proves that the deltoid ligament is ruptured or avulsed.

Compression is achieved by a doughnut of foam rubber surrounding the malleolus on the injured side of the ankle (Fig. 11-6). This should be applied over a layer or two of sheet wadding since there is a small incidence of irritation and allergic reaction from the chemicals in the foam rubber. It is held in place with an elastic cotton bandage. The usual open-cell foam rubber three-fourths to one inch in thickness, compressed to half its thickness, exerts a pressure of approximately 50 grams per square centimeter of skin surface. This is adequate to control edema, disseminate clot, but not enough to interfere with arteriolar supply in young adults (Fig. 11-7).

Rest may include a plaster of paris splint applied on top of the compression dressing for comfort. This should be used for no more than a few days for anything less than a grade 3 sprain. Occa-

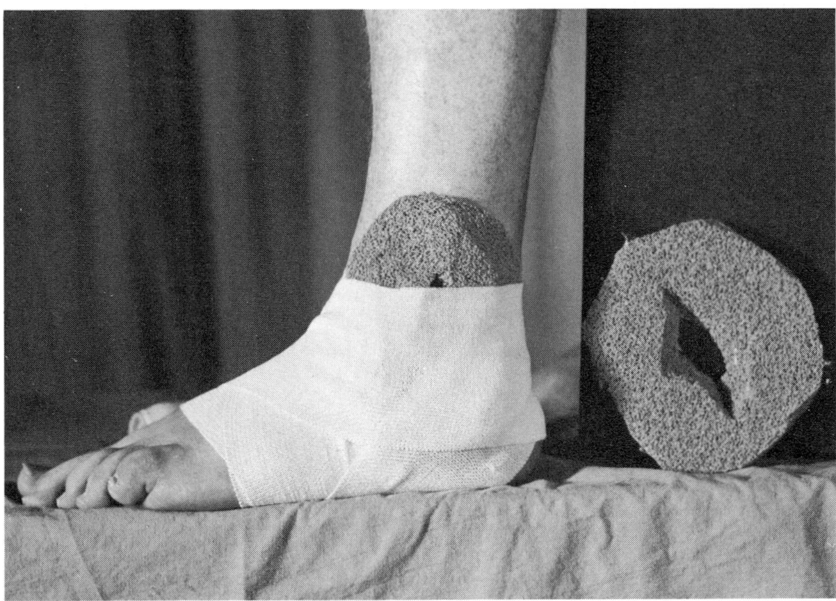

Fig. 11-6. Compression dressing for primary treatment of ankle sprain. (From Quigley, T. B.: Nebraska State Med. J. 42:435, 1957.)

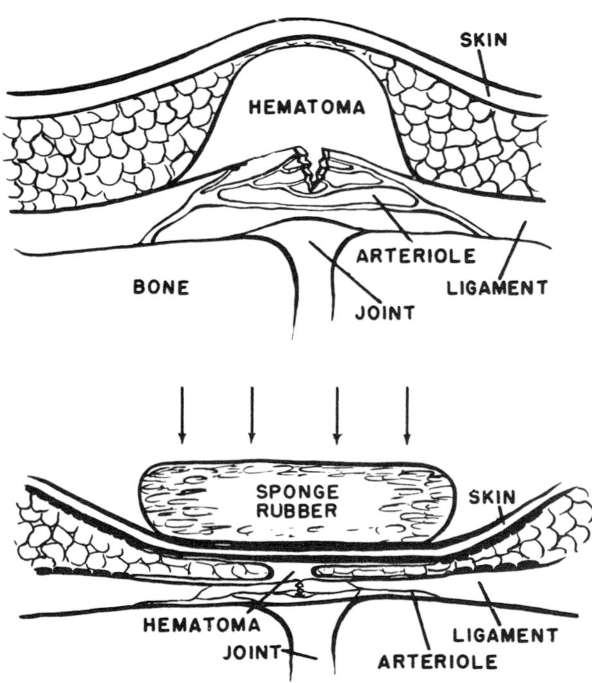

Fig. 11-7. The effect of compression on an ankle sprain. The hematoma is disseminated and its absorption facilitated. (From Quigley, T. B.: Nebraska State Med. J. 42:435, 1957.)

sionally a grade 3 sprain will require a plaster of paris walking boot, but this should never be skin tight and should be applied with due consideration of the fact that it constitutes a closed box beneath which further edema might prove disastrous from the point of view of nutrition of the soft tissue.

Crutches, properly fitted, with instruction in their use, are, of course, essential for all but the most trivial sprain. Instruction in the use of crutches cannot be overemphasized. A crutch palsy is a severe price to pay for imposition of rest on an injured ankle. Crutches should be discarded only when normal walking is possible.

Twenty-four hours after injury when the source of bleeding at the site of partial ligament rupture has clotted, heat can be applied in the form of a hot bath, and gentle massage is useful if available. Active exercise within the limits of pain can then be initiated.

A sprain is a sterile wound. No wound can heal faster than nature intends. There are, however, many ways of interfering with the normal process of healing, notably the injection of local anesthetics and the imposition of active motion and use beyond the threshold of pain, the "running it out" concept of the uninitiated.

Other modalities of treatment advertised to "speed the healing process" come and go. Most of these do no positive harm but benefit only the manufacturers of the equipment or drugs involved. Oral enzymes of various sorts, concentrated vitamin C pills, and a host of expensive electrical and electronic devices to provide heat are examples of this illogical and unscientific thinking.

When edema, pain, and tenderness have subsided and normal function is possible, the injured portion of the ligament is replaced by scar. This is adequate for all ordinary activities, but on stress such as running and certainly in sports it is weaker than the ligament it replaces. Scar is inelastic and reinjury is a real possibility if not a probability before the disorderly arrangement of collagen fibrils has been replaced by the orderly pattern of normal ligament. Therefore, for athletic activities the injured ligament should be protected by adhesive taping for at least 6 months.

Complete rupture or avulsion of the *anterior tibiofibular* or *fibulotalar ligaments,* as has been mentioned, is difficult to define with precision, but treatment is as has been described for incomplete rupture or sprain, and surgical repair is unnecessary. The diagnosis usually becomes clear when the period of convalescence is prolonged, but the eventual result is almost invariably functionally satisfactory.

Complete rupture of the *deltoid ligament* should be treated when possible by precise surgical repair.

Rupture or avulsion of the fibular collateral ligament can and probably should be primarily treated as a severe sprain. Immobilization for a month in a walking plaster of paris cast when the initial edema has subsided is advisable.

If further sprain with decreasing provocation occurs, reconstruction of the fibular collateral ligament by the elegant peroneus brevis tenondesis described by Watson Jones[7] is an eminently satisfactory solution to the problem.

Acceptable reduction of ankle fractures depends, of course, on the patient and the function to be expected of the injured ankle after healing has occurred. In the young and vigorous, little less

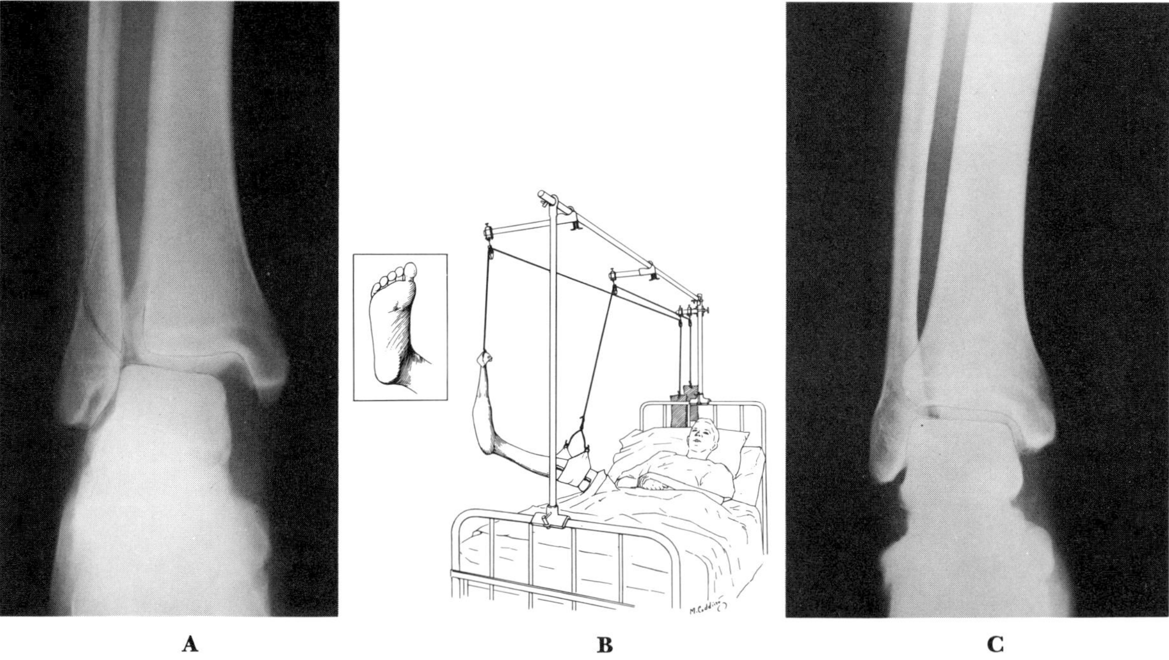

Fig. 11-8. A, Supination-external rotation fracture of the ankle with lateral displacement of the talus. The deltoid ligament obviously is ruptured or avulsed. **B,** Suspension in stockinette imposes pronation, adduction, and internal rotation on the ankle, reversing a common mechanism of injury. **C,** Supination-external rotation fracture of the ankle after suspension overnight. The ruptured or avulsed deltoid ligament probably does not lie trapped in the joint since the mortise is normal, but the positions of its torn ends are unknown. (From Quigley, T. B.: Amer. J. Surg. **97**:488, 1959.)

than perfection, as far as it can be achieved, can be accepted. In the aged and infirm, the standards need be much less rigorous.

The following case histories will illustrate these concepts of diagnosis and management of ankle injuries.

Case 1. A 20-year-old lacrosse player, with his cleated foot fixed to the ground, was struck by another player and sustained the supination-external rotation fracture of the distal fibula seen in radiographs taken a few moments after injury (Fig. 11-8, *A*). The lateral displacement of the talus

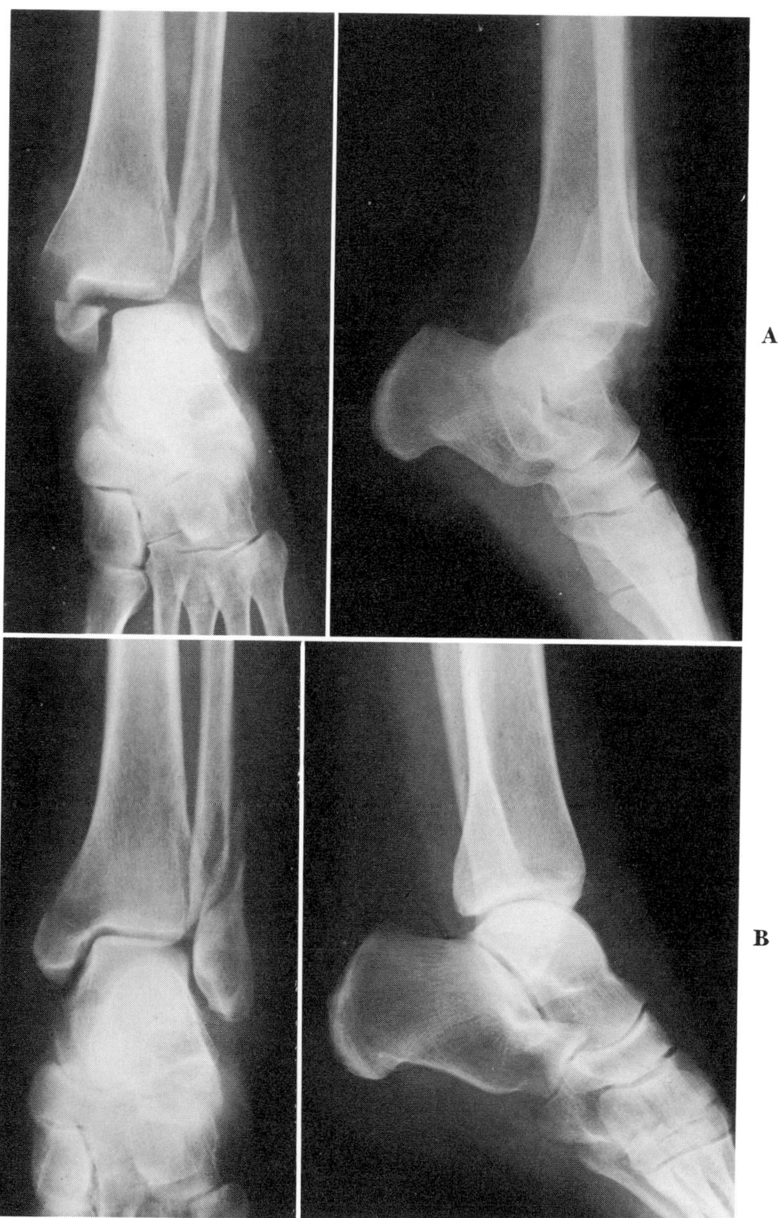

Fig. 11-9. A, A bimalleolar fracture from abduction-supination and external rotation. The patient is obese, skin is of poor quality, and there is an incipient stasis ulcer above the medial malleolus. **B,** The ankle shown in **A** after a few days of suspension in stockinette. This reduction was accepted, and the end result was satisfactory for the patient's needs. (From Quigley, T. B.: Amer. J. Surg. **97**:488, 1959.)

made it obvious that the deltoid ligament was ruptured.

This injury was treated by a simple method of suspension overnight, until permission for definitive treatment could be obtained from his parents.[5] This consisted of the application of stockinette from the upper thigh to beyond the toes and suspension of the stockinette from an overhead frame with a sling beneath the distal thigh to keep the knee moderately flexed. When the body is supine, the lower extremity lies in external rotation. Therefore, such suspension imposes on the injured ankle pronation and internal rotation, reversing the mechanism of injury (Fig. 11-8, *B*). Portable roentgen-ray films taken the next morning (Fig. 11-8, *C*) show what appears to be a perfect reduction of the fibula. However, the state of the deltoid ligament is unknown. It probably does not lie within the joint since the space between the medial malleolus and the talus is normal. However, the ends of the ruptured deltoid ligament may or may not lie in the most advantageous position for healing.

Diagnostic manipulation under anesthesia and operation were therefore carried out, gross rupture of the ligament was encountered, suture was easily accomplished, and the eventual result 4 months after injury was perfect function.

Case 2. An obese 66-year-old woman fell on icy pavement, sustaining a bimalleolar fracture from pronation, abduction, and external rotation forces Fig. 11-9, *A*. Circulation was feeble, the skin of the lower extremities was of poor quality, and there was an impending stasis ulcer on the medial lower leg. Operation was obviously contraindicated. The limb was suspended in stockinette for a few days. Edema subsided, and the fragments fell into fairly satisfactory alignment (Fig. 11-9, *B*). A plaster cast from toes to upper thigh was applied over the suspension stockinette without moving her from the bed. The eventual result was satisfactory for her needs.

Case 3. A 19-year-old intramural football player sustained the pronation external rotation injury seen in Fig. 11-10, *A*. Injuries of this severity cannot be treated with any expectation of a good functional result by any other method than open surgical repair. The only question is whether to carry

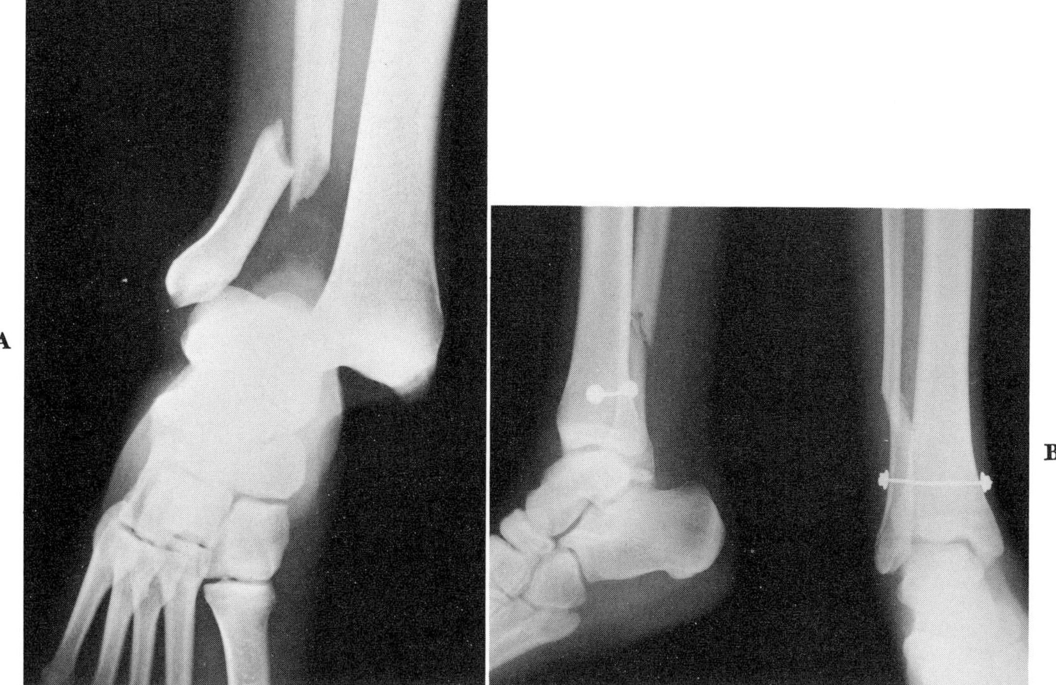

Fig. 11-10. A, A severe pronation–external rotation injury sustained in intramural football. Both the anterior and the posterior tibiofibular and the deltoid ligament are ruptured or avulsed. **B,** Postoperative film of ankle injury seen in **A.** The tibiofibular ligaments are approximated by the bolt. The deltoid ligament is repaired by suture.

out operation immediately or to delay repair until edema has subsided after a preliminary reduction. In this case operation was carried out within 3 hours of injury. Complete rupture of both the anterior and posterior elements of the tibiofibular ligament does not lend itself to suture, which is comparable to sewing two paint brushes together end to end. However, the frayed and torn ligaments can be approximated after evacuation of clot by a bolt, as was done in this case (Fig. 11-10, *B*). The bolt was tightened with the foot in moderate plantar flexion, so that the mortise is well snugged. After suture of the deltoid ligament and debridement of the ruptured anterior capsule, immobilization was carried out with the foot and ankle in slight plantar flexion. Needless to say, no weight bearing was permitted until the bolt was removed 4 months after injury. The minor contracture of the heel cord was easily remedied by appropriate exercise, including walking upstairs backwards. Five years later this man was tennis champion of his community.

The question naturally arises, "What sort of results can be expected in these ankle injuries involving ligament rupture if operation is not carried out?" Unquestionably many of them are satisfactory if not good, but enough disability does occur to lend considerable weight to the argument that precise surgical reconstruction is the treatment of choice, particularly in the young and vigorous.

Case 4. Here is seen the end result of an injury that was treated surgically but from the wrong point of view. A fracture of the fibula sustained by a vigorous young man of 25 while skiing was precisely reconstructed and fastened with screws, but the hematoma in the ruptured tibiofibular ligament was not evaluated and the operative intervention may well have contributed to the cross union that now exists (Fig. 11-11). The calcified fragments of the ruptured deltoid ligament are clearly seen on the medial side of the joint. This young man was unable to dorsiflex his ankle beyond 90°, he was unable, therefore, to ski, run, play golf, or even go up and down stairs with comfort. Reconstructive surgery was advised, but apparently with not enough enthusiasm for him to accept it. It is probable that if this original injury had been treated by a medial approach to the ankle and suture of the ruptured deltoid ligament, the fracture of the fibula would have fallen into acceptable position, the hematoma in the ruptured tibiofibular ligament system would have absorbed without event, and function would have been better.

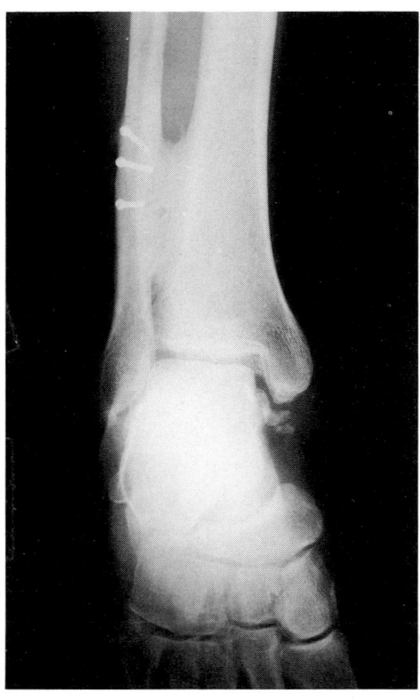

Fig. 11-11. The result of the wrong surgical approach. If the deltoid ligament, seen as a calcified mass, had been sutured, the fibula may have fallen into position, and cross union enhanced by operative intervention might not have occurred.

Case 5. This 18-year-old woman fell on a skating rink. She was treated by her family doctor by immediate application of a plaster of paris walking boot. When first seen 18 months later she complained of pain in her ankle. Radiographs showed a laterally displaced healed fracture of the fibula and an obvious old deltoid ligament rupture (Fig. 11-12). The fibula fracture was recreated, the scar tissue was removed, but the result was only fairly satisfactory. How much simpler the solution to this problem would have been had the deltoid ligament been sutured soon after injury. It is likely that this woman will eventually come to fusion of her ankle, since in the 10 years since injury she has become obese, the mother of several children, and her ankle is increasingly uncomfortable.

The plaster of paris walking boot is a treacherous method of management for all but the simplest of ankle injuries.[2] It imposes not only rotational stresses in external rotation, particularly if weight

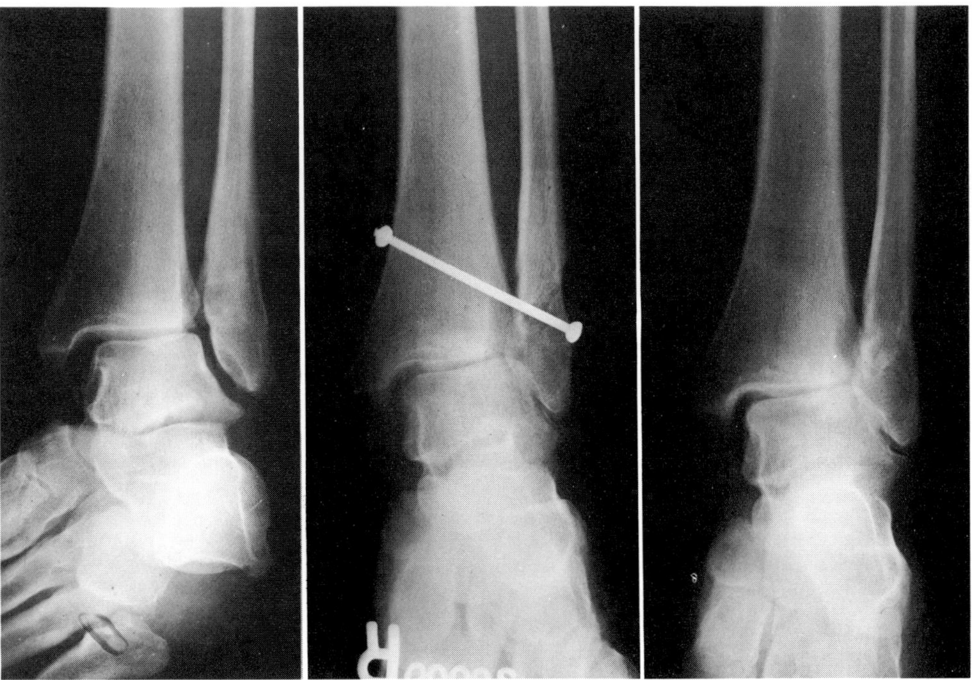

Fig. 11-12. A painful ankle in a young woman first seen 18 months after primary treatment with a walking boot. Recreation of the fibular fracture and realignment of the talus were only partially successful, anatomically and symptomatically.

bearing is on a crutch tip, but also potential displacement of fracture fragments by direct pressure even in the most carefully applied, lightly padded, plaster.

SUMMARY

1. Precise diagnosis is essential to treatment.
2. Ligament rupture is at least as important as fracture.
3. Ankle fractures and ligament injuries produced by rotatory, abduction, and adduction forces fall into predictable patterns.
4. Ligament rupture or avulsion can be suspected from the pattern of fracture when present and proved by arthrography and diagnostic manipulation.
5. Surgical repair of rupture or avulsion of the deltoid ligament is better than immobilization and hope.
6. Surgical repair of rupture of the anterior tibiofibular ligament is not necessary.
7. Primary repair of rupture of the fibular collateral ligament is rarely necessary. Peroneus brevis tenondesis is excellent when needed.
8. Little less than perfection in reduction of ankle fractures can be accepted in the young and vigorous. There should be little hesitation in carrying out operative treatment, when necessary and not contraindicated, to achieve this goal.

REFERENCES

1. Lauge-Hansen, N.: Fracture of ankle: Clinical use of genetic roentgen diagnosis and genetic reduction, Arch. Surg. **64**:488, 1952.
2. Quigley, T. B.: Indications and contraindications for the plaster of paris walking boot, Amer. J. Surg. **83**: 281, 1952.
3. Quigley, T. B.: Management of ankle injuries sustained in sports, J.A.M.A. **169**:1431, 1959.
4. Quigley, T. B.: Diagnosis and treatment of ankle injuries sustained in sports, Amer. Acad. Orthop. Surg. Lect. **16**:35, 1959.
5. Quigley, T. B.: A simple aid to the reduction of abduction-external rotation fractures of the ankle, Amer. J. Surg. **97**:488, 1959.
6. Thorndike, A.: Athletic injuries: prevention, diagnosis and treatment, ed. 4, Philadelphia, 1956, Lea & Febiger.
7. Watson-Jones, R.: Fractures and joint injuries, ed. 4, Edinburgh, 1955, E. & S. Livingstone, pp. 821-823.

Chapter 12

Early care of severe extremity wounds: a review of the Vietnam experience and its civilian applications

KRISTAPS J. KEGGI, M.D.
WAYNE O. SOUTHWICK, M.D.
New Haven, Connecticut

War has always been a school for surgeons. The present conflict is no exception to this rule. The lessons that are learned in Vietnam will lead to better care of the injured among our civilians. Many advances will have to be made in civilian communications, first aid, and transportation. It may also be necessary to think of a chain of evacuation leading to trauma centers. On the scale of our future growth, these administrative measures could be the most productive, but we cannot minimize the surgical principles that are applied in the treatment of large numbers of severe war wounds. We would like to cover the management of these wounds and emphasize the fact that all of the principles of military surgery have immediate application in individual civilian injuries and mass disasters. We intend to focus on the wounds of the extremities. These represent approximately 75% of all combat wounds and the great majority of civilian injuries. They are also the ones that require the greatest number of reconstructive procedures following the initial lifesaving measures, and their rehabilitation can span a period of several years.

GOALS

The goals of surgery are to save life and limb. Injuries and wounds that represent a threat to the patient's life must be treated without delay. Wounds of the chest and abdomen demand immediate attention, but the wounds of the limbs cannot be overlooked even during the initial phase of lifesaving procedures. A lacerated femoral artery may be fatal in a matter of minutes. An inadequately treated wound of an extremity can also progress to a delayed but equally fatal septicemia or clostridial infection.[27] Life before limb is a cardinal principle,[15,32] but whenever possible the wounds of the extremities should also receive immediate attention. It is a matter of judgment at the first surgical facility.

Lifesaving measures include:

1. Immediate control of hemorrhage by compression dressings or tourniquets.
2. Establishment of an airway and adequate oxygenation.
3. Rapid transfusion through multiple catheters passed through the peripheral veins into the central circulation.
4. Thoracic and abdominal operations.
5. Repair of major arteries.

As soon as it is apparent that the patient's life has been secured, all efforts should be directed at preservation of limb. Extremity wounds must be treated with the full knowledge that once the patient survives he will probably be most concerned about his ability to use his arms and legs. They represent life.

PATHOLOGY OF WAR WOUNDS

War wounds are characterized by extensive tissue devitalization and heavy bacterial contamination.* It is a combination almost certain to produce an infection that can kill the patient or lead to the immediate loss of a limb. An infection can also delay reconstruction and may lead to a chronic osteomyelitis and the late loss of limb. Some of these late amputations are frequently the most tragic, since they come after many years of false hope and multiple surgical procedures.

Wound size depends on multiple factors. The most important one is the velocity of the missile doing the damage.†

The following formula expresses the importance of velocity in the determination of kinetic energy:

$$E = \frac{m\,V_2}{2}$$

Such other factors as missile size, missile course, missile disintegration, and secondary missiles are also important. Tissue resistance to devitalization is also of note. Skin, fascia, and ligaments are less affected by a high-velocity missile than the large muscles of the extremities. As the missile passes through tissues, the kinetic energy that it has gathered is transmitted to them. With high-velocity missile, extensive cavitation takes place (Fig. 12-1), and on subsequent dissection it becomes obvious that the path of the missile is surrounded by a wide tract of devitalized tissue. Low-velocity missiles represented by most civilian weapons cause a small core of devitalized tissue and represent a simpler therapeutic problem that can frequently be handled without extensive debridement.[15]

The wounds encountered in a combat zone are extremely dirty. The soil on which the soldier fights covers his body and gets into his wounds. Recent bacteriologic studies have shown the following organisms in the soil in Vietnam: *Bacillus sporogenes, Bacillus subtilis, Bacillus myocardis, Bacillus pumilus,* hemolytic and nonhemolytic streptococci, *Aerobacter aerogenes, Escherichia* coli, *Clostridium perfringens, Clostridium paraputrificum, Clostridium tertium, Clostridium sporogenes, Clostridium novyi,* fungi, and yeasts. Even without bacteriologic studies, the facts of contamination are obvious at the time of the initial surgery. The following foreign bodies were removed from the wounds debrided at the Third Surgical Hospital during its first year in Vietnam (1965-1966):

Bullets	Worms
Shell fragments	Nails
Grass	Nuts and bolts
Grease	Screws
Leaves	Pieces of wire
Sand	Pieces of tin (can)
Stones	Glass fragments
Clothing	Water buffalo feces
Insects (dead and alive)	

In addition to this gross contamination by the hostile environment, many of the soldiers have a variety of skin infections. There is also the routine contact with medical personnel. Thus, by the time the wounds are cultured in Japan, *Staphylococcus aureus* can be identified in 19% of the cases,[41] and *Pseudomonas* becomes the most troublesome organism in the large wounds that cannot be closed very rapidly.[25,29]

This general picture of wound contamination is similar to the World War II and Korean experience. It is also typical of the civilian wounds in which the initial contamination is by the wide spectrum of organisms found in the general environment and soil, but the troublesome infections are due to the hospital *Staphylococcus* or *Pseudomonas*.

In addition to tissue devitalization and heavy contamination, there are several other factors that determine the severity of wounds. These are arterial injury, venous injury, decreased venous return, presence of hematoma, depth of wounds, compression of tissue by tight fascial compartments, the patient's general condition, and the presence of shock and septicemia. All of these deserve some individual consideration.*

Arterial injury when associated with an extremity wound has been shown to contribute to a higher rate of fatal clostridial infections and a greater incidence of wound suppuration. Thus missile wounds that penetrate a limb or transect or contuse an artery present a greater threat to life and limb than wounds without vascular damage. It is also important to realize that major arterial injuries can be masked and difficult to identify in the presence of shock, decreased peripheral pulses, and multiple wounds. Some of these hidden injuries can occur without compromising the entire

*See references 7-10, 14, 25, 29, 37, 38, 45, and 46.
†See references 7-10, 30, 32, and 38.

*See references 7-10, 14, 17, 41, and 44.

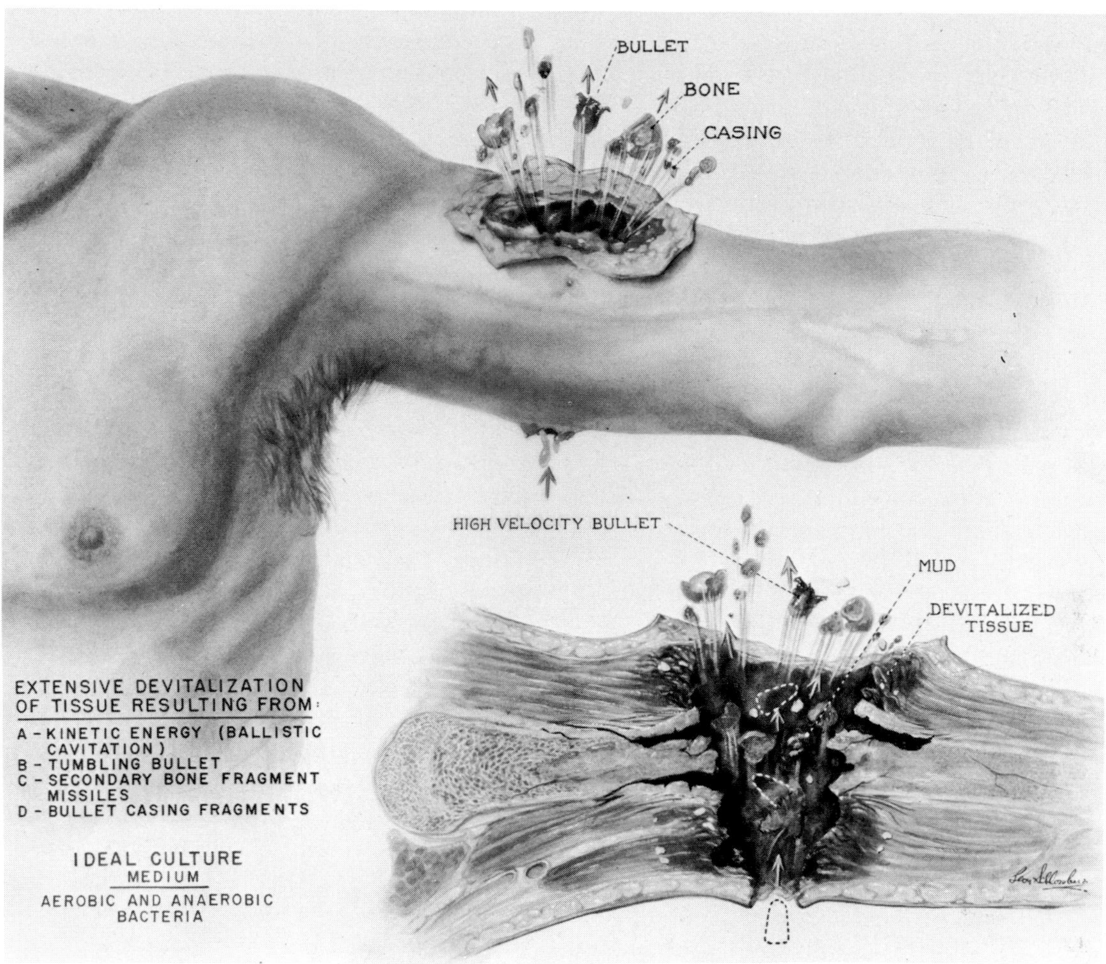

Fig. 12-1. These drawings are based on a through-and-through high-velocity missile wound treated and photographed in Vietnam. The first picture of this sequence shows ballistic cavitation and the extensive tissue devitalization inflicted by the high-velocity bullet. It also depicts bullet deformation and fragmentation. Mud is represented to show heavy bacterial contamination. The piece of bone emerging from the exit wound must be described as a secondary missile that can inflict additional damage to the soft tissues of the extremity.

blood supply to the distal segments of the extremity. Thus, a missile wound passing through the proximal leg may injure the anterior tibial artery without impairing the arterial flow to the foot through the posterior tibial and peroneal vessels. A wound of this type presents a major threat to the viability of the muscles in the anterior tibial compartment, and it may well contribute to the the rapid progression of an infection in this area. The wound itself may be "benign" in appearance. It may have been caused by a low-velocity missile with minimal tissue devitalization around its path, but the secondary muscle "infarction" caused by the transected artery is an easy focus for a massive infection.

The delayed restoration of arterial flow to an extremity may also contribute to the danger of an overwhelming infection. The delays in transportation are always obvious, but the delays caused by such prolonged lifesaving procedures as thoracoabdominal explorations can lead to the loss of a limb due to neglect. By the time the lifesaving surgery is completed, the limb with a major arterial injury may have to undergo amputation because of distal tissue death. Tissue devitalization may be recognized at the time of surgery, but it can be missed. The skin may remain viable and hide the underlying muscle necrosis. Thus reexploration of an extremity following a delayed arterial repair may show liquefaction of all muscles distal to the vascular injury. As the edema of the ischemic necrosis sets in, its devitalizing effect is compounded by tight fascial compartments. Thus, if there is an arterial injury, even the most minor extremity wounds must be debrided adequately.

It is also imperative that fasciotomies of all the muscle compartments be performed to alleviate tissue compression by progressive edema. These fasciotomies will also contribute to better venous return through the edematous extremity. Fasciotomies should always be performed on the muscle compartments that have been injured and are being debrided. They may also be necessary in areas distal to the actual injury. Thus, a leg with extensive vascular injuries at the level of the thigh may well require fasciotomies distal to the knee. This situation is most likely to arise in delayed vascular repairs and arterial injuries with associated damage to the venous system. Fasciotomies through several longitudinal incisions can be performed, but in the leg, resection of the fibular shaft allows decompression of all four fascial compartments through one incision.

Injury to major extremity veins can occur alone or in conjunction with arterial wounds. From observation in a combat zone and along the chain of evacuation, an extremity with venous injuries represents a problem prone to serious complications. Inadequate venous return contributes to pooling of blood in the peripheral veins. The increased venous pressure is responsible for greater blood loss from the wound and the accumulation of hematoma. It is also a factor in the formation of interstitial edema and greater compression of tissues in fascial compartments that are already tight. It tends to decrease tissue oxygenation. All of these factors contribute to muscle devitalization and increase the chances of infection.

The presence of a hematoma in a wound without adequate drainage is an extremely hazardous situation. It is not a "clean" hematoma. There has been contamination from the outside. The hematoma deep within necrotic muscle represents the ideal culture media at an ideal temperature for bacterial proliferation. Without adequate drainage and debridement, massive infection is the most likely result.

Finally, it is important to speak of the patient and his general condition. Septicemia, electrolyte imbalance, and poor nutrition may be detrimental to wound healing. The patient's age cannot be neglected. An aging noncommissioned officer should be treated with much greater caution than the 18-year-old recruit.

Another critical aspect of wound pathology is the understanding and visualization of the path that the missile took through its target. There are times when it seems impossible to relate two wounds to the same missile. That is a common problem if the surgeon thinks of his patient in terms of rigid anatomic position. The soldier moves. His trunk and extremities can be in the most contorted positions. Most bullets and shell fragments move in a straight line. The path of a missile through the target must be visualized in terms of the soldier's position at the time of wounding. For example, a leg could present with wounds over the anterior aspects of the thigh and the tibia. These wounds could be associated with extensive destruction of the posterior femoral condyles. As this leg is examined in an extended, anatomic position, it is impossible to visualize the path of the missile. Flexion of the knee, however, shows very clearly the straight line between the two skin wounds and through the fractures of the femoral condyles.

An understanding of the missile path and extremity position is important in the planning of surgical approaches for debridement. It is of greatest importance in wounds close to the major joints (shoulder, hip, and knee). It may determine the need for joint exploration. An understanding of the missile path also makes it easier to follow the core of devitalized tissues.

TREATMENT

The prognosis of war wounds without treatment is severe. The facts of tissue devitalization and gross contamination are such that overwhelming infections seem inevitable. The history of wounds in our wars of the past tells the story of these infections.

Our treatment of casualties follows well-established and extremely successful patterns. These patterns are based on clinical experience accumulated during the two world wars and the Korean war.*

*See references 2, 14, 33, and 46.

The mortality rate of those who reach our hospitals in Vietnam is approximately 2%. It is rare to see a case of gas gangrene or fatal septicemia. It is equally rare to see extensive osteomyelitis or a massive pyarthrosis. Yet, in spite of our success, there are always dangers of inadequate treatment. In spite of all the teaching and the experience accumulated within the last fifty years, the principles of wound care are often forgotten and relearned by clinical experience under combat conditions. Our own approach to the wounds in Vietnam was based on the principles outlined by Hampton.[14] His culminative experience from World War II is still the basis for all military surgery, but only by direct experience with adequate and inadequate treatment did we come to believe and understand the problems discussed by Dr. Hampton. This presentation on wound care is based on our experience in Vietnam. It is a reaffirmation of the staged management of wounds from first aid and debridement to reconstructive surgery in the major hospitals of the continental United States.

FIRST AID

The treatment of wounds begins at the scene of the injury. The basic rules of first aid apply in all cases. The patient's airway is cleared and his breathing established. Major hemorrhage is stopped by compression dressings or tourniquets. Wounds of the chest and abdomen are covered. Extremities with fractures are splinted.[28,33,34] The local application of an antibiotic ointment (oxytetracycline) has been shown to be of value in controlling bacterial growth.[19] A dressing that covers the wound prevents further contamination.

TRANSPORTATION AND DISTRIBUTION OF PATIENTS

Following first aid, rapid transportation to a hospital becomes very crucial. The hospital must also be ready to receive the patient and to deliver care without delays. In Vietnam, both helicopter evacuation and patient distribution to the well-established hospital is controlled via radio by a team that has full information about the number and the location of casualties, along with the receiving capabilities of the hospitals. In this manner, the times from injury to evacuation, and from arrival in the hospital to definitive surgery are kept at a minimum. It is a system that should be an example for civilian planning of emergency care and transportation.

EMERGENCY CARE—ANTIBIOTICS

As soon as the patient arrives in the hospital, attention should be directed to lifesaving measures. These principles have been reviewed in the introductory section of this course. They should be followed with care. Tetanus prophylaxis must be routine for any patient with a dirty wound. Antibiotics should be started as soon as possible. Penicillin and streptomycin were the drugs used at the Third Surgical Hospital between 1965 and 1966. Chloramphenicol was given to patients with penicillin allergies, extensive abdominal wounds, or liver injuries. It is our impression that antibiotics started in the Emergency Room should also be a part of the routine in the care of major extremity wounds seen in our civilian hospitals. The antibiotics may have to be changed in the course of wound care and closure, but these changes should be based on serial cultures and sensitivity determinations.[29]

RADIOGRAPHS

Preoperative radiographs are of importance in multiple fragment wounds and in wounds that are in proximity to the major joints. Under condition of relative calm, all extremity wounds should have preoperative films in two planes. If there is a large influx of casualties, most extremity wounds can be treated without preoperative radiographs. This is especially true in the case of through-and-through bullet wounds, in which the damage is obvious on initial examination.

ANESTHESIA

Following preoperative evaluation and first aid measures, the patient is taken to the operating room. It was our experience in Vietnam that even though blood transfusions were started, it was not necessary to restore a normal blood pressure in most of the major extremity wounds. Blood transfusions can be continued during anesthesia, and frequently it was impossible to stop hemorrhage until the bleeding vessels had been exposed. Restoration of blood pressure can cause heavier bleeding, which can be stopped only by identification and ligation of the lacerated vessels. The ligation of open arteries also reestablishes a closed system necessary for an effective blood pressure. Thus, in the

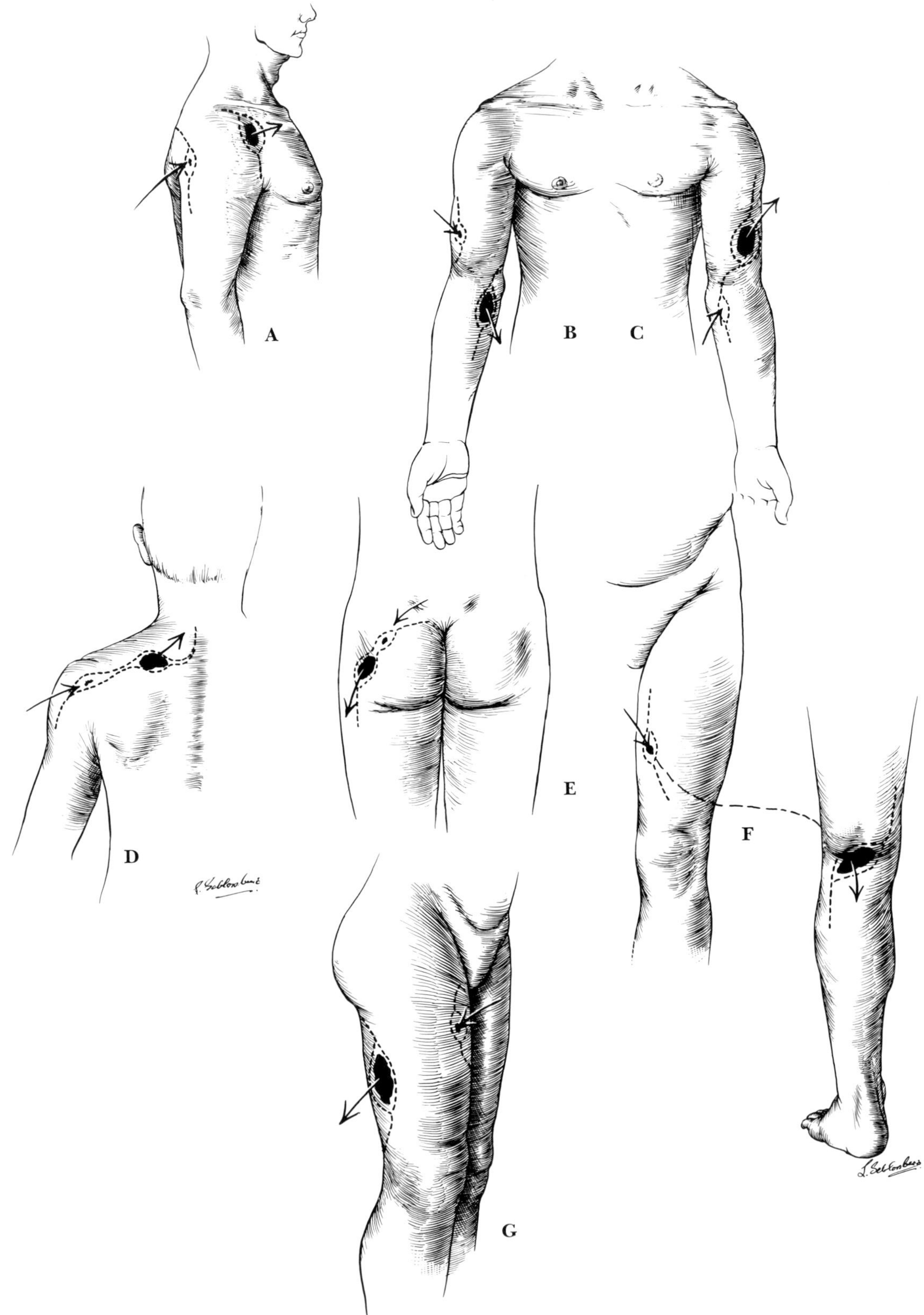

Fig. 12-2. A-D, Skin incisions are usually in line with the long axis of the extremity. **E-G,** Skin incisions are usually in line with the long axis of the extremity or **S** shaped at the major flexor creases, **F.**

presence of major extremity wounds, it was our experience that the dangers of anesthesia did not justify any delays in the surgery intended to correct the cause of the patient's hypotension. This was specifically the case in high-velocity wounds of the proximal thigh and the upper arm, in which compression dressings and tourniquets were relatively ineffective.

Whenever possible, the initial surgery was performed under spinal block or local anesthesia. At the Third Surgical Hospital between 1965 and 1966, this type of anesthesia was possible in approximately two thirds of the patients with primary extremity wounds.

SKIN PREPARATION

Under mass casualty conditions, skin preparation may have to be minimized, but most of the time the surgeon and his assistants should be prepared to do a thorough job of washing and shaving the entire extremity. PHisoHex and Aqueous Zephiran were the agents most commonly used. Under combat conditions, the patients are covered with dirt from toes to groin and from fingertips to axilla. Such weapons as antipersonnel mines, mortars, and other explosives may produce multiple superficial penetrations of the skin with superficial wounds that can be sufficiently cleaned by shaving and scrubbing the extremity with a brush. Even a solitary wound of the thigh should be prepped to the toes.

Following the initial shaving and scrubbing, the extremity should be reprepped with more specific attention to the skin at the level of the wound. At this time, the wound should also be irrigated with large amounts of sterile saline. It may also be

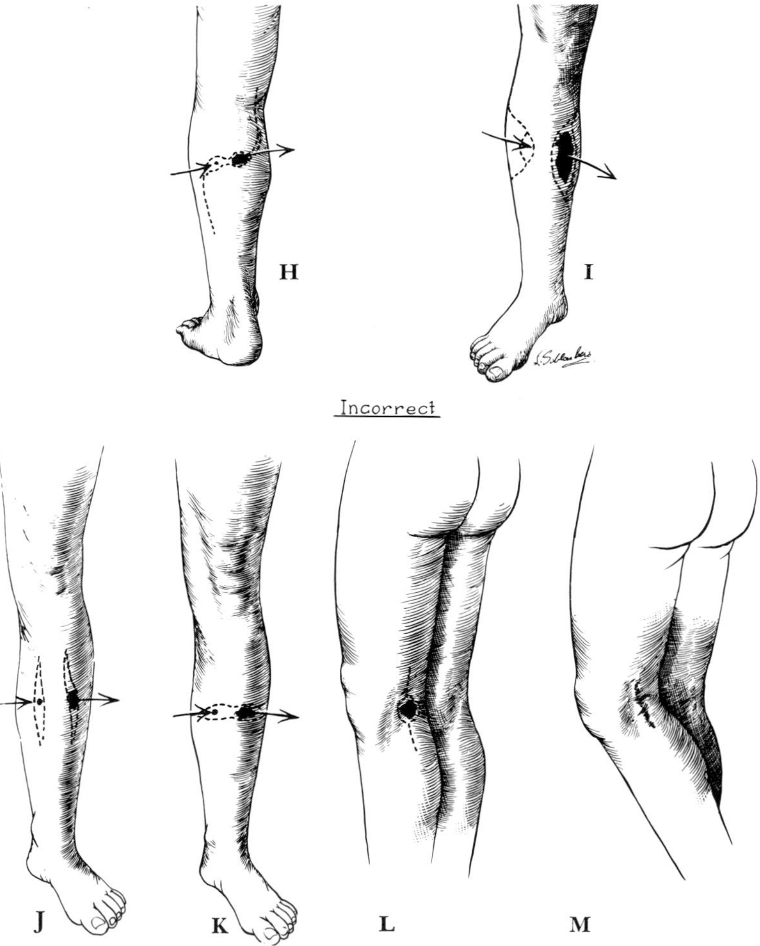

Fig. 12-2, cont'd. S-shaped incisions for maximum exposure, **H.** Preservation of blood supply by leaving broad bases to narrow strips of skin, **I. J-M,** Incorrect incisions.

practical to do some preliminary debridement of the dirtiest tags of skin and muscle. Following the second prep, the extremity is draped. It should be draped free to allow a variety of incisions. Different positions of the extremity may also be necessary to facilitate exposure of all the contaminated and devitalized tissues.

SKIN INCISIONS

Whenever possible, the skin incisions should follow the standard incisions used to expose the long bones and major joints. They should usually be in line with the long axis of the extremity (Fig. 12-2). In the case of wounds that are too close to each other (Fig. 12-2, *G* and *I*), they should be slightly curved to allow a broad base for the skin between the wounds. If this strip of skin is very narrow in spite of the curved incisions, if it is contused or completely devitalized, it may be wiser to connect the two wounds with a gentle S-shaped incision (Fig. 12-2, *C* and *H*). This type of incision will give good exposure, preserve the blood supply to the skin flaps, and allow for relatively easy closure at a later time. Incisions such as those shown in Fig. 12-2, *J* and *K* are unacceptable because they will not allow good exposure and debridement (especially Fig. 12-2, *K*). They may also compromise the skin between the incisions (Fig. 12-2, *J*). A long transverse incision (Fig. 12-2, *K*) can not only cut across the blood supply of the distal skin but also gives inadequate exposure of the tissues. If it is necessary to cross a flexor crease, the incision

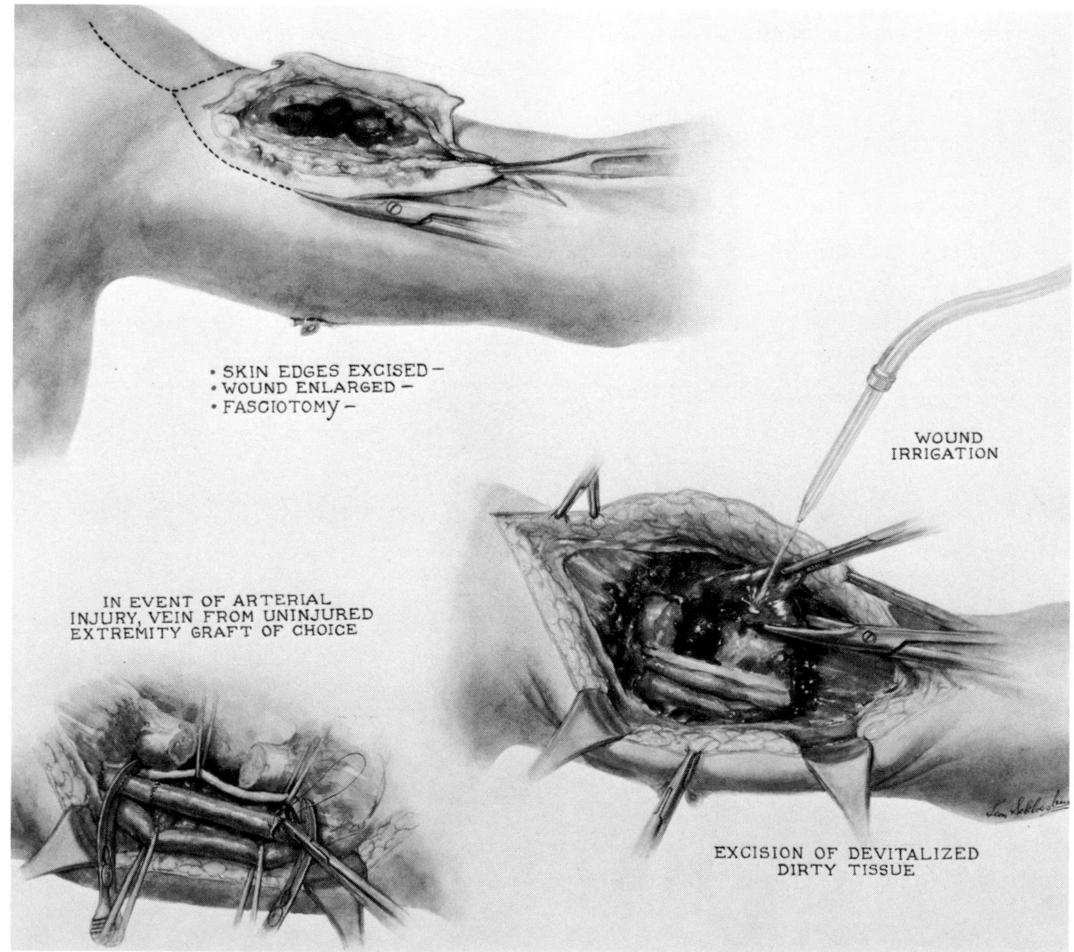

Fig. 12-3. The dirty skin edges must be excised and the wound extended in line with the long axis of the extremity. Debridement of devitalized tissues must be followed by irrigation. If end-to-end repair of injured arteries is impossible, a vein graft may have to be performed.

must be S-shaped (Fig. 12-2, *F*). A vertical incision across the flexor crease of a joint is unacceptable since it will produce a scar that impairs function and is difficult to treat (Fig. 12-2, *L* and *M*).

The dirty wound edges should be excised (Figs. 12-2 and 12-3). This is best performed with a pair of sharp scissors, but a scalpel may also work. The incision can also be extended with the scissors (Fig. 12-3). It is preferable to make a skin incision that seems too long than one that hinders exposure and adequate debridement. In the staged management of extremity wounds, it is imperative to realize that the goals of initial surgery are to prevent infection. This surgery should be performed with confidence and the full realization that delayed closure or skin grafts can be performed in any size wound as long as the wound is not infected. Thus, if you must err it is best to err on the side of longer incisions and larger wounds.

FASCIOTOMIES

As soon as the skin incision has been made, the underlying fascia should be slit. This fasciotomy should extend proximally and distally to the skin incision. Again, it is best to err on the side of excessive fasciotomies than to risk compression of an edematous, partially devitalized muscle by a band of tight fascia. Fasciotomies may also have to be performed in segments of the limb distal to the wound to allow arterial flow and venous return. This has been discussed in the section on pathology and must be kept in mind at all times. It may mean the survival of a limb below the knee and distal to the elbow. In these areas, collateral vessels, if they remain open, may supply enough blood to the foot or hand in spite of extensive arterial injuries. Fasciotomies are also important in restoring venous return and thus preventing tissue edema. Fasciotomies can be per-

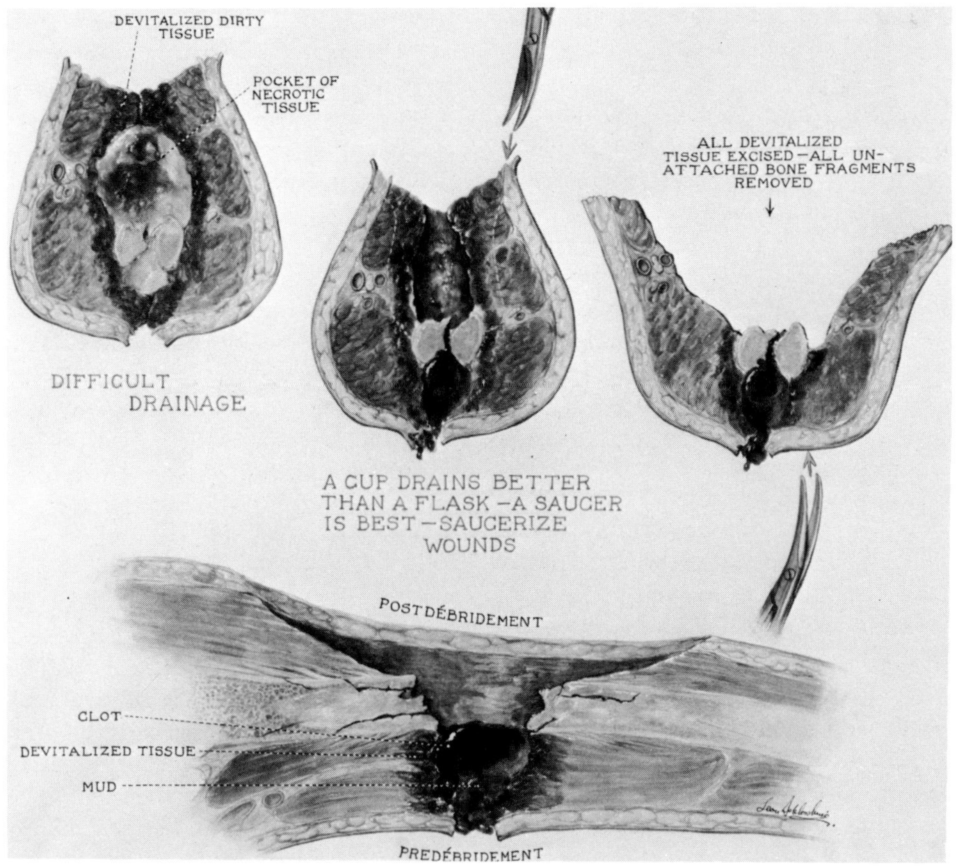

Fig. 12-4. All devitalized tissues must be excised. Even some normal muscle mass may have to be sacrificed to achieve a shallow, saucerized wound. Large, curved scissors are probably the most effective instrument for this procedure.

formed through multiple longitudinal incisions. If total fascial release is needed in the leg, it may be accomplished by resection of the entire fibular shaft. This procedure allows the release of all four compartments through one incision (anterior, lateral, superficial posterior, and deep posterior).

DEBRIDEMENT OF SOFT TISSUES

Debridement means the surgical excision of all dirty and devitalized tissue. It also implies saucerization of the wound (Fig. 12-4). As in the case of skin incisions, it is best to err on the side of excessive debridement than to risk an infection that may lead to an amputation or the loss of a life. It is not a gamble with what may be safe. In civilian life with relatively clean wounds, minimal tissue devitalization, and ideal conditions of postoperative follow-up, it may be possible to "get away" with a limited debridement, but even then it is a matter of critical judgment and extreme caution. In combat or during civil disasters, it is best to follow the principles of the staged management of wounds. This means the complete removal of all foreign bodies and devitalized tissue without any attempt to close the wound. All tags of subcutaneous fat, shredded fascia, and devitalized muscle must be excised. All muscles that are brown and friable, do not contract, and do not bleed must be excised. It may even be necessary to excise some normal muscle to obtain a shallow saucerized wound. Undermining of normal-looking tissues to excise a pocket of devitalized muscle is unacceptable. The overlying tissues must be incised (skin), split (fascia or muscle), or excised (muscle). The wound should be in the shape of a saucer.

These principles are shown in Fig. 12-4. This illustration shows the saucerized wound after debridement. It also shows how some of the normal muscle has been sacrificed to fashion the shallow wound. This sacrifice of normal muscle would not affect the ultimate function of the extremity since the involved biceps, coracobrachialis, brachialis, and triceps have already been compromised by the high-velocity missile. The task is to prevent infection in those portions of the muscle that will remain. This excision of some normal muscle avoids the risk of infection in a pocket of necrotic tissue covered by a "ledge" of normal muscle. Major nerves and blood vessels must be preserved. Shredded tendons must be trimmed or excised if the damage is extensive. Even though ultimate function and the steps of reconstruction must be kept in mind, these should not become an obsession that keeps the surgeon from doing an adequate debridement. Complete debridement and saucerization should be the only goals of the initial operation.

DEBRIDEMENT OF BONE

In general, bones should be preserved. The debate on removal of large pieces of cortical bone without soft tissue attachments exists as it did during World War II. It was our approach to remove any fragments of bone that fell from the wound with irrigation. This included bone fragments of all sizes. We did not replace pieces of bone that fell out of the wounds in the course of debridement. That seems equivalent to doing a primary bone graft in a dirty field. It was and is our impression that if bone grafting must be done, it is best done under ideal conditions after soft tissue healing. The contaminated bone ends should be cleaned with a curet and occasionally may need to be debrided with a rongeur. Maximum preservation of bone without replacement of contaminated and devitalized fragments seems to be the course of choice in avoiding osteomyelitis but preserving potential healing with skeletal stability.

INTERNAL FIXATION OF BONES

Internal fixation of fractures in large and dirty wounds should be avoided unless it seems the only way to save the injured extremity. It has many indications after uncomplicated healing of the soft tissues has occurred, but its indications are extremely rare during the initial care of the contaminated wound with extensive tissue devitalization. It is usually considered to protect the relatively delicate repair of an artery or a vein graft from a major fracture. It is extremely fortunate that most of the major fractures can be well splinted by external means and that there are very few anatomic areas in which the large vessels are right next to the bones. All fractures distal to the elbow and the knee can be immobilized with a simple splint or a cast. Most of the elbow fractures can be splinted adequately by external means. The humerus can always be strapped to the chest with or without an additional plaster splint. Most of the femoral shaft fractures are well controlled with a traction splint of the Thomas type. Only the fractures of the distal femur present a major problem. The distal fragment with its gastrocnemius attachment is pulled into flexion, and the major vessels are very close to the bone. Even simple fractures through this area can cause lacerations of normal vessels. Thus, if a vessel has been transected and repaired at the level of a fracture of the distal femur, it is very susceptible to reinjury by the bone fragments that are not properly fixed. This is the one area in which internal fixation of the fracture must be considered.

The risk of infection is well worth taking if internal fixation means a chance to save a useful extremity. Rush rods driven through the femoral condyles, a simple plate, or a blade-plate combination can be used. Alas, in high-velocity wounds, the fractures are often so comminuted that any thought of internal fixation must be abandoned. Occasionally, it may be possible to pass a Küntscher nail from the femoral shaft through the comminuted fracture fragments into the proximal tibia. This kind of fixation obviously would not provide stability of the fracture fragments, but it would immobilize them long enough to allow good healing of the vascular repairs. It may be the only solution in some of the severe popliteal injuries with unstable fractures through the femoral condyles and the distal femur. Even though we feel that there are indications for internal fixation, it must be reemphasized that these indications are rare in the presence of a dirty wound. During the first year of the Third Surgical Hospital in Vietnam (1965-1966), there were only three instances in which internal fixation of a long bone seemed indicated. All three were in fractures of the distal femur associated with major vascular injuries of that area.

The radiographs (Fig. 12-5) show the fracture and vascular injury of a Vietnam veteran who,

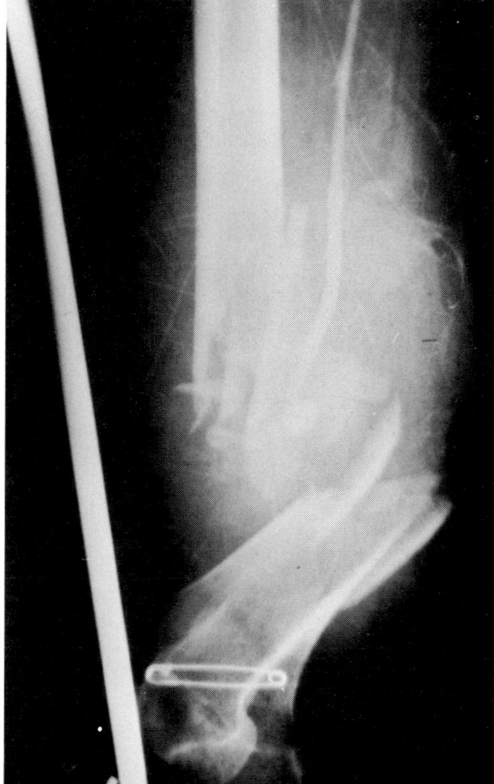

A

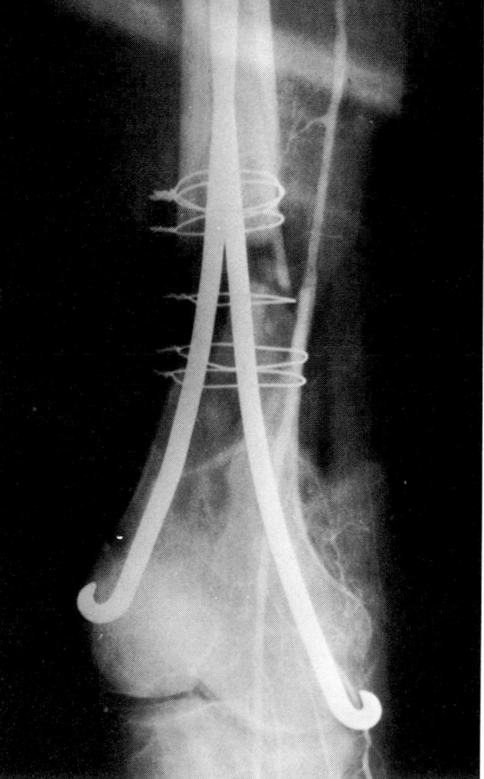

B

Fig. 12-5. A, A severe civilian injury with extensive skin wounds, massive comminution of the femur, and a complete transection of the femoral artery. The flexed position of the distal femoral fragment is typical of fractures through this area. **B,** The fracture fragments have been stabilized, and the femoral artery has been repaired. The arteriogram obtained on the operating table demonstrates the fixed bones and the patent artery. The wounds were left open and grafted at 5 days. The femur healed, and the patient regained full use of his extremity. The indications for internal fixation of open fractures are rare, but there are times when it means limb survival.

after his return from the combat zone, impaled himself on a steel fence while attempting to fly under the influence of LSD. He had a large, dirty wound, but after examination of the fracture and its associated vascular injuries, we felt it wise to use internal fixation. It was accomplished as shown with two Rush rods and circumferential wires. Following this stabilization of the bones, the femoral artery was repaired in an end-to-end fashion. The deep veins were ligated; the wounds were left open and closed with skin grafts 5 days following the initial surgery. The extremity went on to uncomplicated healing, and the patient was doing well 1 year after injury. This is a rare case, but we feel that without internal fixation, the vascular repair may well have been compromised by the many bone fragments that were moving out of control in the patient's leg. If internal fixation is to be done in the presence of vascular injuries, it should be performed before the vessels are reconstructed. It is impossible to fix a long bone without the application of significant force. This can tear a freshly repaired artery.

VASCULAR INJURIES

The success of the treatment of vascular injuries depends on early recognition, early repair, adequate wound debridement, and fasciotomies at the level of the injury and quite often in the distal muscle compartments.* Arterial repairs are indicated and feasible in those injuries proximal to the elbow and to the knee. Most of the recent series of vascular injuries show this, and the success rate for these repairs is between 80% and 90%. The worst results are consistently in the popliteal area, in which one half of the repairs seem to end in failure.[13]

If possible, the transected arteries are repaired in an end-to-end fashion,[39] but in the presence of a large devitalized segment, vein grafts are used (Fig. 12-3). These grafts should be taken from the superficial system of another extremity. If a major artery has been transected or injured, it is likely that the deep veins that run with the arteries are damaged. By taking a superficial vein from the same extremity, the surgeon may be depriving the extremity of its only effective venous channel. The vein graft must be placed with its valves in a reversed position to allow the peripheral flow of the arterial blood. As stated previously, the success of the repairs depends on adequate debridement. Infection is one of the main causes of failure in vascular repairs, and debridement of dirty, devitalized tissue is the best way to prevent infection.

After the repair has been completed, the blood vessel should be covered by soft tissues. This may be difficult at times, but usually it is possible to mobilize some fascia or viable muscle to cover the large vessels (Fig. 12-6). A skin flap can be used as long as large portions of the wound are left open for drainage. If nothing is available, a moist dressing may be the last resort. Large veins should also be repaired,[20,21] especially in popliteal injuries and in extremities in which it is obvious that there is extensive damage to both the deep and superficial systems. Following repair of the vessels, the extremity should be splinted or casted for adequate immobilization. In very rare instances, internal fixation of a concomitant fracture is also indicated. (See previous section.)

JOINT INJURIES

All joint injuries should be carefully explored, debrided, and irrigated. The principles of debridement outlined for soft tissue wounds and bones also apply to the joints. If there is any suspicion that there has been penetration of a joint by a missile or a foreign body, this joint should be explored. If possible, this should be done through standard incisions with minor modifications dictated by the wound location. After thorough exploration, debridement, and irrigation of the joint, the synovium should be closed with loose interrupted catgut sutures. The capsule, muscles, and skin should be left open. These principles are specifically designed for the knee but apply whenever possible to all other joints. Primary fusions or major reconstructions have no place in the early management of these injuries. Occasionally internal fixation (with K wires, screws, or staples) can be considered if this procedure restores a major articular fragment to its normal position. Again, it must be emphasized that this must be done with extreme care in any wound with gross contamination.

NERVE INJURIES

In major wounds of the extremities, there are no indications for primary nerve repair.[26] The extent of nerve injury and of the local damage

*See references 1, 12, 13, 20, 21, 37, and 39.

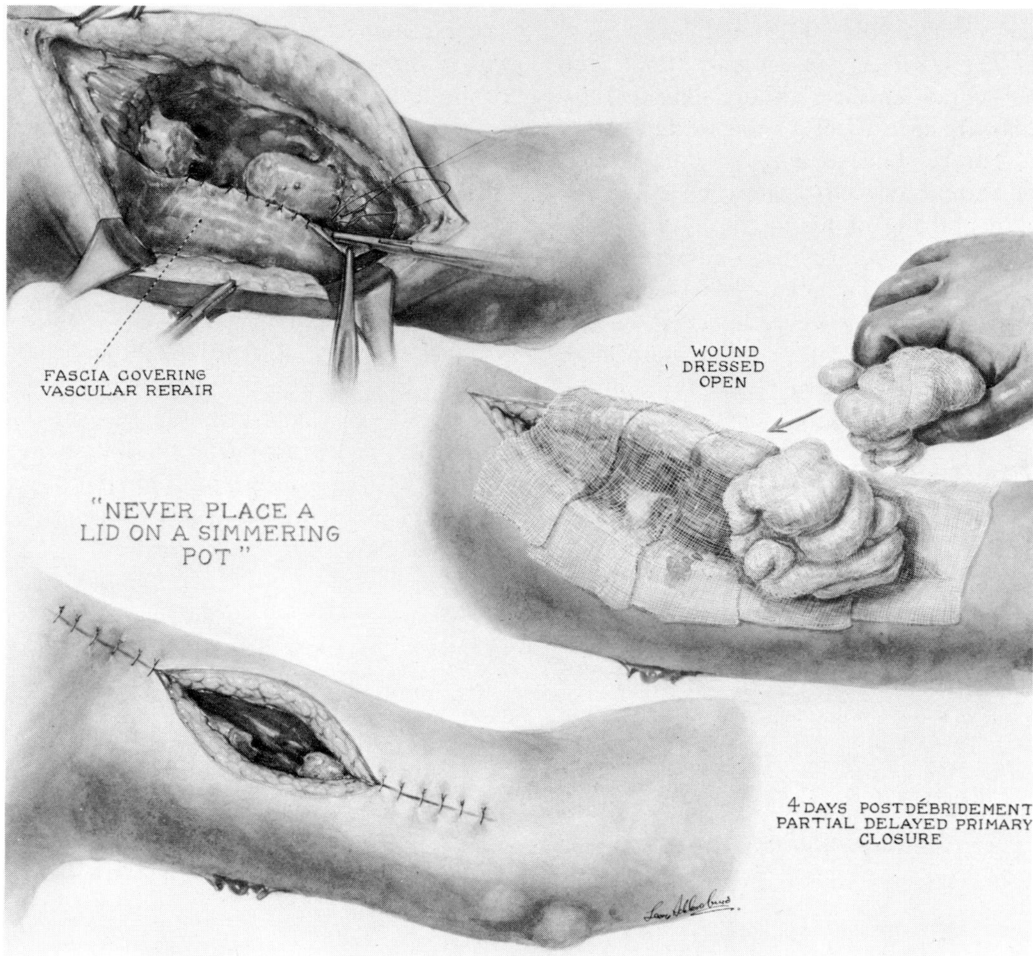

Fig. 12-6. Large vessels and nerves should be covered by soft tissues prior to the open dressing of the wound with fine mesh gauze and loose fluffs. Primary delayed closure can be performed after 4 days if there is enough skin and if the wound is clean. If the wound is large, if closure is under tension, and if there is any fear of infection, the wound should remain open.

cannot be estimated during the initial debridement. There is little time to do a meticulous repair even if it is a "clean" transection. Nerves should not be debrided even though they may look devitalized. Dirt should be removed by irrigation and with a fine, smooth forceps. After this cleansing, the nerve ends should be left where they lie. If possible, they should be covered with some soft tissue to avoid desiccation by a dressing. It is not necessary to tag them since all secondary explorations, repairs, and grafts will start by identification of the nerve in its normal tissues, both proximally and distally to the site of the wound. These secondary procedures should be performed only after there has been complete soft tissue healing. During the initial operation, the major nerves passing through the wound site should be identified, protected, cleaned but not debrided, covered by soft tissue, and left for late reconstruction.

DRESSINGS OF WOUNDS

After adequate debridement, the wound should have a saucerized appearance (Fig. 12-4). Its deepest portion should be fully visible. Only after this type of debridement has been accomplished should a dressing be applied. The dressing should not be a "plug" to contain a hematoma. It should not be a "pack" to control hemorrhage (as in the nose or the uterus). A layer of fine mesh gauze (Fig. 12-6) is placed over the surface of the shallow wound. The wound is then filled with very loose gauze fluffs (Fig. 12-6) to absorb any blood and serum from the raw surfaces of the debrided tissues. The fluffs are covered by bandages that gently compress the limb. The dressing should be left on until the patient is ready for delayed primary closure or skin grafting of his wound.[3,6] It should not be changed and contaminated under the semiclean conditions of the average ward. The indications for early dressing change are massive hemorrhage (not controlled by gentle compression), high fever, cellulitis of the extremity, purulent drainage, and an obviously "infected" odor.

IMMOBILIZATION OF EXTREMITIES

Rest and immobilization have been recognized since Hippocrates as important factors in patient care. After the adequately debrided wound has been dressed, the extremity must be immobilized. Immobilization is imperative in the presence of fractures and multiple wounds, but it must also be considered in lesser injuries of the skin and soft tissues. Immobilization is accomplished by splints or casts (Fig. 12-7). If the injury is distal to the knee or elbow, a long leg or long arm cast is an excellent form of immobilization. The application of a cast in a major wound should be followed immediately by the univalving of that cast (Fig. 12-7). This should be done in the operating room or at the very latest in the recovery area. There are those who advocate the bivalving of a cast as the only means to prevent and treat extremity swelling, inadequate venous return, arterial insufficiency, and nerve compression.

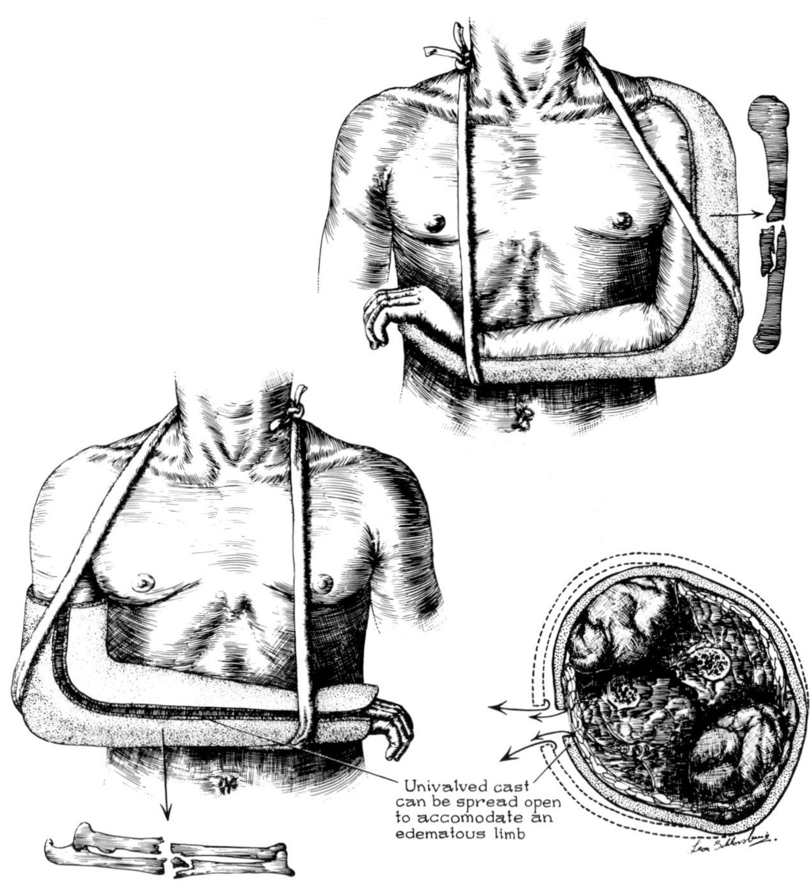

Fig. 12-7. Immobilization of the injured extremities is extremely important. The variety of splints and casts that can be used for this purpose taxes the imagination. Only two types of devices are shown. All casts must be univalved as shown. The plaster, the padding of the cast, and all strands of dressing must be cut to accommodate an edematous limb.

In our experience, a single longitudinal cut extending from one end of the cast to the other is sufficient if all the layers of the cast, cast padding, and dressing are transected. This is accomplished by removing a ½″ strip of plaster extending the entire length of the cast. The removal of this plaster strip allows the easy insertion of scissors for the cutting of all padding and circumferential dressings. The plaster cut can be placed in various positions on the cast and should avoid (if at all possible) major wounds. After the cast has been univalved in this fashion, it should be possible to pass a finger over the patient's skin without touching any residual bands of dressing, cast padding, or any other material. If swelling occurs, it is possible to spread the cast at will without losing its stability and its immobilizing properties (Fig. 12-7). This is essential in a combat situation in which the patient may be in transit along the chain of evacuation. It is equally important in the civilian situation in which, during the long hours of the night, the patient's extremity may be under the observation of an inexperienced nurse.

In fractures of the humerus and femur, a simple cast of the extremity is not sufficient. The humerus can be splinted against the chest with a sling and swathe or Velpeau dressing. These can be supplemented by a molded splint that gives additional and rigid support to the humerus. This splint can be hooked over the shoulder for further immobilization of the extremity (Fig. 12-7). The femur can be splinted in traction with a Thomas splint. Strips of adhesive from the knee to the ankle can be attached in traction to the foot piece. The entire leg and splint are then incorporated in plaster or heavy circumferential bandages for additional support and immobilization (Tobruk splint). A spica cast is usually unacceptable because of the length of time that it takes to apply and the difficulties encountered in transporting a patient with such a device. It is impossible in helicopters with narrow doors and narrow stretchers.

AMPUTATIONS

Even under the most ideal conditions, an amputation can turn into a surgical disaster through such complications as edema, wound infection, and skin sloughs. Amputations of extremities that are severely traumatized and grossly contaminated are extremely risky. They should be approached with the greatest of care. The principles of debridement, open dressing, delayed closure, and late reconstruction apply in all of these cases. It is our experience that the open circular amputation[14] is fast and safe. It avoids the risk of sloughing and infected skin flaps. Even in a civilian situation these risks are not worth taking. It is difficult to do an adequate skin prep with a dirty stump distal to the level of the elective incisions. It is much safer to do a good amputation in the presence of a healed scar, or a skin graft distal to the operative site.

The open circular amputation must be performed at the lowest possible level. As much skin as possible should be preserved. The incision should be circular down to the fascia. The skin and subcutaneous tissues should be stripped from the fascia for a short distance (1″ to 1½″) proximal to the incision. The skin sleeve should then be allowed to retract, and the fascia should be cut at this level (Fig. 12-8, *A*). It should be handled like the skin, and after it has retracted, the muscles should be cut at the retracted fascial level. The bone is cut at the level of the retracted muscles (Fig. 12-8, *B*). All of the major vessels are ligated. The nerves are pulled down and transected. They retract into the muscle mass. The stump, if it is cut in this manner, will present a loose sleeve of skin that easily pulls over the muscles of the wound. It should be placed in traction with a stockinette fixed to the very edge of the amputation (Fig. 12-8, *C*). A spreader should also be used to allow for traction in line with the skin sleeve of the amputated extremity.

The skin can now be kept in traction until it becomes fixed over the stump and heals it over without any further procedures. Skin traction can be discontinued at the end of several weeks, and the granulating surface that remains can be covered with a skin graft. If there is much loose skin, a delayed closure of the wound can also be done. If the amputation is performed in this open circular manner, it should lead to early healing without infection. If the amputation is done without regard for tissue retraction, the result is a stump with the naked bone protruding through a stump of retracted muscles and skin (Fig. 12-8, *D*).

The word guillotine implies the ablation of an extremity in one swift motion of steel passing through all the tissues at the same level. Fig. 12-8, *D* shows this and shows the poor result of this method. It is probably impossible to strike "guillotine amputation" from the surgical lexicon, but an effort

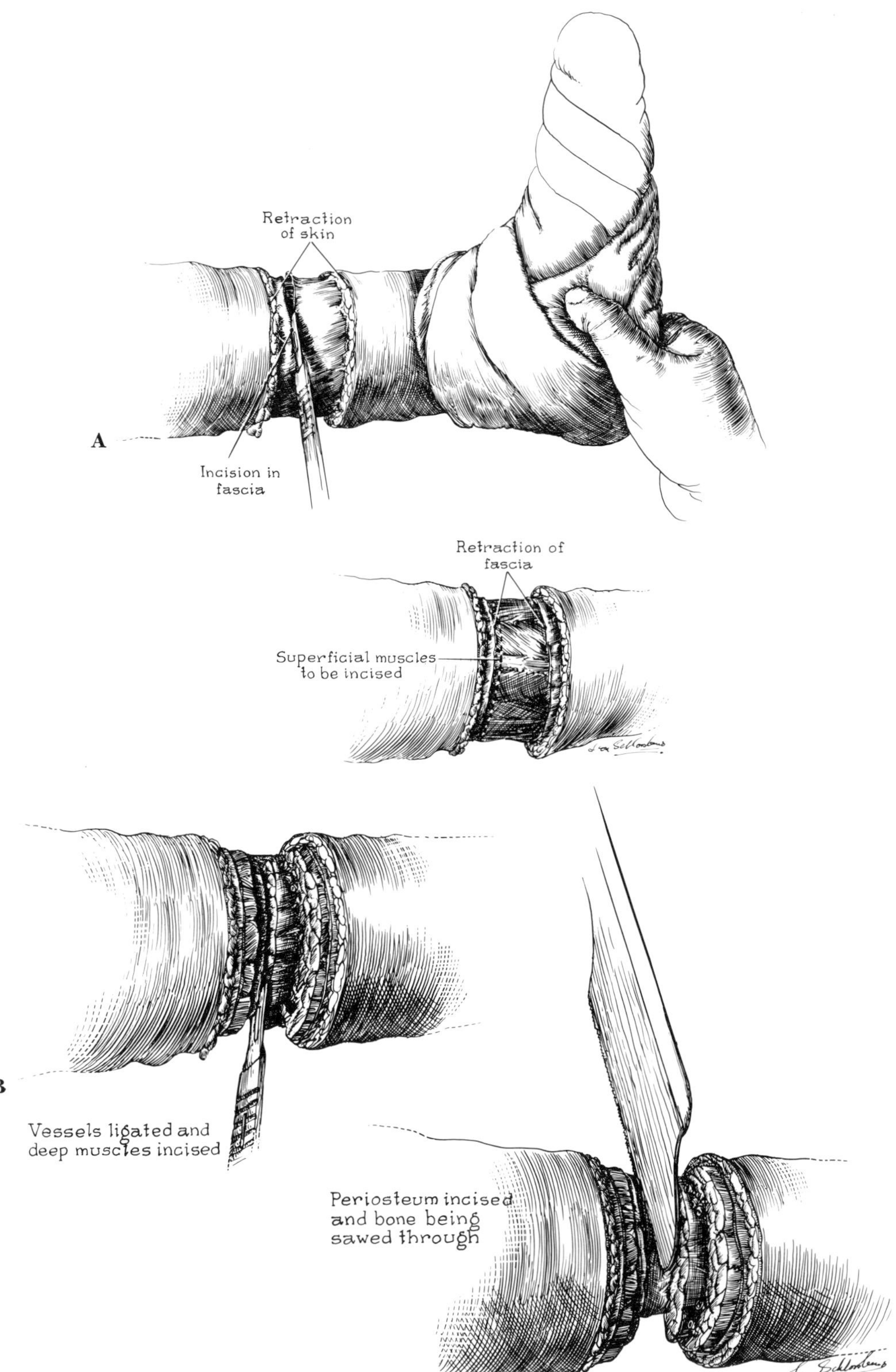

Fig. 12-8. A, The open circular amputation means that every layer of skin, fascia, and muscle is freed and allowed to retract prior to the transection of the next layer. This assures a sleeve of skin that will cover the stump. **B,** After all the soft tissues have been transected and allowed to retract, the amputation is completed by sawing the bone.

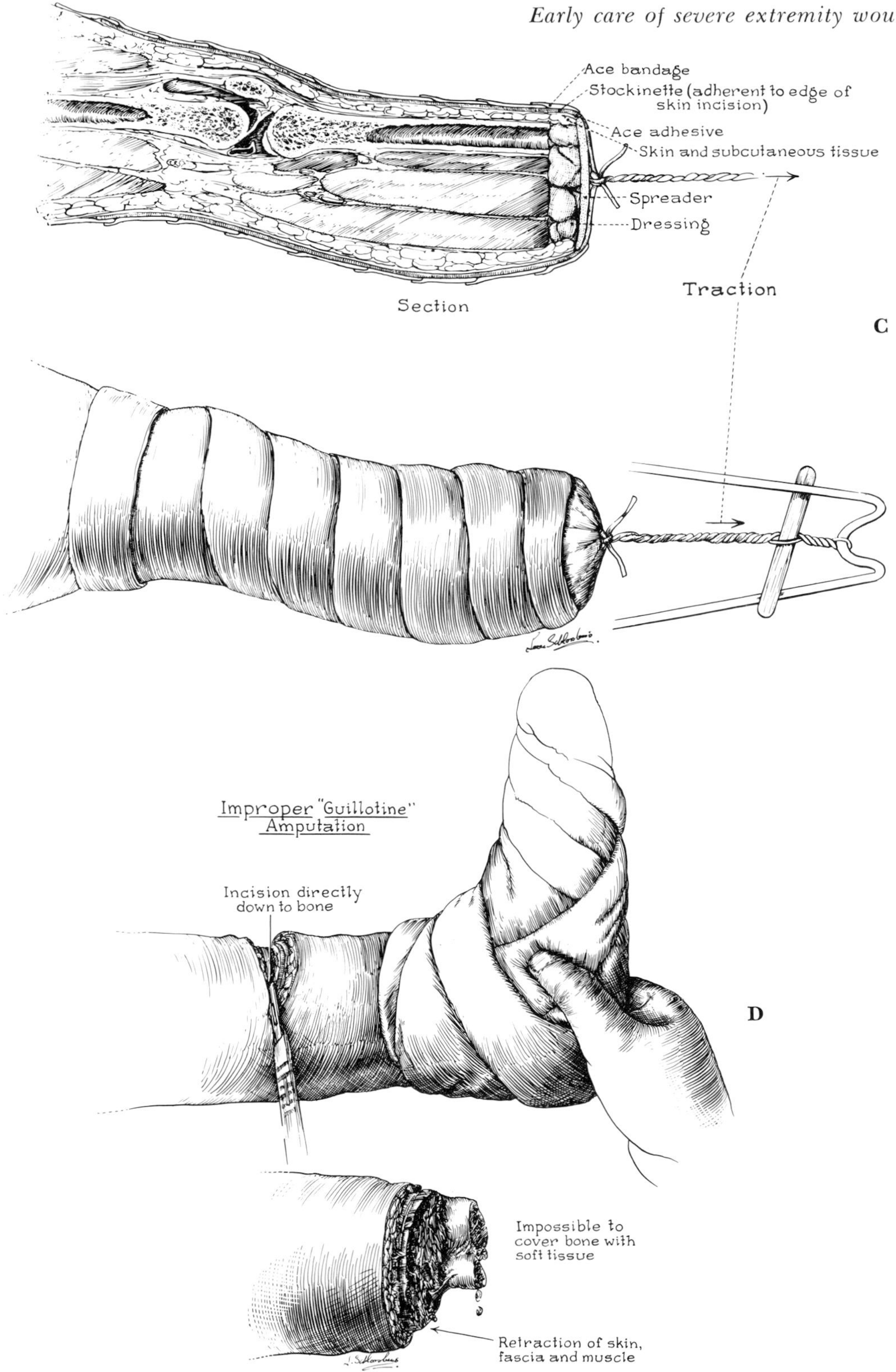

Fig. 12-8, cont'd. C, Skin traction is the final essential step of the open circular amputation. The stockinette must be fixed down to the skin edge, and a spreader assures evenly distributed traction without compression of the stump. **D,** A guillotine amputation without proper attention to sequential tissue retraction should not be done. The end result is bony stump without muscle and skin coverage.

should be made to teach the proper technique of the open circular amputation and its postoperative management in skin traction. This latter point cannot be neglected. The stump must remain in traction at all times. If the patient is in bed, this can be accomplished by attaching the stockinette to a rope with pulley and weight. If the patient is moved, the extremity can be placed on a splint with the stockinette in traction, as shown in Fig. 12-8, *C*. The skin traction should not be removed until there has been solid fixation of the skin to the distal stump. The open circular amputation provides the safest way of handling a dirty devitalized extremity in its initial phases. It is also the safest way to a carefully planned revision of a well-healed stump during the reconstructive phase of total rehabilitation.

POSTOPERATIVE WOUND CARE, CLOSURE, AND SKIN GRAFTS

As outlined in the section on wound dressings, there are few indications for frequent exposure of the debrided area. The dressing applied in the operating room should stay on the patient's extremity until 4 to 6 days after surgery. At that time, the patient should be taken to the operating room for an inspection of the debrided area. It is a constance source of amazement to see how little edema and inflammation there is in a wound that has been adequately debrided. After the old blood has been washed away with saline, the skin edges look clean, and the muscles are red with early granulations. If that is not the case, a secondary debridement must be performed. At this time it is much more obvious what skin and which muscles must be debrided. The tissues are no longer devitalized —they are necrotic.

The gross appearance of the dead muscles is now an obvious brown or a very dark red. There is no fresh blood in the tissues. Once more the debridement must be down to normal muscle. The wound should be left open. If at the time of wound inspection it is clean and if the skin edges can be approximated without tension, a closure of the wound can be done. Usually it is possible to close the wound and obliterate dead space with large interrupted sutures through the skin alone. These sutures are placed loosely and wide apart to prevent the accumulation of hematomas, seromas, and tissue debris. We prefer this technique to the insertion of an ordinary drain. If a drain must be used, we favor the suction irrigation systems with a continuous flow of antibiotics through the closed wound.

Occasionally it may be impossible to close the entire wound, but a few sutures at each end of the incision can decrease its size without compromising drainage (Fig. 12-6). If there is any worry about contamination, hematoma accumulation, insufficient skin or wound depth, the safest approach is to redress the wound and to apply a split-thickness skin graft at a later time. Split-thickness grafts with or without multiple perforations (or meshing) have been advocated at the time of initial debridement and can be performed weeks after injury.[35,36,43] In our experience they seem to be the most successful at 7 to 10 days after the initial surgery (Fig. 12-9). There are many ways to fix these grafts and to handle them postoperatively. Our own preference is to tack them down with a few sutures and to treat them open without a postoperative dressing. The extremity must be splinted during this procedure, but by allowing continuous inspection of the graft it is possible to prevent accumulation of fluid underneath the graft.

The greatest advantage of the split-thickness grafts is that they allow coverage of very large wounds and do not mask infections. If there is any infection, it will push away the graft and drain without abscess formation. If the tissues have been closed, the infection can be missed in its early phases, and by the time it is discovered it may have formed an abscess, it may have spread along the fascial planes (the "path of least resistance"), and the patient may have a septicemia with all its secondary complications. At this point, it should be mentioned that excellent results can also be obtained in some debrided wounds by simply allowing them to heal without surgical closure or skin grafts. This was one of the great contributions of Dr. Orr during World War I and has recently been vindicated by Dr. Brown.[3]

LATE CARE OF WOUNDS

After skin closure has been obtained, the patient can be considered for any reconstructive surgery that seems indicated. It may take from 3 to 6 months before all soft tissues have healed to the point where such procedures as bone grafts, nerve repairs, and tendon transfers can be done (Fig. 12-10). An exact time cannot be given. It depends

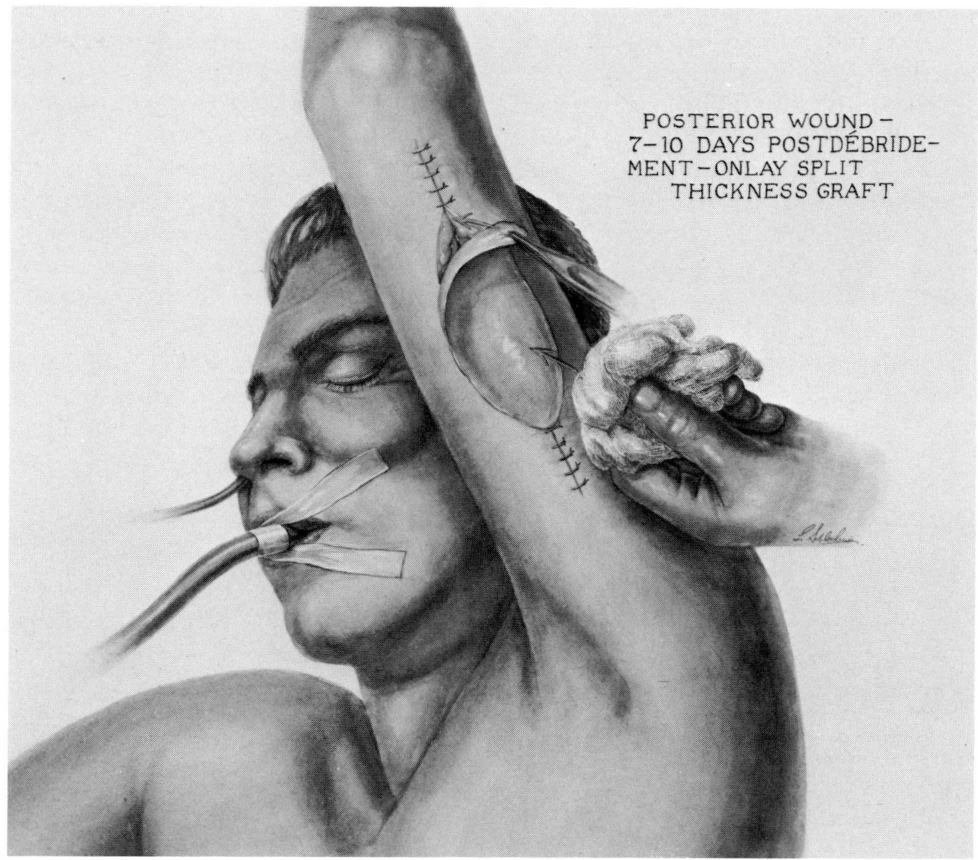

Fig. 12-9. Split-thickness skin grafts are the safest way to obtain early wound coverage. It is the method of choice in all large wounds.

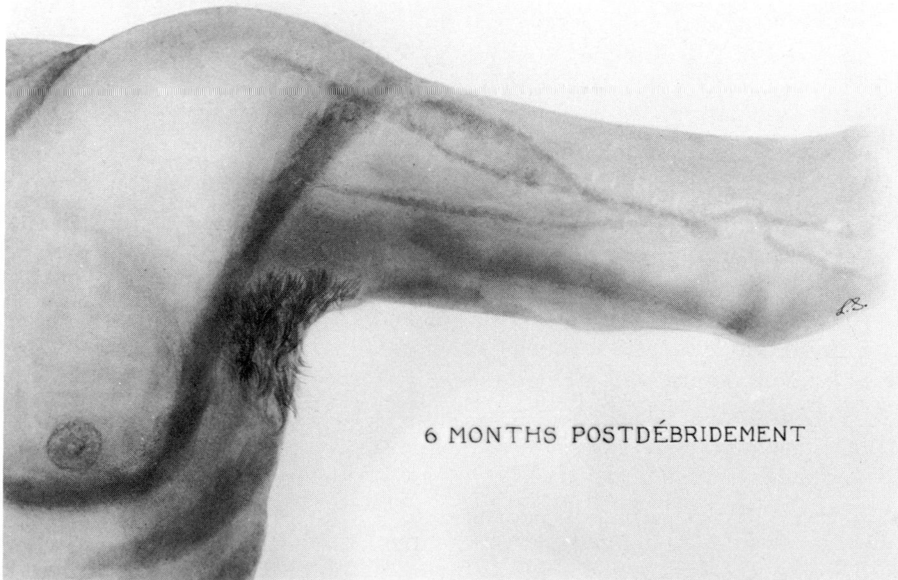

Fig. 12-10. There must be complete soft tissue healing before such reconstructive procedures as nerve repairs, bone grafts, and tendon transfers can be considered with safety.

on the location of the wound, the size of the wound, and such other problems as infection, vascular injury, and fractures. It depends on the appearance of the scar and its underlying tissues. If induration, swelling, and redness have subsided rapidly, if the tissues are soft and the skin is normal in appearance, the area may be ready for secondary procedures before 3 months. It is a matter of careful clinical judgment.

Prior to bone, tendon, and nerve work, the patient's scars may need revision, and split-thickness grafts may have to be replaced by full-thickness pedicles. It may take years to perform all the indicated procedures. During the months of waiting, all efforts should also be directed at maintaining the patient's muscle function and joint motion. The patient cannot be left in a cast without thought for function. All the forms of extremity immobilization in wounds with complex reconstructive problems should be planned to allow maximum motion of all joints and muscles. Skeletal traction provides the best opportunity for this type of approach, but, if possible, the patients should be ambulated. The patient's general adjustment to his injury must also be considered. Psychiatric support can be of help. Social and economic problems should be resolved. We should never forget the patient.

WAR WOUNDS VERSUS CIVILIAN WOUNDS

The principles of debridement, open dressing, and delayed closure are fairly well established in the care of the wounded in a combat (military) situation. The organization of hospitals is also designed for the staged management of all the major wounds. It is the continuous topic of conversation among military surgeons who are continuously faced with the large and dirty extremity wounds seen in a combat situation. In a civilian hospital, these wounds are less common, but if we consider the entire country, we find that they represent a major health hazard. The individual surgeon sees relatively few of these wounds, and when he gets them, he tends to take risks in their management. He knows that a single procedure will minimize the patient's hospitalization. He is also familiar with the difficulties of scheduling a dressing change or skin graft in the midst of an elective surgical schedule that has been arranged several months before.

In the face of all these factors, it is easy to rationalize a primary closure. The other conditions that predispose a wound to complications consist of delays in transportation, delays in the emergency room, and delays with the operating room. With hospitals and surgeons working at full capacity, there is no good time for an emergency. Such a shortage of time can lead to inadequate skin preparation and minimal debridement. If these errors are compounded by primary skin closure, the risk of complications is high. In civilian disasters (tornadoes, floods, collapsing buildings), the wounds should never be closed—a debridement is the only indicated procedure. The management of large and dirty civilian wounds should be patterned after military principles—they should be debrided and left open. Skin closure or coverage should be performed 4 to 10 days following initial surgery. Reconstructive procedures should be considered only after adequate wound healing has been obtained.

CONCLUSION

The early care of major extremity wounds should be aimed at the prevention of surgical disasters. Wound infection is the worst of the complications because it not only compromises the patient's limb, but it also may threaten his life. Our military experience has taught us that debridement with delayed wound closure has a very low incidence of complications. It should not be forgotten in the management of similar civilian wounds.

REFERENCES

1. Bizer, L.: Peripheral vascular injuries in the Vietnam war, Arch. Surg. **98**:165, 1969.
2. Brav, E. A., Hughes, C. W., and McDonald, W. F.: The importance of proper early management of wounds of the extremities. Instructional course lectures of the American Academy of Orthopaedic Surgeons, Ann Arbor, Mich., 1955, J. W. Edwards, Publisher, Inc., vol. 12.
3. Brown, P. W., and Urban, J. G.: Early weight-bearing treatment of open fractures of the tibia, J. Bone Joint Surg. **51A**:59, 1969.
4. Burkhalter, W. E., Butler, B., Metz, W., and Omer, G.: Experiences with delayed primary closure of war wounds of the hand in Vietnam, J. Bone Joint Surg. **50A**:945, 1968.
5. Butler, B., Jr.: Initial management of hand wounds, Milit. Med. **134**:1, 1969.
6. Davis, G. L.: The infrequent dressing change. Procedure in association with primary delayed closure of compound extremity wounds of war, Arch. Surg. **96**:795, 1968.
7. DeMuth, W. E., Jr.: Bullet velocity and design as

determinants of wounding capability. An experimental study, J. Trauma **6**:222, 1966.

8. DeMuth, W. E., Jr.: Bullet velocity as applied to military rifle wounding capacity, J. Trauma **9**:27, 1969.
9. DeMuth, W. E., Jr., and Smith, J. M.: High velocity bullet wounds of muscle and bone: The basis of rational early treatment, J. Trauma **6**:744, 1966.
10. Dziemian, A. J., Mendelson, J. A., and Lindsey, D.: Comparison of the wounding characteristics of some commonly encountered bullets, J. Trauma **1**:341, 1961.
11. Eiseman, B.: Combat casualty management, J. Trauma **7**:53, 1967.
12. Fisher, G. W.: Acute arterial injuries treated by the United States Army Medical Service in Vietnam, 1965-1966, J. Trauma **7**:844, 1967.
13. Gorman, J. F.: Combat arterial trauma. Analysis of 106 limb-threatening injuries, Arch. Surg. **98**:160, 1969.
14. Hampton, O.: Wounds of the extremities in military surgery, St. Louis, 1951, The C. V. Mosby Co.
15. Hampton, O. P., Jr.: The indications for debridement of gun shot (bullet) wounds of the extremities in civilian practice, J. Trauma **1**:368, 1961.
16. Hampton, O. P., Jr.: Management of open fractures and open wounds of joints. Editorial, J. Trauma **8**:475, 1968.
17. Hardaway, R. M.: Clinical management of shock, Milit. Med. **134**:643, 1969.
18. Heaton, L. D., et al.: Military surgical practices of the U. S. Army in Vietnam, Curr. Probl. Surg., 1-59, November, 1966.
19. Heisterkamp, C., et al.: Topical antibiotics in war wounds: a re-evaluation, Milit. Med. **134**:13, 1969.
20. Hewitt, R. L.: Technical considerations in acute military vascular injuries of the extremities, Milit. Med. **134**:617, 1969.
21. Hewitt, R. L., Collins, D. J., and Jamit, H. F.: Arterial injuries at a surgical hospital in Vietnam, Arch. Surg. **98**:313, 1969.
22. Jackson, F. E.: Wounding agents in Vietnam, Milit. Med. **133**:904, 1968.
23. Jones, E. L., Peters, A. F., and Gasior, R. M.: Early management of battle casualties in Vietnam, Arch. Surg. **97**:1, 1968.
24. Kadis, L. B., et al.: Clinical considerations in the anesthetic management of Vietnam casualties, Arch. Surg. **97**:16, 1968.
25. Kovaric, J. J., et al.: Bacterial flora of one hundred and twelve combat wounds, Milit. Med. **133**:622, 1968.
26. Leaver, R. C.: Neurosurgery in Vietnam 1967-1968, Milit. Med. **134**:604, 1969.
27. Matsumoto, T., and Dobek, A. S.: Systemic antibiotic(s) in contaminated crush wound, Arch. Surg. **99**:103, 1969.
28. Matsumoto, T., et al.: Antibiotic topical spray in a simulated combat wound, Arch. Surg. **96**:786, 1968.
29. Matsumoto, T., et al.: Combat surgery in communication zone. I. War wound and bacteriology (preliminary report), Milit. Med. **134**:655, 1969.
30. Mendelson, J. A., and Glover, J. L.: Sphere and shell fragment wounds of soft tissues: experimental study, J. Trauma **7**:889, 1967.
31. Metz, C. W., Jr., and Barclay, W. A.: Management of war wounds in the continental United States, Arch. Surg. **97**:707, 1968.
32. Morgan, M. M., Spencer, A. D., and Hershey, F. B.: Debridement of civilian gunshot wounds of soft tissue, J. Trauma **1**:354, 1961.
33. NATO handbook on emergency war surgery, United States Government Printing Office, 1958.
34. Noyes, H. E., et al.: Delayed topical antimicrobials as adjuncts to systemic antibiotic therapy of war wounds: bacteriologic studies, Milit. Med. **132**:461, 1967.
35. Omer, G. E., Moll, J. H., and Bacon, W. L.: Combined fractures of the femur and tibia in a single extremity. Analytical study of cases at Brooke General Hospital 1961 to 1967, J. Trauma **8**:1026, 1968.
36. Pollock, W. J., and Parkes, J. C.: Open skin grafting of war wounds, J. Bone Joint Surg. **51A**:926, 1969.
37. Rich, N. M.: Vietnam missile wounds evaluated in 750 patients, Milit. Med. **133**:9, 1968.
38. Rich, N. M., Johnson, E. V., and Dimond, F. C., Jr.: Wounding power of missiles used in the Republic of Vietnam, J.A.M.A. **199**:157, 1967.
39. Rich, N. M., Manion, W. C., and Hughes, C. W.: Surgical and pathological evaluation of vascular injuries in Vietnam, J. Trauma **9**:279, 1969.
40. Robson, M. C., and Heggers, J. P.: Bacterial quantification of open wounds, Milit. Med. **134**:19, 1969.
41. Seidenstein, M., Newman, A., and Tanski, E. V.: Some clinical factors involved in the healing of war wounds, Arch. Surg. **96**:176, 1968.
42. Shepard, G. H., Rich, N. M., and Dimond, F. C., Jr.: Punji stick wounds: experience with 342 wounds in 324 patients in Vietnam, Ann. Surg. **166**:902, 1967.
43. Shuck, J. M., Pruitt, B. A., and Moncrief, J. A.: Hemograft skin for wound coverage. A study in versatility, Arch. Surg. **98**:472, 1968.
44. Trueblood, H. W., Nelsen, J. S., and Oberhelman, H. A., Jr.: The effect of acute anemia and iron deficiency anemia on wound healing, Arch. Surg. **99**:113, 1969.
45. Trueta, J.: Principles and practice of war surgery, St. Louis, 1943, The C. V. Mosby Co.
46. Ziperman, H. H.: The management of soft tissue missile wounds in war and peace, J. Trauma **1**:361, 1961.

Chapter 13

The articular cartilages: a review*

HENRY J. MANKIN, M.D.
New York, New York

INTRODUCTION

The articular cartilages comprise a unique and extraordinary body tissue, whose structural, biochemical, and metabolic characteristics were, until recent years, virtually unexplored. The accessibility of the joints to investigation and the striking gross appearance of the tissue attracted the attention of early anatomists, and the "hyaline" cartilages were distinguished many centuries ago. With the introduction of the microscope, the unique histologic appearance of the tissue was established, and cartilage was known to have a high matrix to cell ratio,[59,63] peculiar staining characteristics,[55,59,63] no blood, nerve, or lymphatic supply,[55,59,98] and almost no potential for repair[63,98] long before the turn of the century.

Paradoxically, however, some of the same characteristics that made the tissue attractive to scientists and accessible to study by gross and microscopic techniques created enormous problems when the more sophisticated approaches of modern biochemistry and metabolism were attempted. The extraordinarily low cell population and the polyanionic character of the matrix made it difficult to apply standard histochemical stains or perform metabolic studies, and the complexity of the matrix components made separation and identification impossible by standard biochemical techniques. Articular cartilage is difficult to degrade physically, and the water insolubility of the collagen fraction and marked viscosity and hydrophilic character of the protein polysaccharides discouraged chemists and led them to seek answers to their questions in tissues that more readily yielded to their methods.

In the last three decades, a small group of intrepid scientists have worked tirelessly at development of new techniques and applications of old ones to shed light on this mysterious and enigmatic tissue. The pieces of the puzzle are falling into place, and new concepts have emerged in the last ten years regarding the structure, biochemistry, and metabolism. This article will attempt to review the current state of knowledge about the hyaline articular cartilages but, in a sense, is a testimonial to the vigor and consummate skill of investigators such as Meyer, Schubert, Dorfman, Chrisman, Mathews, Dziewiatkowski, Eichelberger, Muir, MacConnaill, and the Silberbergs. This review is dedicated to them.

STRUCTURE OF ARTICULAR CARTILAGE

One of the most remarkable characteristics of articular cartilage is the structural preponderance of the extracellular materials.[10,34] The chondrocytes are sparse, even in very young cartilage,[10,79,116] and most of the mass consists of the macromolecular proteinaceous matrix (Figs. 13-1 and 13-2). A number of investigators have performed cell counts or DNA determinations, and these have varied considerably depending on the species, the anatomic site, the technique of study, and the age of the animal.* Such a study, performed in rabbits of various ages, is illustrated in Fig. 13-11. It can be seen that in the adult animal the counts are in the range of 2×10^5 cells/mm.^{3}, considerably less than the population density of many other tissues.

*Supported in part by U.S. Public Health Service Research Grant #AM 11382-03 from the National Institute of Arthritis and Metabolic Diseases.

*See references 77, 79, 92, 107, 116, and 123.

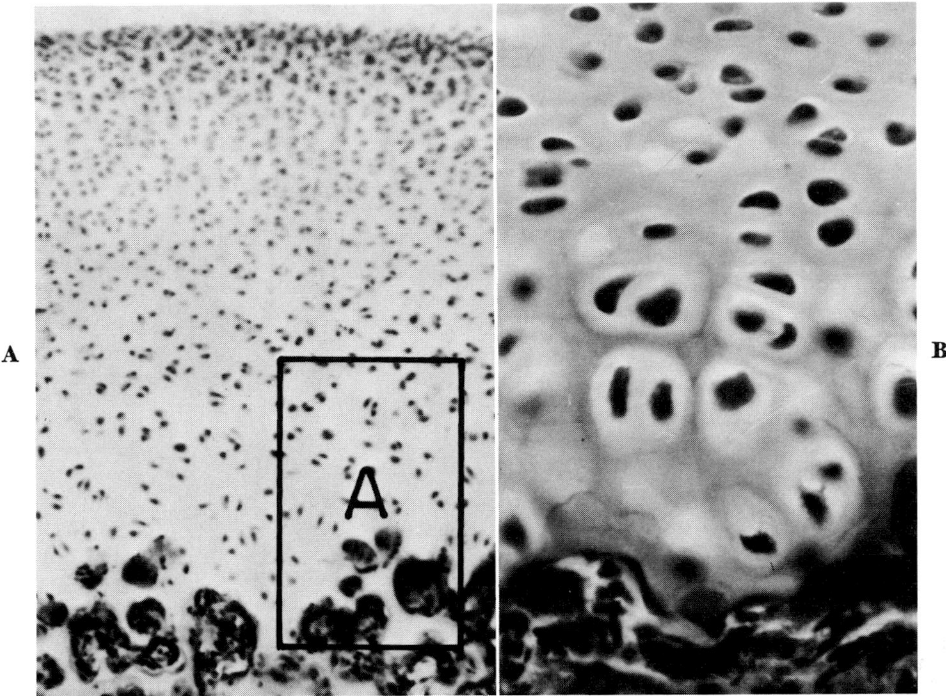

Fig. 13-1. Photomicrographs of the articular cartilage from the distal femur of an immature rabbit (aged 2 months). Note the relatively cellular pattern and the absence of a well-developed basilar calcified zone. Vascular buds are seen to "invade" from the metaphysis, **A.** Columnar arrangement of the cells in the basal area, **B,** and the pattern of vascular invasion suggest that the lowermost part of the articular cartilage is in reality a "micro"epiphyseal plate for endochondral ossification of the underlying nucleus of the bony epiphysis. (×100; ×430.) (From Mankin, H. J.: Anat. Rec. **145:**73, 1963.)

Early microscopists defined four distinct zones in adult cartilaginous tissues, and noted differences not only in the spatial arrangement but also in the cellular morphology within the zones. The classical description of these zones includes: a *tangential or gliding zone* consisting of flattened or markedly ovoid cells lying adjacent to the surface with the long axis of the cells parallel to the articular margin; a *transitional or intermediate zone* in which the cells are plump and ovoid with a more or less random orientation; a *radial zone,* in which the cells tend to be small, round, and basophilic and arranged in short, irregular columns perpendicular to the joint surface; and a *calcified zone,* in which small irregular cells with pyknotic nuclei lie in lacunar spaces totally surrounded by massive incrustations of apatitic calcium salts (Fig. 13-3). This last zone, the calcified layer, is separated from those above by a thin, wavy, bluish line (on hematoxylin and eosin stain), which was designated as the "tidemark" by Collins[27] (Fig. 13-4). The exact nature of this basophilic area at the margin of the calcification is unknown, but speculation ranges from an artifact of preparation associated with the exposed surface of the calcium salts to a local increase in concentration of acid mucopolysaccharides.[44]

Cartilage from mature animals is totally avascular, aneural, and alymphatic.[10] Cartilage canals are described in immature animals and presumably convey blood vessels through the cartilage to the epiphyseal nucleus, but probably provide little if any nutrient material to the chondrocytes.[10] The surface of the cartilage is not covered by a perichondrium in adult animals, nor has a synovial layer or reflection been seen.[34,93,110,126] Electron microscopic studies have failed to show any form of a limiting membrane,[90,126] but a zone of tightly packed tangentially arranged bundles of collagen fibers running parallel and slightly subjacent to

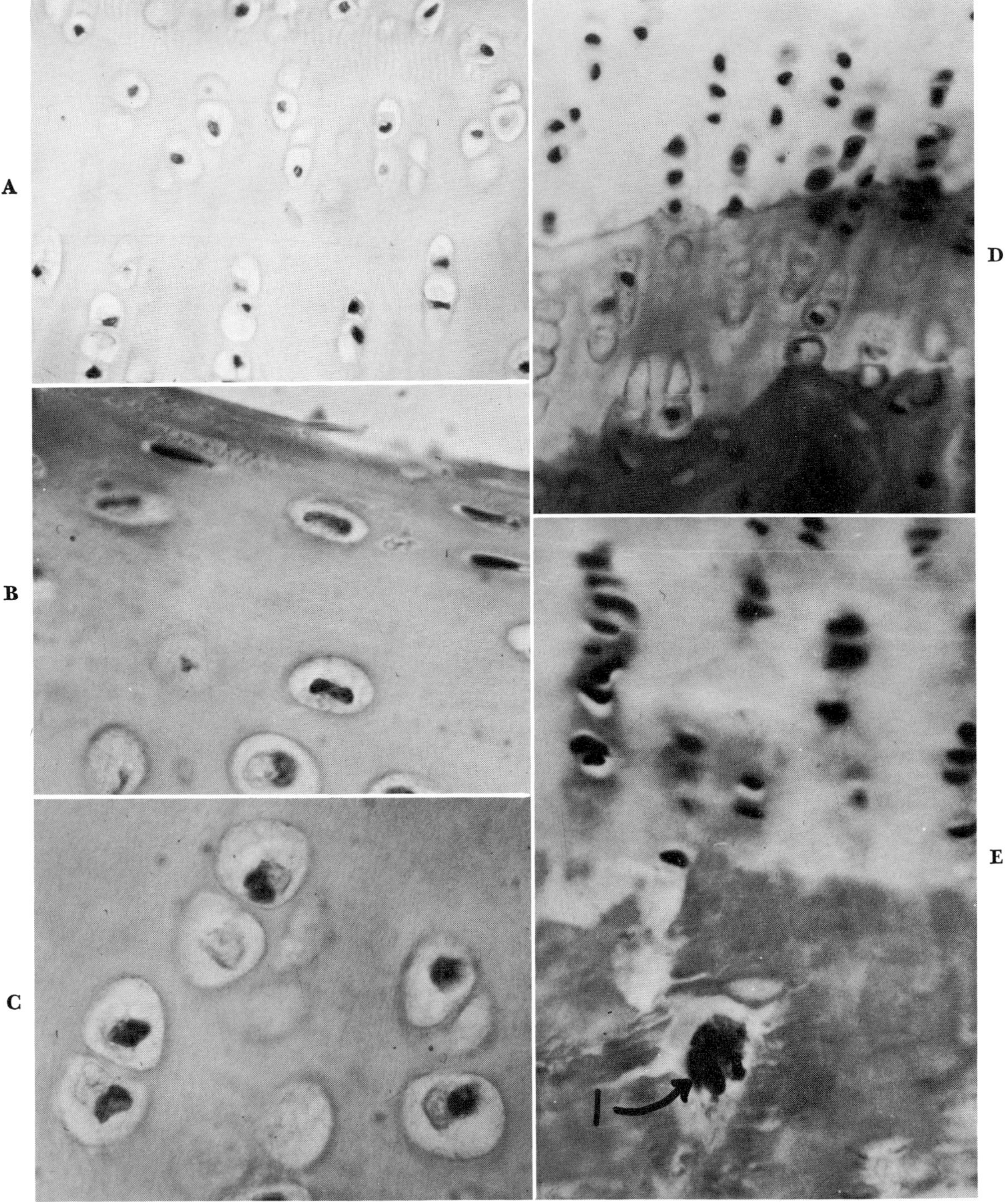

Fig. 13-2. Photomicrographs of the articular cartilage of adult rabbits. **A** shows the sparse cell population with relative preponderance of the smooth amorphous-appearing matrix. **B** and **C** show cellular detail under oil immersion in the superficial zone, **B,** and the transitional zones, **C.** (See text.) **D** demonstrates the appearance with hematoxylin and eosin staining of the basal layer, showing the lower radial zone, calcified zone, and underlying bony end plate. **E** is specially stained with murexide, a calcium-chelating dye, to demonstrate the heavy deposition of apatitic salts surrounding and enclosing the cells, **1.** (**A,** ×430; **B** and **C,** ×950; **D,** ×500; **E,** ×750.) (**D** and **E,** From Mankin, H. J.: Anat. Rec. **145:**73, 1963.)

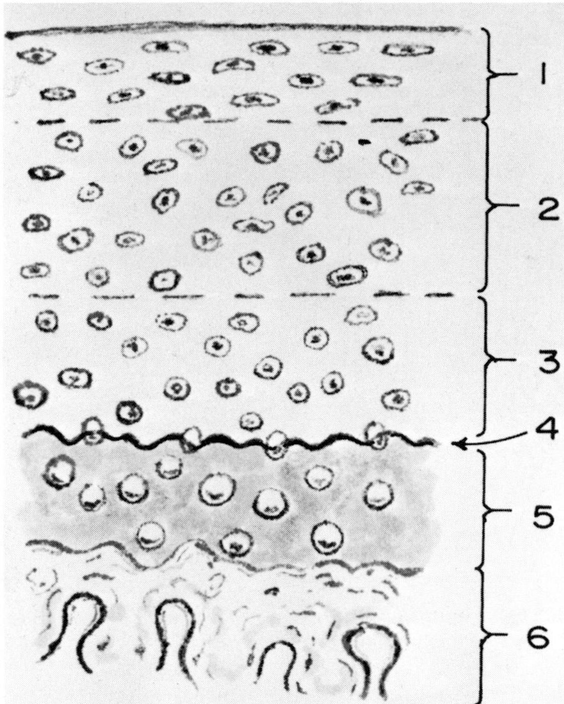

Fig. 13-3. Diagrammatic representation of the zones of mature articular cartilage. At the surface is a narrow layer of flattened cells called the *gliding or tangential zone,* **1.** Beneath this is the *transitional zone,* **2,** in which ovoid-to-rounded cells are randomly distributed. Deep to this are the short, irregular columns of the *radial zone,* **3,** which is separated from the *zone of calcified cartilage,* **5,** by the "tidemark," **4,** a thin, wavy basophilic line seen best on hematoxylin and eosin staining. The bony end plate below the cartilage consists of mature cortical bone with well-defined haversian systems, **6.** (From Mankin, H. J.: Bull. Rheum. Dis. **17**:447, 1967.)

the surface has been described.[34,126] This zone, originally thought to be a collagen-free "pure" hyaline cartilage, was called the "lamina splendens"[10] and consists, according to Weiss, Rosenberg, and Helfet,[126] of a dense network of randomly oriented, delicate fibers of 40 to 120 Å in diameter; this network overlies bundles of closely spaced unit collagen fibers approximately 350 Å in thickness (Fig. 13-5). The zone is deficient in polysaccharide as compared with deeper areas[6,67,126] *(vide infra)* and is believed to serve a protective function.

Examination of the articular cartilage by gross inspection suggests that the surface is extraordinarily smooth, but on histologic or electron microscopic studies, pits, depressions, and irregularities are noted.[34,93,126] Recent studies by Walker and

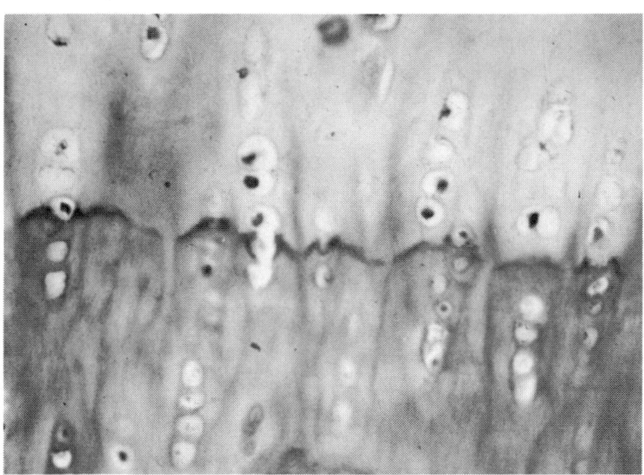

Fig. 13-4. High-power photomicrograph of the articular cartilage of an adult rabbit, demonstrating the irregular wavy bluish line marking the junction of the radial and calcified zones of the cartilage. The line is best seen on sections stained with hematoxylin and eosin, and was named the "tidemark" by Collins.[27] Its significance and nature are unknown. (×400.)

associates,[124,125] using the scanning electron microscope, clearly demonstrated an irregularly corrugated pattern, believed by these authors to be necessary for a complex lubrication system involving synovial fluid entrapment and condensation. The biochemical studies of Balazs, Bloom, and Swann[6] corroborated this concept in that they suggested that the outermost layer, which on the electron micrograph appears as a fine filamentous-amorphous network, is primarily made up of adsorbed hyaluronic acid presumably from synovial fluid.

It has been known for many years that the cartilage contains collagen fibers responsible in large part for the stiffness of the matrix.[11,44] The arrangement of these collagen fibers has been the subject of considerable study and speculation. In 1925, Benninghoff[11] demonstrated histologically that the collagen fibers form bundles arranged in arcades. The fibers were thought to be anchored in the zone of calcified cartilage, then to run vertically toward the surface through the radial zone, turning obliquely in the transitional zone to follow the tangential orientation of the gliding layer, and then turning once again, perpendicularly, to run back to the calcified zone. The chondrocytes lying between the limbs of the arcades were thought to be arranged in clusters called "chrondones" (Fig. 13-6). The Benninghoff arcades, which can be visualized on phase-contrast microscopy of adult cartilage,[10,18] were thought to be important to the

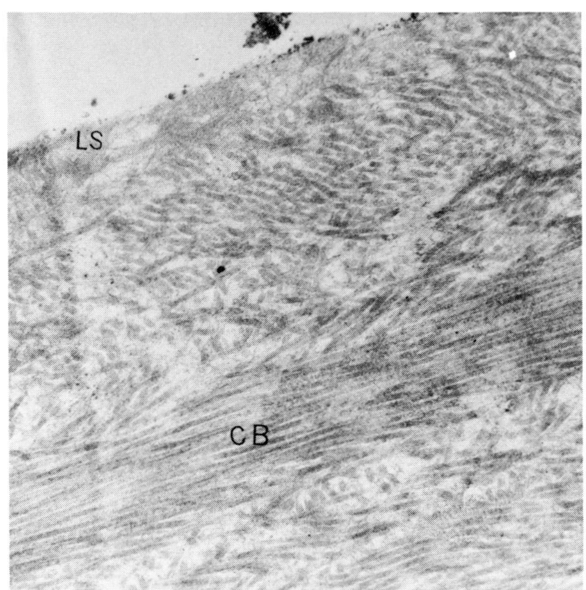

Fig. 13-5. The surface of normal human articular cartilage is covered by a filamentous layer corresponding to the lamina splendens, **LS.** Collagen fibers of the superficial zone are arranged in closely packed bundles, **CB,** which run parallel to the surface. Individual fibers are 320 Å ± 50 Å diameter and show 640 Å periodicity. (×28,000.) (Courtesy Dr. Charles Weiss, New York, N. Y.)

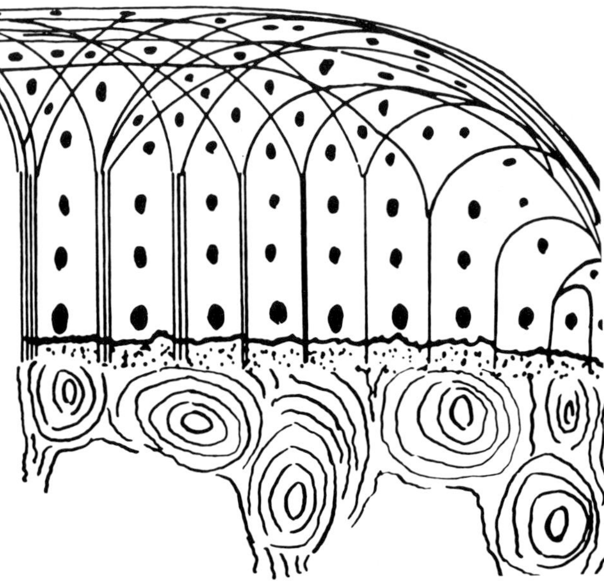

Fig. 13-6. Illustration of the Benninghoff concept of the arrangement of the collagen fibers in mature articular cartilage. Fiber bundles are considered to be in arcades, anchored in the calcified zone, and sweeping jointward, running obliquely, tangentially, and then obliquely to once more descend in a direction perpendicular to the surface to the calcified zone. Groups of cells between the arcades were called "chondrones." (Illustration is a copy of original by Benninghoff[11] and was graciously supplied by Dr. Thomas D. Brower, Lexington, Ky.)

resiliency of the articular surface, providing a system of tension resistors similar to an old-fashioned innerspring mattress. With the introduction of the electron microscope, a number of investigators have demonstrated a more random orientation of the fibers, virtual absence of continuous arcades, and a lack of chondrone type of organization.* The fiber diameter and distance between adjacent fibers appear to increase with depth from the articular surface.[86,126] It has been postulated that the arrangement of these fibers does indeed serve as an important aid to resiliency, but probably does so in a fashion similar to ticking in a straw mattress rather than as the organized "bedspring" arcade system of Benninghoff.

CHONDROCYTES OF ARTICULAR CARTILAGE

In their general characteristics, the chondrocytes resemble connective tissue cells in both light and electron microscopic features. They are round to oval to flattened, depending on the zone in which they are found, and measure up to 20 μ in their longest diameter.[10,34] The nucleus is often eccentric, rounded, and strongly basophilic on hematoxylin and eosin staining, measuring 4 to 6 μ in long diameter.[77] The cell occupies a rounded lacuna in the matrix and probably fills this in vivo, but appears to shrink away from the walls in fixed preparations[10] (Fig. 13-2).

The ultrastructure of these cells has been extensively studied in recent years, and the reader is referred to the excellent studies of Davies and associates,[34] Silberberg,[110] Silberberg and associates,[111,112] Meachim,[90,91] and Weiss, Rosenberg, and Helfet.[126] The characteristics vary considerably, depending on the zones in which the cell is found, but the typical cell from the transitional zone demonstrates an eccentrically placed, often reniform or somewhat lobulated, nucleus with one or more prominent nucleoli (Fig. 13-7). The nuclear membrane is well defined. There is often a conspicuous Golgi apparatus with closely packed agranular lamellae with dilatations, small vesicles, and vacu-

*See references 20, 66, 69, and 126.

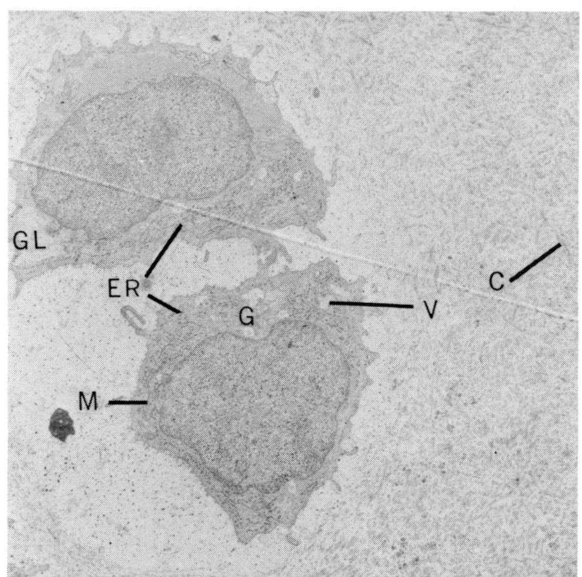

Fig. 13-7. Collagen fibers, **C,** of the deeper zones are arranged in a random fashion, except in the immediate vicinity of the chondrocytes. The individual fibers are spaced more widely apart and are of greater diameter (300 Å to 600 Å). The ovoid chondrocytes of the deeper zone have extensive endoplasmic reticulum, **ER,** abundant glycogen, **GL,** well-developed Golgi, **G,** and mitochondria, **M.** Vacuoles, **V,** containing filamentous material, and often merging with the cell membrane, are common. (×5,000.) (Courtesy Dr. Charles Weiss, New York, N. Y.)

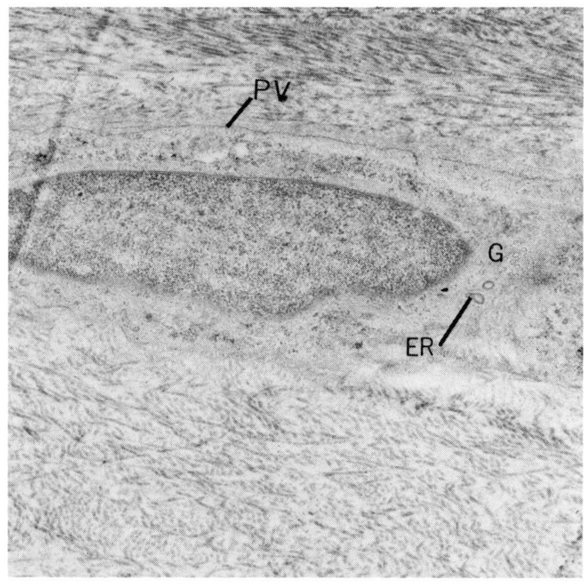

Fig. 13-8. The elongated cells of the superficial zone contain numerous pinocytosis vesicles, **PV,** few mitochondria, and a poorly developed endoplasmic reticulum, **ER.** Small, empty vesicles and saccules comprise the Golgi apparatus, **G.** (×15,000.) (Courtesy Dr. Charles Weiss, New York, N. Y.)

oles. A number of large vacuoles containing moderately dense amorphous material and intracellular fibrils are present in the region of the Golgi complex.[126] There are numerous mitochondria,[34,110,126] and the endoplasmic reticulum is well developed with numerous cisternae whose contents are more electron-dense than the surrounding material.[111,112,126] Small pinocytic vesicles are often present in the cytoplasm, particularly near the cell surface.[126] Lipid drops are seen fairly frequently throughout the cytoplasm,[28] and there are numerous aggregations of glycogen, which in some cells form large deposits.* Intracytoplasmic filaments have been noted, and, when present in excessive number, appear to be correlated with cell degeneration.[90,91,94] An occasional microtubule may be seen.[126]

The plasma membrane, although well defined, is irregular in contour, but, unlike osteocytes, does not show long protoplasmic processes under normal conditions. Instead, there are noted numerous short, footlike processes[110-112] and indentations in a scalloped pattern, suggesting that there has been a recent discharge of vacuolar contents from the surface.[126] Immediately around the cell is a "halo" or "moat" that has been shown to be rich in polysaccharide but poor in collagen[20,126] and that demonstrates a high concentration of chloride.[16]

The characteristics of cells in other zones may differ considerably. The flattened, elongated cells of the superficial zone show a far less developed endoplasmic reticulum, with many large cisternae[34,110,126] (Fig. 13-8). The mitochondria are small, and the Golgi apparatus forms numerous flattened saccules, apparently devoid of electron-dense material.[126] In the deeper layers, cells frequently show evidence of degeneration, and the intracellular cytoplasmic filaments are more abundant.[110-112] Cell death may be seen in any zone but is most frequent in the lower radial and calcified zones.* Cells in the basilar layers in adult animals do not incorporate cytidine-^{3}H, an indicator of RNA synthesis, suggesting that they are either dead or in an inert phase.[74]

*See references 34, 110-112, and 126.

*See references 90, 91, 93, 94, and 110.

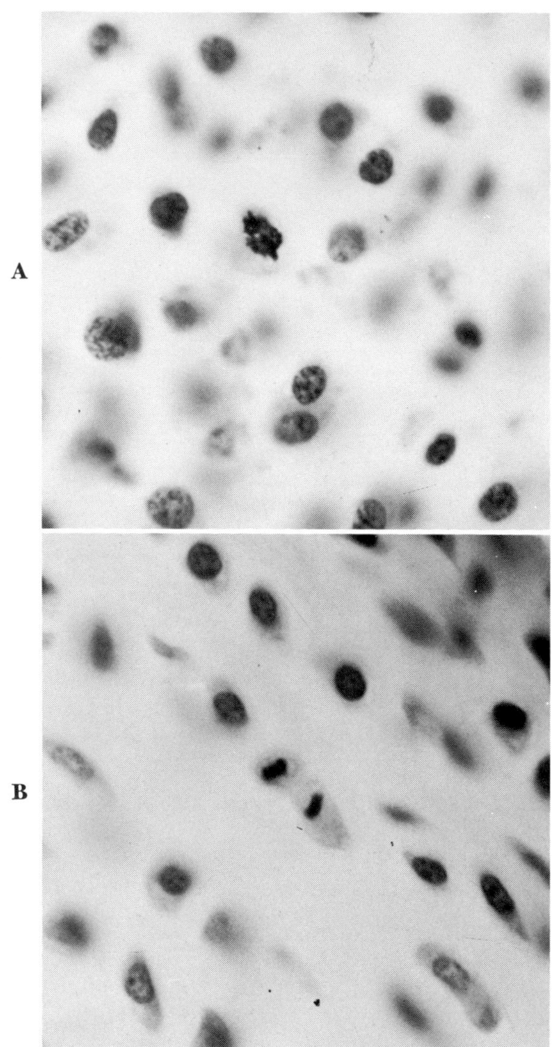

Fig. 13-9. Oil immersion photomicrographs of articular cartilage from immature rabbits (aged 2 months) demonstrating cells undergoing mitotic division. A cell in metaphase is seen in **A** and one in telophase is seen in **B.** (×950.)

One of the areas of considerable confusion in the past has been related to the kinetics of chondrocyte proliferation. Mitotic figures were noted in cartilage from immature animals (Fig. 13-9), and this suggested that at least during the phase of net synthesis growth is occurring by standard methods of cell replication.[42,73,79] With cessation of length growth and epiphyseal closure, the articular cartilage chondrocytes assume an "inert" appearance, and mitotic figures have not been seen in normal articular cartilage from adult animals.* Under states of abnormal stress, such as lacerative injury[72,78] or mild compression,[31,32] mitotic figures are occasionally seen, but in normal cartilage of the human adult there is no evidence for mitotic activity in the chondrocytes.

Despite the low-friction character of joint motion,[8,124] it is certainly likely that attrition occurs, and it seems extraordinary that there is no apparent mechanism for mitotic compensation for this attritive loss. As the animal ages, cartilage cells with irregularly shaped nuclei are more frequently noted, and these were thought by several previous investigators to represent evidence of "amitotic" division.[10,42,76] This mysterious process was considered to be an important feature of the metabolism of aging cartilage despite several inconsistencies in its basic theory when viewed in the light of modern genetic knowledge.[76]

In recent years, mitotic counts, studies with tritiated thymidine (an indicator of desoxyribonucleic acid replication), and cytophotometric determinations of nuclear DNA content have established the pattern of cellular proliferation of the articular cartilages.[71,73,75,76,104] In immature cartilage there are two separate zones of cell division (Fig. 13-10): a superficial zone beneath the tangential layer, presumably for growth of the articular cartilage mass, and a deeper zone adjacent to the zone of calcification, which probably represents the proliferative focus of a short epiphysial plate for ossification of the bony nucleus of the underlying epiphysis.[73] With aging, the more superficial area of proliferation disappears, leaving only the deep zone (Fig. 13-11).

The total number of mitotic figures and thymidine-label cells decreases and, finally, at maturity, with the development of the "tidemark," all evidence of mitotic activity ceases[76,79] (Fig. 13-11). Thymidine-incorporation studies[76] and cytophotometric determinations in adult cartilage[71] have failed to show any evidence of either DNA synthesis or polyploidy. These experiments would suggest that amitotic division does not occur and that there is no compensation for normal cell death and attrition with aging. Such a concept would predict that the cell count in articular cartilage would decrease with age, and this has been shown to be true for rabbits[77] (Fig. 13-12) and cattle.[107,123] Similar studies with human material[92,116] have indicated, however, that there is little or no decrease in cell counts with even advanced years. In view

*See references 25, 73, 76, and 79.

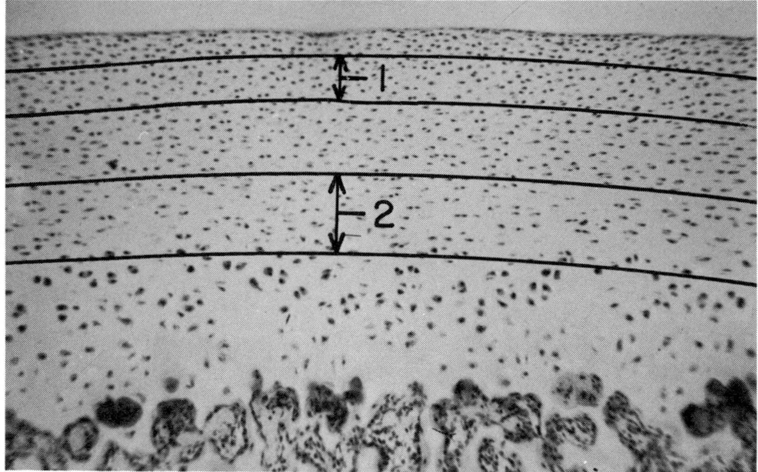

Fig. 13-10. Zones of cell division indicated on a low-power photomicrograph of cartilage from an immature rabbit (aged 2 months). The superficial zone, **1,** lies subjacent to the gliding surface and is considered to contribute to the size of the cartilage mass. The deeper layer, **2,** lies in proximity to the underlying bony epiphysis and is thought to be the proliferative zone of a "micro"epiphyseal plate for endochondral ossification of the epiphyseal nucleus. (×100.)

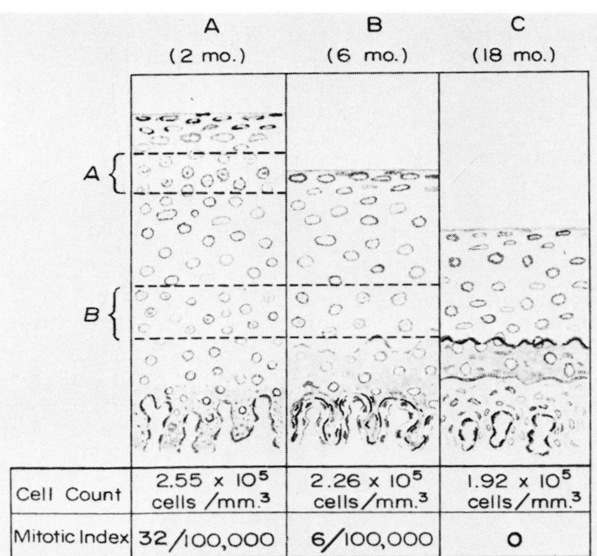

Fig. 13-11. Diagrammatic representation of the changes occurring in the articular cartilage of rabbits with aging. In the immature animal (**A,** 2 months), the cartilage is thick, has a relatively high cell density, and is mitotically active. Mitoses are not uniformly distributed but are found in two zones (**A** and **B,** see text). As the animal ages (**B,** 6 months) the cartilage thins, cell and mitotic counts decrease, and the mitoses are mostly confined to one area, **B.** With maturity (**C,** 18 months), the cartilage is considerably reduced in thickness, and there is a well-developed calcified zone and "tidemark." The cell count is diminished, and there is no mitotic activity observed. (From Mankin, H. J.: Bull. Rheum. Dis. **17:** 447, 1967.)

of the frequency of cell death seen on electron microscopic studies, and the absence of mitotic activity, these findings are as yet unexplained.

It should be pointed out that, unlike the cells from other tissues, such as brain or muscle, the articular cartilage chondrocyte appears to "turn off" the switch for DNA synthesis at maturity rather than "breaking" the switch. Thus, under conditions such as acromegaly, continuous mild compression,[31,32] osteoarthritis,[82] and lacerative injury,[72,78] the cartilage cell is apparently capable of reversion to a "chondroblastic" state and exhibiting mitotic division. The results of such activity have been somewhat disappointing in that the response is limited and appears to be insufficient to heal lacerative defects in the surface[72,78] or regenerate cartilage destroyed by osteoarthritis or other pathologic processes.

CHEMISTRY OF ARTICULAR CARTILAGE

One of the most extraordinary features of the chemical composition of articular cartilage is its hyperhydrated state. Measurements of the water content of fresh articular cartilage from many sites of many species of virtually all ages range from 65% to 80%.* Most of this water is not tightly bound, but

*See references 14, 40, 64, 65, 95, and 123.

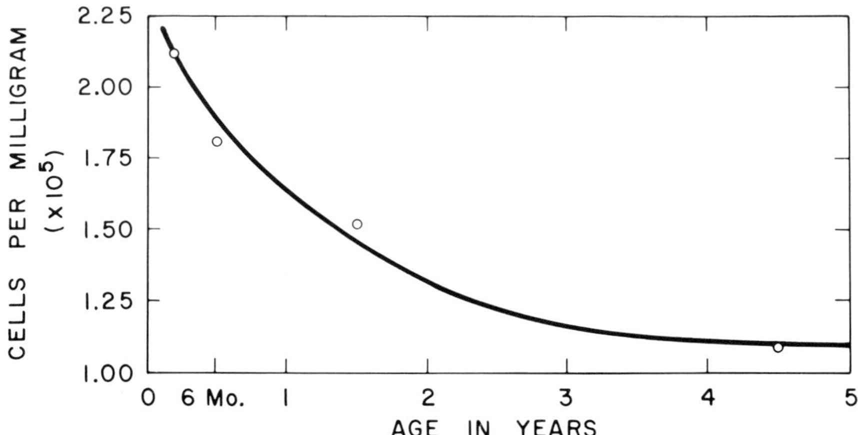

Fig. 13-12. Effect of aging on cell count per unit wet weight of articular cartilage from rabbits of various ages. Cells were counted for four age groups, as indicated, and after appropriate corrections[77] were expressed as cells per milligram wet weight. Note the decline with advancing age. (From Mankin, H. J.: Bull. New York Acad. Med. **44:**545, 1968.)

forms a gel in combination with the mucopolysaccharides and can be readily removed by drying or heating[65] (unlike bone, in which a large percentage of the water is tightly bound to the collagen fiber or the mineral crystal). The concentration decreases only slightly with aging, but appears to be increased in cartilage from osteoarthritic joints.[12,14,65] Several studies have suggested that the elastic behavior of cartilage is to a large extent dependent on the water content,[43,114] but this effect may be considerably modified by the presence of bivalent or trivalent cations.[114]

The concentration of electrolytes is essentially the same as one finds in intracellular and extracellular fluids of the tissues,[40,95] with two exceptions: both free and bound sulfate concentrations are extraordinarily high[5,83,113] (as one might anticipate in view of the concentration of sulfated polysaccharide); and there is an increase in the concentration of sodium, which serves as the principal cation for the polyanionic matrix.[40,95] Studies by Maroudas and her coworkers[85,87,88] have indicated that the electrolytes traverse the cartilage matrix rapidly, but the diffusion coefficients are approximately 40% of that for an aqueous solution. The diffusion rate is equal in fresh cartilage to that in tissue obtained at autopsy, indicating that the process is passive rather than dependent on cellular activity. According to additional experiments, diffusion is primarily dependent on fixed charge density and agitation of the fluid medium.[85,87] Larger molecules do not traverse as rapidly, and glucose has a diffusion coefficient approximately 30% of that in aqueous solution.[87] Cationic dyes traverse more rapidly than anionic ones, indicating the affinity for the polyanionic matrix and the importance of charge in predicting the rate of diffusion.[17,57,87]

Over 50% of the dry weight of articular cartilage and about 90% of the protein content is in the form of collagen (Table 13-1). Despite repeated attempts to separate this molecule chemically from the protein polysaccharide, all but drastic extraction techniques have failed to produce a "clean" collagen.[96,108] It has been shown that most of the collagen in cartilage is insoluble in water or dilute acid, and only about 1% to 2% can be extracted by solutions of 5-molar guanidine hydrochloride.[96] The amino acid composition appears to be identical with that of other collagens, although a recent report by Miller, Vanderkorst, and Sokoloff[96] suggested an increased quantity of hydroxylysine. Mathews[89] indicated that there is a complex interaction of acid mucopolysaccharides and collagen that is quite stable and probably associated with side chain interactions between the chondroitin sulfates and the collagen fibrils. The stability of the complex seems dependent on electrostatic forces and is increased with increase in polysaccharide chain length.

Table 13-1. Reported results of studies of the composition of the organic solids of articular cartilage*

Investigator	*Tissue studied*	*Collagen* %	*GAG*† %	*Noncollagen protein* %	*Ash* %	*Sialic acid* %	*DNA* %	*Total nitrogen*	*Kerato-sulfate* %
Anderson et al.[5]	Human	56.4	20.3	22.8	4.3			14.9	
Smith et al.[113]	Bovine	72.4	12.3‡						
Campo and Tourtelotte[22]	Calf	55.1	22.2	8.4	5.8	0.44		12.2	3.2
Herring[52]	Calf	63.7	25.3	9.6	6.2	0.52			3.7
Bollet et al.[13]	Human	45.2‡	4.9‡	(shoulder)					
		39.2‡	7.0‡	(knee)					
Mankin and Lippiello[82]	Aged human	48.8	14.1				0.53		
Miles and Eichelberger[95]	Human	68.7‡	12.0	23.1‡				14.7	

*All values are expressed as percentages of the dry weight and, where indicated, have been determined by conversion of data reported as hydroxyproline, collagen nitrogen, uronic acid, or hexosamine to collagen or GAG (as chondroitin sulfate) by standard conversion factors.
†As chondroitin sulfate (estimated from hexosamine or uronic acid values.)
‡Estimation by conversion of reported data.

As indicated in the previous discussion of the structure of cartilage, the distribution and size of the collagen fibers vary according to the level studied. In the "moat" area, smaller, more soluble, unbanded fragments have been seen on electron-microscopy and are considered by some investigators to represent tropocollagen fragments.[20] The majority of the fibers are considerably larger, varying from 250 to over 900 Å in width and exhibiting the banded periodic pattern of native collagen[110-112,126] (Fig. 13-13).

The other major components of the organic solids of articular cartilage are the protein polysaccharides (Table 13-1). These complexes are highly viscous, hydrophilic, high molecular weight macromolecules, consisting of a protein core to which is attached a large number of chains of sulfated polysaccharides* (Fig. 13-14). The protein core varies considerably in size and amino acid composition, but the basic unit is thought to be about 4,000 Å long with about 60 polysaccharide side chains.[97,109] The elegant physical studies of Schubert and his co-workers[106,108,109] have demonstrated that the protein polysaccharides are heterogeneous and can be separated by the ultracentrifuge into two major groups, PP-L and PP-H, with different physical and chemical properties. The PP-L molecule has been further divided into a series of materials of slightly varying characteristics.[106,108,109] The polysaccharide molecule consists of a chain of repeated dimeric "glycosaminoglycan" (GAG) units, and this expression (GAG) is preferred by some investigators as being the more descriptive. The number of saccharide units in a macromolecule may range between 50 and 50,000.[108] In articular cartilage, only three of the many dimeric GAG units have been found, and these are chondroitin-4 sulfate (N-acetyl-galactosamine with a $SO_4^{=}$ on

*See references 23, 97, 108, and 109.

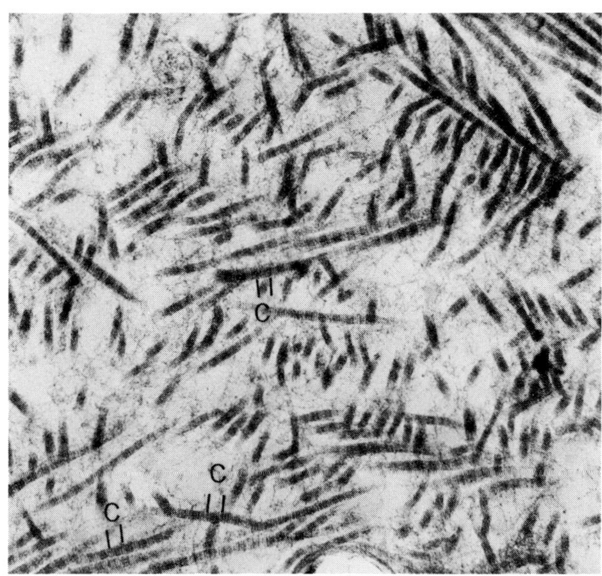

Fig. 13-13. Randomly oriented collagen fibers, **C,** of the deeper zones are approximately 600 Å in diameter and have typical 640 Å periodicity. (See markers.) (×40,000.) (Courtesy Dr. Charles Weiss, New York, N. Y.)

the 4-carbon position and glucuronic acid [Fig. 13-15]), chondroitin-6 sulfate (N-acetyl-galactosamine with a $SO_4^=$ on the 6-carbon position and glucuronic acid), and keratin sulfate (N-acetyl glucosamine with a $SO_4^=$ at the 6-carbon position and galactose).[97,108,109] The long-chain polysaccharide molecule is attached to the protein core by an O-glycoside linkage to serine, and the linking unit is thought to be in the form of a glucuronyl-galactosyl-galactosyl-xylosyl serine.[51,100,105]

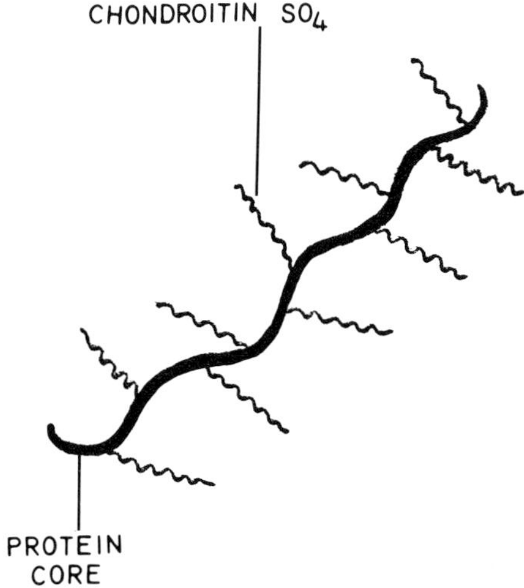

Fig. 13-14. Diagram indicating the current concept of the structure of the protein-polysaccharide complex of cartilage. The protein core is about 4,000 Å long and is linked to about sixty polysaccharide side chains, most of which are chondroitin sulfate. The number of saccharide units in each side chain may vary from 50 to 50,000, but they are arranged in the repeating dimeric units illustrated in Fig. 13-15.

The protein polysaccharides are not diffusely distributed throughout the cartilage but are found to occur in highest concentrations immediately surrounding the cells (the perilacunar areas or territorial zones).[7,67,118] The concentration is decreased in the superficialmost portion of the gliding zone[6] and is also significantly less in the interterritorial regions, except for keratin sulfate, which is primarily located interterritorially.[118] The most prevalent GAG in articular cartilage is chondroitin-6 sulfate. The concentration of chondroitin-4 sulfate is increased in embryonic tissues but decreases rapidly in the postnatal period and may undergo a further slow decline with old age.[71,97] Keratin sulfate occurs in very low concentrations in young cartilage,[61] but slowly increases with age, and accounts for a small percentage of GAG[53,61] (unlike rib cartilage, where there is a rapid and progressive increase in keratin sulfate with age[58]).

The protein polysaccharides have a number of physical and chemical properties considered to be important to the resiliency of the articular surface and probably aid materially in providing water for surface lubrication. These properties are related to the viscosity, water binding capacity, and polyelectrolytic character of this complex macromolecule.[88,97,109] As indicated previously, the protein polysaccharide is closely linked to the collagen and may serve to direct or maintain the spatial position of the fibrous protein as well as possibly prevent calcification.[54] Another property imparted to the cartilage by the polysaccharides is that of metachromatic staining.[103,109,115] Dyes such as alcian

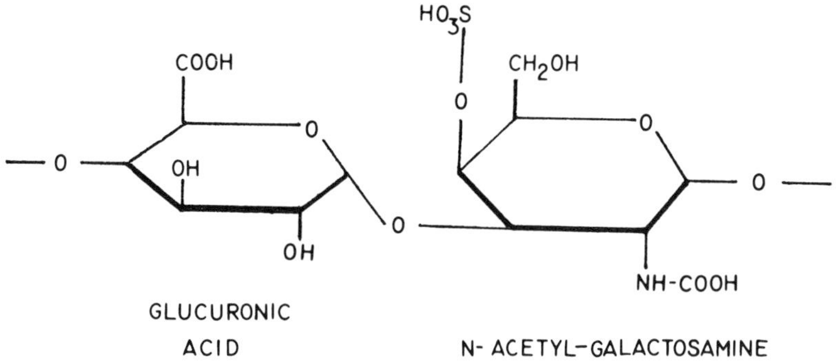

Fig. 13-15. Repeating dimeric unit found in chondroitin-4 sulfate. A glucuronic acid molecule is linked by a 1-3 ester linkage to an N-acetyl galactosamine, to which is attached a sulfate at the C_4 position. Chondroitin-6 sulfate is identical, except that the sulfate is linked to the C_6 position. Keratin sulfate is similar in structure, but the unit saccharides are an N-acetyl glucosamine with a sulfate on C_6 and galactose. Another terminology calls these units glycosaminoglycans (GAG).

blue, toluidine blue, azure A, crystal violet, and others serve as the counterions (cations) to the polyanionic protein polysaccharide. Minute crystals of dye polymerize in a spatial relationship dictated by the loci of the available sulfates, and with a critical concentration and arrangement will change the spectrum of transmitted light from the "orthochromatic" color to the "metachromatic" color. This phenomenon is reasonably specific for the polysaccharide, and it may be used as an indicator of the concentration and distribution of this material within the cartilage.[103,109,115]

Several other organic materials are found in small quantities in cartilage. These include sialic acid, probably in the form of sialoprotein, and most likely in combination with the protein polysaccharide complexes[4,52] (Table 13-1). In addition, Collins and his coworkers[28,48] described lipids within the cell and matrix of human cartilage, detectable by stains with specific fat-soluble dyes. The concentration is very low, accounting for less than 4% of the wet weight, and the exact nature of this material is unknown.[117] A variety of enzymes has been described in the articular cartilages, but these will be discussed in greater detail under the sections concerned with metabolism.

NUTRITION OF ARTICULAR CARTILAGE

The source of nutritive materials for the cartilaginous surfaces has been one of the oldest and most controversial puzzles associated with this peculiar tissue. Since the tissue is avascular, it has been thought that much or all of the nutritive materials diffuse through the matrix from the synovial fluid that bathes the surface of the cartilage, but the evidence for this was sparse, and Hunter[55] and Virchow[122] expressed divergent opinions centuries ago. In 1920, Strangeways[119] reported on experiments suggesting that the synovial fluid is the *only* source of nutrients for adult cartilage, and studies by Collins[27] yielded data that led him to agree strongly with this opinion. The dye diffusion studies of Brower, Akahoshi, and Orlic[17] and studies using other substrates[74,87] are considered confirmation of this view. In the past 20 years, however Ingelmark and Sääf,[56] Ekholm,[41] and McKibben and Holdsworth[70] presented experimental evidence suggesting that at least a portion of the substrates entering the articular cartilage arrive by diffusion from the underlying bony end plate. It is apparent from review of these studies that in the immature animal, in which the calcified zone is not well developed, the basal layers of the cartilage are partially nourished by diffusion from the vascular buds (Fig. 13-1) of the underlying bony nucleus.[70] However, in the adult, at the time of appearance of the "tidemark," heavy deposition of apatites in the calcified zone (Fig. 13-2) must considerably limit this type of diffusion, and current thinking suggests that very little, if any, nutrient traverses from the basilar bone after maturity is reached.

METABOLISM OF ARTICULAR CARTILAGE

Until 15 years ago, little was known about the metabolism of articular cartilage. The earliest studies included measurements of respiratory activity, and these suggested that cartilage had a low metabolic rate.[19] Several later reappraisals of these data pointed out that the rate per unit mass was indeed low, but because of the sparse cell population, the rate per cell was considerably higher and approached that seen in other tissues.[36,107] Several studies of glycolysis in cartilaginous tissues have demonstrated the presence of most of the glycolytic enzymes in large quantity.[60,68] Articular cartilage has been shown to be relatively tolerant to high concentrations of potassium cyanide,[84] only minimally affected by short periods of oxygen deprivation,[71] but very sensitive to monoiodoacetate.[84] These data, plus the finding of a high concentration of lactic acid,[60,68] suggested that the metabolic pattern is consistent with the avascular character of the tissue and that the anaerobic pathway is quite well developed. Recent studies by Krane, Parsons, and Kunin[60] on epiphysial cartilage demonstrated that this tissue has a low oxygen consumption, a high aerobic production of lactate from glucose, a high concentration of lactate, and "anaerobic" character to the constituent lactic dehydrogenase. Although this information applies to a different type of cartilage, it is likely that articular cartilage has a similar pattern and that anaerobic and shunt pathways are quite well developed and probably utilized more readily than the aerobic pathway for energy production.

Early investigators advanced the view that cartilage cells were "inert" and that little synthetic activity was occurring. Almost 20 years ago, however, radiosulfate studies first indicated a surpris-

A

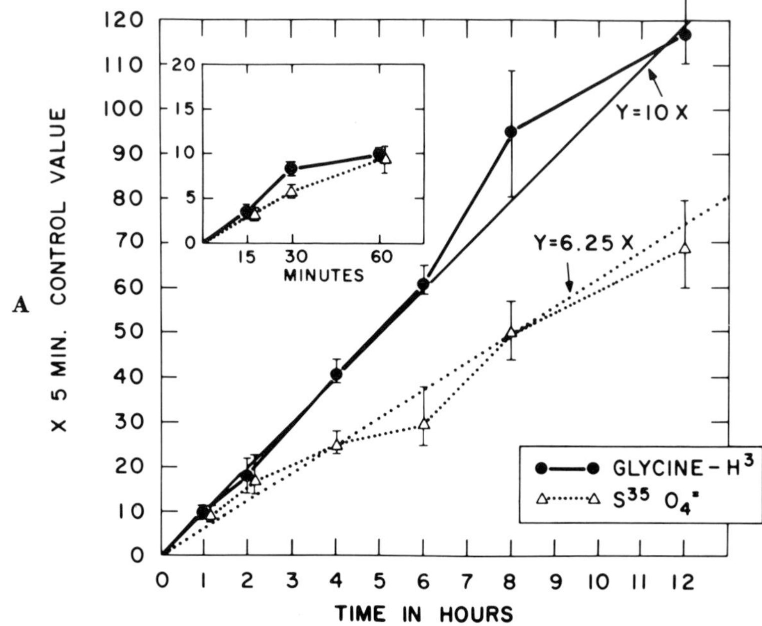

B

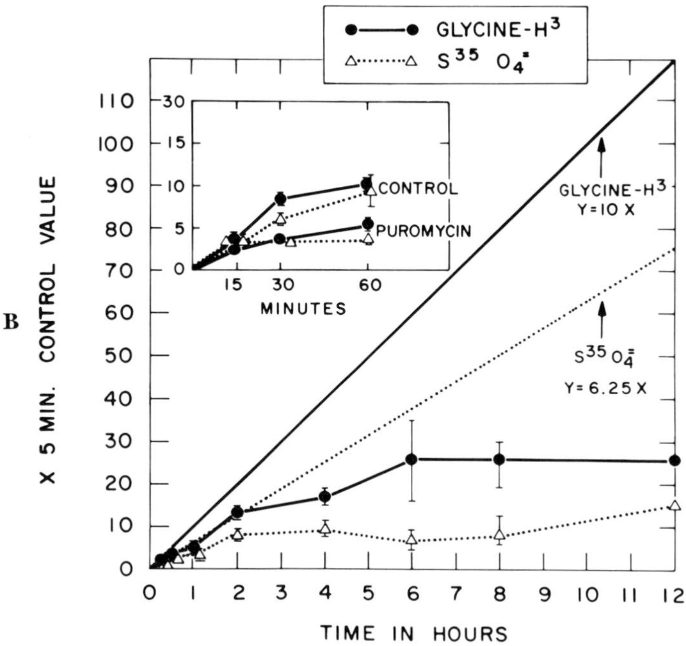

Fig. 13-16. Rates of incorporation of glycine-^{3}H and $^{35}SO_4^=$ by articular cartilage from immature rabbits in an in vitro system. Small segments of articular cartilage were incubated in Eagle's medium containing the isotopes and no inhibitor, **A**, puromycin, **B**, and actinomycin-D, **C**. Samples were harvested at regular intervals and assayed for incorporated activity. Note that the rates of incorporation are linear with time up to 12 hours, **A**. Both glycine-^{3}H and $^{35}SO_4^=$ incorporation are inhibited within 2 hours by puromycin and after 6 hours by actinomycin-D. (See text.) (**A**, From Mankin, H. J.: Bull. Rheum. Dis. **17**:447, 1967.)

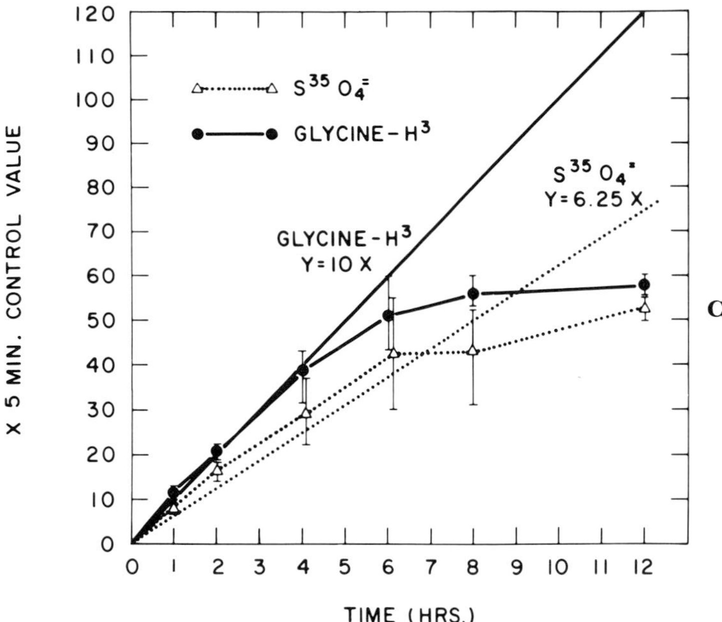

Fig. 13-16, cont'd. For legend see opposite page.

ingly rapid rate of turnover for at least one component of the matrix.* These studies have been enlarged and broadened by a number of investigators.† The pattern that has emerged is one of highly developed and complex activity directed entirely (or almost entirely) to synthesis, maintenance, and degradation of the macromolecules that comprise the extracellular material.‡

The chondrocyte, like many connective tissue cells, supports multiple synthetic processes and activities. It has been shown that there are at least three specific types of synthetic activity carried on by the chondrocyte, that all of these functions are performed by the same unit cell, and that all of these occur either simultaneously or within very short periods.[21,109,120] The three functions include the synthesis of protein of protein-polysaccharide and collagen, the synthesis of polysaccharide (and its polymerization), and the sulfation of the polysaccharide.

The synthesis of the protein of protein-polysaccharide and the collagen appears to conform to the standard molecular genetic scheme. The "message" is carried from the nuclear DNA to the ribosome by messenger RNA; amino acids carried by S-RNA are assembled at the ribosome into collagen chains or protein molecules; and the completed protein unit is then extruded into the external environment. Studies utilizing puromycin, a potent inhibitor of protein synthesis (which acts by interfering with amino-acyl S-RNA condensation) have demonstrated complete inhibition of amino acid incorporation into the cell in a very short period of time[1,71] (Fig. 13-16). When actinomycin-D, an inhibitor of messenger RNA, is introduced to the tissue in vitro, synthetic activity continues without apparent decline for approximately 6 hours, and then ceases. (The 6-hour span is consistent with the whole life of messenger RNA in other tissues, Fig. 13-16). These studies and others would support the validity of the concept that at least that portion of the synthetic activity of the cell devoted to synthesis of protein is occurring by the standard genetic pathway.

A second complex synthetic process carried on by the cell is that of synthesis and polymerization of the polysaccharide.* The formation of this macromolecule is performed through a complex series of steps in which a glucose molecule is bonded to uridine diphosphate (UDP) and, through one of several enzymatic pathways, is converted into uridine diphosphate—N-acetyl-galactosamine (Fig.

*See references 3, 15, 38, and 39.
†See references 21, 26, and 29.
‡See references 12, 21, 37, 50, and 83.

*See references 37, 97, 109, and 120.

A. 1) N-Ac-Glucosamine-1-P + UTP → UDP-N-Ac-Glucosamine + UDP
2) UDP-N-Ac-Glucosamine → UDP-N-Ac-Galactosamine

B. 1) Glucose-1-P + UTP → UDP-Glucose + UDP
2) UDP-Glucose → UDP-Glucuronic acid

C. UDP-N-Ac-Galactosamine + UDP-Glucuronic acid → Chondroitin + 2UDP

Fig. 13-17. Steps in the synthesis and polymerization of the polysaccharides of cartilage. The process is considerably more complex than is indicated in these expressions, and involves a number of discrete steps catalyzed by specific enzyme systems.[37,97,120] (Abbreviations used include: **Ac,** acetyl; **P,** phosphate; **UTP,** uridine-triphosphate; **UDP,** uridine-diphosphate.)

1. ATP + Sulfate ⇌ AMP-Sulfate + PP
2. AMP-Sulfate + ATP → Phospho-AMP-sulfate + ADP (PAPS–"active sulfate")
3. PAPS + Chondroitin → Chondroitin sulfate + Phospho-AMP

Fig. 13-18. Steps in "sulfation" (addition of a sulfate molecule to the C_4 or C_6 position of N-acetyl galactosamine of the glycosaminoglycan unit[33,101] of the polysaccharide). (See text.) Abbreviations used include: **ATP,** adenosine-triphosphate; **AMP,** adenosine-monophosphate; **P,** phosphate; **ADP,** adenosine-diphosphate; **PAPS,** 3′ phosphoadenosine 5′ phosphosulfate ("active sulfate").

13-17). Glucuronic acid is synthesized from glucose by a similar system also using UDP, and the two sugars are united by an ether link to form the first dimeric glycosaminoglycan unit of the polymer. A number of enzymes have been found associated with these complex processes and include nucleoside diphosphokinase, UDP glucose pyrophosphorylase, UDP glucose dehydrogenase, and a variety of transferases and isomerases.[120]

A third activity is that of sulfation, that is, addition of a sulfate to the appropriate sites of the polysaccharide. The method is quite different from those of the other two synthetic processes and involves a combination of ATP and free sulfate to form 3 phosphoadenosine 5 phosphosulfate, known as "active sulfate."[33,101] A sulfate molecule from this high-energy material is then linked to the N-acetyl-galactosamine molecule at the C_4 or C_6 position[120] (Fig. 13-18).

As indicated previously, there is evidence to suggest that the entire protein polysaccharide molecule is synthesized almost simultaneously by the cell.[1,37,71] There may be some temporal delay in sulfation,[37,49,102] but recent biochemical studies suggest that this is minimal.[1,71] The electron microscopic studies of Godman and Lane[49] demonstrated autoradiographically that the radiosulfate is bound and concentrated in the vesicles of the juxtanuclear Golgi apparatus of the chondrocyte within 3 minutes of its presentation to the cell.

The information derived from the qualitative molecular observations just described has been used to study quantitatively the metabolic activity of the tissue as a whole. One of the most useful techniques for such studies utilizes isotopic tracers specific to the macromolecular products of synthesis. In this fashion, both synthesis and degradation rates may be determined by measuring the rates of incorporation or disappearance of these specific labels from the cartilage. Thus, it is possible to establish a rate for protein synthesis by scintillation spectrometric assay of cartilage labeled with glycine-^{3}H,[84] and polysaccharide may be similarly studied after exposure to radiosulfate or ^{14}C-labeled acetate or ^{14}C glucosamine. A number of experiments of this type have been performed and demonstrate: that the rates of synthesis are rapid and linear with time[71,84] (Fig. 13-16); that they are more rapid in immature animals but after the initial decline remain constant despite aging,[77,79] (Fig. 13-19); that they are inhibited by cortisol,[80,81] nitrogen mustard, and a series of antimetabolites (Fig. 13-16)[71]; that they are moderately increased for a short period of time by lacerative injury[78]; and that they are more rapid in the cartilage from osteoarthritic joints.*

*See references 12, 28, 29, and 82.

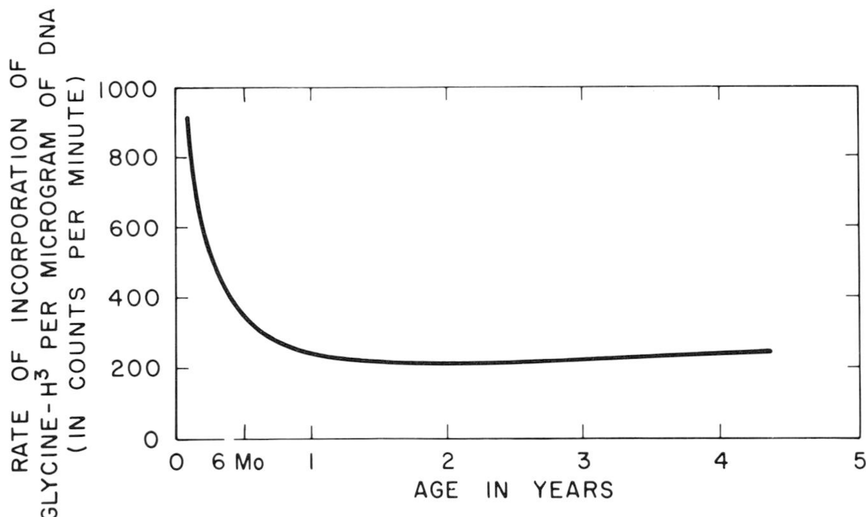

Fig. 13-19. Effect of aging on rate of incorporation of glycine-^{3}H per unit DNA of rabbit articular cartilage. Articular cartilage from rabbits of different ages was incubated with glycine-^{3}H in vitro; samples were harvested at 2 hours and assayed for incorporated radioactivity. DNA determinations were also performed, and the results were expressed as CPM per microgram of DNA. As can be noted, the rate per cell is rapid in young animals but declines rapidly until maturity is reached. At this point until senescence, the rate of glycine-^{3}H incorporation per cell remains constant. This suggests that the rate of protein synthetic activity of the cartilage cell is not altered by age after maturity. (From Mankin, H. J.: Bull. New York Acad. Med. **44**:545, 1968.)

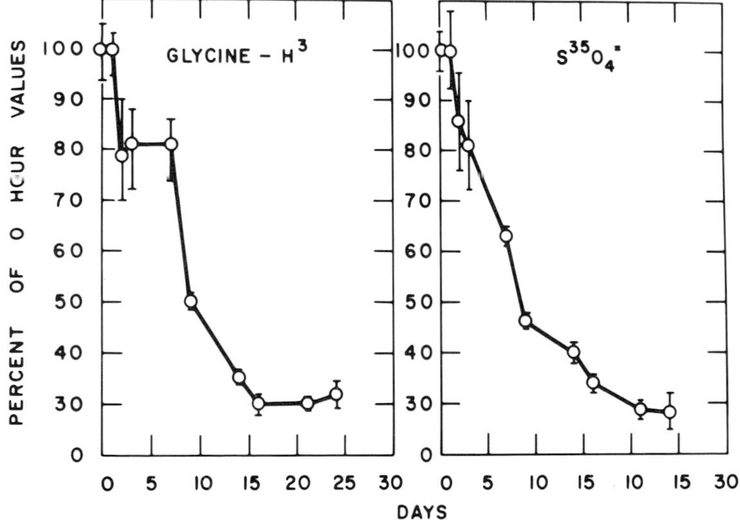

Fig. 13-20. Rates of disappearance of incorporated glycine-^{3}H and $^{35}SO_4^{=}$ in articular cartilage from adult rabbits following intra-articular administration of the isotopes. The cartilage of the knee joints of rabbits was flash-labeled by the intra-articular route; animals were serially killed and their cartilage assayed for incorporated isotopes. It can be seen that there is a rapid disappearance of both isotopes from the cartilage with a half-life of approximately 8 days. This suggests a rapid turnover of a large portion of the protein-polysaccharide of the matrix. (From Mankin, H. J.: Bull. Rheum. Dis. **17**:447, 1967.)

Degradation studies for the articular surfaces have demonstrated that, once incorporated, both glycine-^3H and $^{35}SO_4$ have a rapid disappearance rate with a half-life in cartilage from adult animals of approximately 8 days.[83] (Fig. 13-20.) Recent studies have demonstrated that these data describe the metabolic behavior of a "fast fraction" of the protein polysaccharide, which is greater than one fourth of the total content of this material in the articular cartilage.[83] This would suggest that the degradative rate for the tissue is extraordinarily rapid and far in excess of that which might be considered necessary to compensate for normal attrition. The rapidity of both rates of synthesis and degradation in a tissue that probably experiences only minimal attritional loss (by virtue of almost frictionless joint motion) suggests the presence of an active internal remodeling system.

It has been known for years that certain degradative enzymes act on articular cartilage to degrade the matrix. Papain, a crude material extracted from the papaya plant, was noted to cause a loss of basophilia and metachromasia histologically, and a profound depletion of the polysaccharide on biochemical analysis.[46,121] This enzyme is presumed to act on the protein core of the protein polysaccharide. Vitamin A, in large doses, was also noted to have a profound chondrolytic effect, similar to that observed with papain.[45,46,121] This was thought to occur by stimulation or activation of the lysosomes and discharge of their proteolytic contents into the matrix.[45] Hyaluronidase, another enzyme normally present in certain body tissues, also causes degradation of cartilage, but presumably acts to split the polysaccharide chain, leaving the protein core intact.[12,97,109]

In recent years, a number of investigators have described a heat-and cyanide-sensitive degradative system operating within the cartilage and capable of splitting the protein polysaccharide at or near the protein-sugar bond site.* At least one of these has been identified as a lysosomal acid protease that resembles other series of cathepsins and has been identified by its chemical characteristics as cathepsin-D.[2,128] This material has been seen on specially stained electron micrographs to be not only lysosmal but also distributed intracellularly and extracellularly as well.[47] There is also some evidence for a locally occurring hyaluronidase type of enzyme, but this agent has not as yet been isolated.[12,14]

The enzyme systems just described suggest a remodeling system capable of "turning over" a large fraction of the articular cartilages in a relatively short period of time.[83] The purpose of this type of system is as yet unknown, but one possible explanation is that the rapid turnover is necessary for maintenance of the normal high affinity of the protein polysaccharide for water. This would suggest that mature, more extensively cross-linked protein polysaccharide, or protein polysaccharide tightly bound to collagen, is less hydrophilic than the nascent macromolecule, and this has not yet been shown.

SUMMARY

In this short essay an attempt has been made to define the current state of knowledge about the articular cartilages. There have been numerous advances made in recent years, and when these are studied in concert, several important concepts regarding the tissue seem to emerge.

Articular cartilage is structurally and biochemically heterogeneous

The ultrastructure and synthetic activities of the cells vary considerably, depending on the level of the cartilage studied, and the matrix components are not homogeneously distributed but vary with the zone. Within the chemical framework of the matrix there are heterogeneous classes of the protein polysaccharide, and presumably analogous differences in the size, orientation, and stereochemical configuration of the collagen fibers.

Articular cartilage is mitotically active only in the immature state

Mitotic activity is present in immature animals, but with the cessation of net synthesis, cartilage cells "turn off" the switch for DNA synthesis (but may "turn it on again" under conditions of stress).

Articular cartilage is metabolically active and synthesizes large quantities of the macromolecular components of the matrix

The synthetic activities are extraordinarily complex, involve at least three separate metabolic pathways, and are supported by a well-developed anaerobic glycolytic metabolism.

*See references 24, 47, 62, 127, and 128.

Articular cartilage has an internal remodeling system

The protein polysaccharides are synthesized and degraded at a rate far too rapid to be attributed to normal attritional loss and compensation. A cathepsin (and possibly other enzymes), probably lysosomal in origin, is believed to be actively involved in degradation of the macromolecule.

In reviewing this current knowledge of articular cartilage, there are obviously many questions still unanswered about this extraordinary tissue. The relationship of the cell structure to function has not been completely established, and control mechanisms for DNA synthesis are unknown. The synthetic mechanisms are still somewhat obscure, and the physical and biochemical interaction of the matrix components is poorly understood. The nature and function of the classes of protein polysaccharides have been only partially investigated to date. The glycolytic pathways have not been completely elucidated, and controversy exists regarding nutritional routes, as well as rates and mechanisms of substrate diffusion. The role of the matrix in lubrication and resiliency is still not clear. Beyond this immediate frontier loom vast uncharted areas of pathologic anatomy, chemistry, and physiology. What are the changes that occur in this "normal" pattern with aging, trauma, osteoarthritis, or rheumatoid disease? It is hoped that newer methods and continued interest will provide some of these answers in the years to come.

I gratefully acknowledge the assistance of Dr. Charles Weiss, Mr. Louis Lippiello, Mr. Cornelius Mead, and Miss Judith Horowitz in the preparation of this essay, together with the collaboration in years past of Dr. Thomas D. Brower, Mrs. Patricia Orlic Baron, Mr. Karl Conger, and Miss Carol Boyle. Without them it would not only have been impossible but also incredibly dull.

REFERENCES

1. Adamson, L., Gleason, S., and Anast, C.: Sulfate incorporation by embryonic chick bone, Biochim. Biophys. Acta **83**:262, 1964.
2. Ali, S. Y., Evans, L., Stainthorpe, E., and Lack, C. H.: Characterization of cathepsins in cartilage, Biochem. J. **105**:549, 1967.
3. Amprino, R.: On the incorporation of radiosulfate into cartilage, Experientia **15**:65, 1955.
4. Anderson, A. J.: Some studies on the occurrence of sialic acid in human cartilage, Biochem. J. **78**:399, 1961.
5. Anderson, C. E., Ludowieg, J., Harper, H., and Engleman, E. P.: The composition of the organic component of human articular cartilage, J. Bone Joint Surg. **46A**:1176, 1964.
6. Balazs, E. A., Bloom, G. D., and Swann, D. A.: Fine structure and glycosaminoglycan content of the surface layer of articular cartilage, Fed. Proc. **25**:1813, 1966.
7. Barland, P., Janis, R., and Sandson, J.: Immunofluorescent studies of human articular cartilage, Ann. Rheum. Dis. **25**:156, 1966.
8. Barnett, C. H., and Cobbold, A. F.: Lubrication within living joints, J. Bone Joint Surg. **44B**:662, 1962.
9. Barnett, C. H., Cochrane, W., and Palfrey, A. J.: Age changes in articular cartilage of rabbits, Ann. Rheum. Dis. **22**:389, 1963.
10. Barnett, C. H., Davies, D. V., and MacConnaill, M. A.: Synovial joints their structure and mechanics, Springfield, Ill., 1961, Charles C Thomas, Publisher.
11. Benninghoff, A.: Form und Bau der Gelenk-Knorpel in ihren Beziehungen zur Funktion, Z. Anat. Entwicklungsgesch. **76**:43, 1925.
12. Bollet, A. J.: Connective tissue polysaccharide metabolism and the pathogenesis of arthritis, Advances Intern. Med. **13**:33, 1967.
13. Bollet, A. J., Handy, J. R., and Sturgill, B. C.: Chondroitin sulfate concentration and protein polysaccharide composition of articular cartilage in osteoarthritis, J. Clin. Invest. **42**:853, 1963.
14. Bollet, A. J., and Nance, J. L.: Biochemical findings in normal and osteoarthritic articular cartilage. II. Chondroitin sulfate concentration and chain length, water and ash content, J. Clin. Invest. **45**:1170, 1966.
15. Boström, H.: On the metabolism of the sulfate group of chondroitin sulfuric acid, J. Biol. Chem. **196**:477, 1952.
16. Brower, T. D.: The localization of chloride in hyaline cartilage by histochemical techniques, J. Bone Joint Surg. **38A**:655, 1956.
17. Brower, T. D., Akahoshi, Y., and Orlic, P.: The diffusion of dyes through articular cartilage in vivo, J. Bone Joint Surg. **44A**:456, 1962.
18. Brower, T. D., and Hsu, Wan-Yi: Normal articular cartilage, Clin. Orthop. **64**:9, 1969.
19. Bywaters, E. C. L.: The metabolism of joint tissues, J. Path. Bact. **44**:247, 1937.
20. Cameron, D. A., and Robinson, R. A.: Electron-microscopy of epiphysial and articular cartilage matrix in the femur of the newborn infant, J. Bone Joint Surg. **40A**:163, 1958.
21. Campo, R. D., and Dziewiatkowski, D. D.: Intracellular synthesis of protein polysaccharides by slices of bovine costal cartilage, J. Biol. Chem. **237**:2729, 1962.
22. Campo, R. D., and Tourtelotte, C. D.: The composition of bovine cartilage and bone, Biochim. Biophys. Acta **141**:614, 1967.
23. Chrisman, O. D.: The ground substance of connective tissue, Clin. Orthop. **36**:184, 1964.
24. Chrisman, O. D., Semonsky, C., and Bensch, K. G.:

Cathepsins in articular cartilage. In Workshop on the healing of osseous tissue, Washington, D. C., N. A. S.-N. R. C., 1967.
25. Clark, E. R., and Clark, E. L.: Microscopic observations on new formation of cartilage and bone in the living mammal, Amer. J. Anat. **70**:167, 1942.
26. Coelho, R. R., and Chrisman, O. D.: Sulfate metabolism and cartilage II ^{35}S sulfate uptake and total sulfate in cartilage slices, J. Bone Joint Surg. **42A**:165, 1960.
27. Collins, D. H.: The pathology of articular and spinal disease, London, 1949, E. Arnold and Co.
28. Collins, D. H., Ghadially, F. N., and Meachim, G.: Intracellular lipids of cartilage, Ann. Rheum. Dis. **24**:123, 1965.
29. Collins, D. H., and McElligott, T. F.: Sulphate ($^{35}SO_4$) uptake by chondrocytes in relation to histological changes in osteoarthritic human articular cartilage, Ann. Rheum. Dis. **20**:117, 1961.
30. Collins, D. H., and Meachim, G.: Sulphate ($^{35}SO_4$) fixation by human articular cartilage compared in the knee and shoulder joints, Ann. Rheum. Dis. **20**:117, 1961.
31. Crelin, E. S., and Southwick, W. O.: Mitosis of chondrocytes induced in the knee joint articular cartilage of adult rabbits, Yale J. Biol. Med. **33**: 243, 1960.
32. Crelin, E. S., and Southwick, W. O.: Changes induced by sustained pressure in the knee joint articular cartilage of adult rabbits, Anat. Rec. **149**: 113, 1964.
33. D'Abramo, F., and Lipmann, F.: The formation of adenosine 3′ phosphate-5′ phosphosulfate in extracts of chick embryo cartilage and its conversion into chondroitin sulfate, Biochim. Biophys. Acta **25**:211, 1957.
34. Davies, D. V., Barnett, C. H., Cochran, W., and Palfrey, A. J.: Electron microscopy of articular cartilage in the young adult rabbit, Ann. Rheum. Dis. **21**:11, 1962.
35. DeLuca, S., and Gilbert, J. E.: Biosynthesis of chondroitin sulfate. II. Incorporation of sulfate ^{35}S into microsomial chondroitin sulfate, J. Biol. Chem. **243**:2725, 1968.
36. Dickens, F., and Weil-Malherbe, H.: Metabolism of cartilage, Nature **138**:30, 1936.
37. Dorfman, A.: Metabolism of acid mucopolysaccharides. In Connective tissue: intercellular macromolecules, Boston, 1964, Little, Brown & Co., p. 155.
38. Dziewiatkowski, D. D.: Effect of age on some aspects of sulfate metabolism in the rat, J. Exp. **Med. 99:283, 1954.**
39. Dziewiatkowski, D. D.: Some aspects of the metabolism of chondroitin sulfate ^{35}S in the rat, J. Biol. Chem. **223**:239, 1956.
40. Eichelberger, L., Akeson, W. H., and Roma, M.: Biochemical studies of articular cartilage. I. Normal values, J. Bone Joint Surg. **40A**:142, 1958.
41. Ekholm, R.: Articular cartilage nutrition, Acta Anat., vol. 11, supp. 15, 1951.
42. Elliott, H. C.: Studies on articular cartilage. I. Growth mechanisms, Amer. J. Anat. **58**:127, 1936.
43. Elmore, S. M., Sokoloff, L., Norris, G., and Carmeci, P.: The nature of "imperfect" elasticity of articular cartilage, J. Appl. Physiol. **18**:393, 1963.
44. Fawns, H. T., and Landells, I. W.: Histochemical studies of rheumatic conditions. Observations of the fine structures of the matrix of normal bone and cartilage, Ann. Rheum. Dis. **12**:105, 1953.
45. Fell, H. B., and Dingle, J. T.: Studies on the mode of action of excess of vitamin A: G. Lysosomal proteases and the degradation of cartilage matrix, Arthritis Rheum. **7**:398, 1964.
46. Bell, H. B., and Thomas, L.: Comparison of the effects of papain and vitamin A on cartilage, J. Exp. Med. **111**:719, 1960.
47. Fessel, J. M., and Chrisman, D. D.: Enzymatic degradation of chondromucoprotein by cell free extracts of human cartilage, Arthritis Rheum. **7**: 398, 1964.
48. Ghadially, F. N., Meachim, G., and Collins, D. H.: Extracellular lipid in the matrix of human articular cartilage, Ann. Rheum. Dis. **24**:136, 1965.
49. Godman, G. C., and Lane, N.: On the site of sulfation in the chondrocyte, J. Cell. Biol. **21**: 353, 1964.
50. Gross, J. I., Mathews, M. B., and Dorfman, A.: Sodium chondroitin sulphate—protein complexes of cartilage. II. Metabolism, J. Biol. Chem. **235**: 2889, 1960.
51. Helting, T., and Roden, L.: The carbohydrate-protein linkage region of chondroitin-6-sulfate, Biochim. Biophys. Acta **170**:301, 1968.
52. Herring, G. M.: The chemical structure of tendon, cartilage, dentin and bone matrix, Clin. Orthop. **60**:261, 1968.
53. Hoffman, P., and Mashburn, T. A., Jr.: Protein polysaccharide of bovine cartilage. II. The relation of keratin sulfate and chondroitin sulfate, J. Biol. Chem. **242**:3805, 1967.
54. Howell, D. S., Pita, J. C., Altman, R., Meuller, F., and Madruga, J.: Micropuncture studies of interstitial fluid from articular cartilage of growing rabbits. Paper read at annual meeting of A. R. A., June, 1969, Boston, Mass.
55. Hunter, W.: On the structure and diseases of articulating cartilage, Phil. Trans. B. **42**:514, 1743.
56. Ingelmark, B. E., and Sääf, J.: Ueber die Ernahrung des Gelenkknorpels und die Bildung der Gelenkflussigkeit unter verschiedenen Funktionellen Verhaltnissen, Acta. Orthop. Scand. **17**:303, 1948.
57. Kantor, T. G., and Schubert, M.: The difference in permeability of cartilage to cationic and anionic dyes, J. Histochem. Cytochem. **5**:28, 1957.
58. Kaplan, D., and Meyer, K.: Aging of human cartilage, Nature **183**:1267, 1959.
59. Kolliker, A.: A manual of human histology, vol. 1, London, 1853, Sydenham Society.
60. Krane, S., Parsons, V., and Kunin, A. S.: Studies of the metabolism of epiphysial cartilage. In

Bassett, C. A. L., editor: Cartilage degradation and repair, Washington, D. C., N. A. S.-N. R. C., 1967.

61. Kuhn, R., and Leppelmann, H. J.: Galaktosamin und Glucosamin im Knorpel in Abhängigkeit vom Lebensalter, Liebig Ann. Chem. **611**:254, 1958.
62. Lack, C. H., and Ali, S. Y.: The degradation of cartilage by enzymes. In Bassett, C. A. L., editor: Cartilage degradation and repair, Washington, D. C., N. A. S.-N. R. C., 1967.
63. Leidy, J.: On the intimate structure and history of articular cartilage, Amer. J. Med. Sci. **17**:277, 1849.
64. Lindahl, O.: Ueber den Wassergehalt des Knorpels, Acta Orthop. Scand. **17**:134, 1958.
65. Linn, F. C., and Sokoloff, L.: Movement and composition of interstitial fluid of cartilage, Arthritis Rheum. **8**:481, 1965.
66. Little, K., Pimm, L. H., and Trueta, J.: Osteoarthritis of the hip: an electron microscopic study, J. Bone Joint Surg. **40B**:123, 1958.
67. Loewe, G.: Localization of chondromucoproteins in cartilage, Ann. Rheum. Dis. **24**:528, 1965.
68. Lutwak-Mann, C.: Enzyme systems in articular cartilage, Biochem. J. **34**:517, 1940.
69. McConnaill, M. A.: The movements of bone and joints. 4. The mechanical structure of articulating cartilage, J. Bone Joint Surg. **33B**:251, 1951.
70. McKibben, B., and Holdsworth, F. S.: The nutrition of immature joint cartilage in the lamb, J. Bone Joint Surg. **48B**:793, 1966.
71. Mankin, H. J.: Unpublished data.
72. Mankin, H. J.: Localization of tritiated thymidine in articular cartilage of rabbits. II. Repair in immature cartilage, J. Bone Joint Surg. **44A**:688, 1962.
73. Mankin, H. J.: Localization of tritiated thymidine in articular cartilage of rabbits. I. Growth and immature cartilage, J. Bone Joint Surg. **44A**:682, 1962.
74. Mankin, H. J.: Localization of tritiated cytidine in articular cartilage of immature and adult rabbits after intraarticular injection, Lab. Invest. **12**:543, 1963.
75. Mankin, H. J.: The calcified zone (basal layer) of articular cartilage of rabbits, Anat. Rec. **145**:73, 1963.
76. Mankin, H. J.: Localization of tritiated thymidine in articular cartilage of rabbits. III. Mature articular cartilage, J. Bone Joint Surg. **45A**:529, 1963.
77. Mankin, H. J., and Baron, P. A.: The effect of aging on protein synthesis in articular cartilage of rabbits, Lab. Invest. **14**:658, 1965.
78. Mankin, H. J., and Boyle, C. J.: The acute effects of lacerative injury on DNA and protein synthesis in articular cartilage. In Bassett, C. A. L., editor: Cartilage degradation and repair, Washington, D. C., N. A. S.-N. R. C., 1967.
79. Mankin, H. J.: The effect of aging on articular cartilage, Bull. New York Acad. Med. **44**:545, 1968.
80. Mankin, H. J., and Conger, K. A.: The effect of cortisol on articular cartilage of rabbits, Lab. Invest. **15**:794, 1966.
81. Mankin, H. J., and Conger, K. A.: The acute effects of intraarticular hydrocortisone on articular cartilage in rabbits, J. Bone Joint Surg. **48A**:1383, 1966.
82. Mankin, H. J., and Lippiello, L.: Biochemical and metabolic abnormalities in articular cartilage from osteoarthritic human hips. To be published.
83. Mankin, H. J., and Lipiello, L.: The turnover of the matrix of articular cartilage, J. Bone Joint Surg. **51A**:1591, 1969.
84. Mankin, H. J., and Orlic, P. A.: A method of estimating the "health" of rabbit articular cartilage by assays of ribonucleic acid and protein synthesis, Lab. Invest. **13**:465, 1964.
85. Maroudas, A.: Physicochemical properties of cartilage in the light of ion exchange theory, Biophys. J. **8**:575, 1968.
86. Maroudas, A., and Bullough, P.: Permeability of articular cartilage, Nature **219**:1260, 1968.
87. Maroudas, A., Bullough, P., Swanson, S. A. V., and Freeman, M. A. R.: The permeability of articular cartilage, J. Bone Joint Surg. **50B**:166, 1968.
88. Maroudas, A., Muir, H., and Wingham, J.: The correlation of fixed negative charge with glycosaminoglycan content of human articular cartilage, Biochim. Biophys. Acta **177**:492, 1969.
89. Mathews, M. B.: The interaction of collagen and acid mucopolysaccharides: a model for connective tissue, Biochem. J. **96**:710, 1965.
90. Meachim, G.: The histology and ultrastructure of cartilage. In Bassett, C. A. L., editor: Cartilage degradation and repair, Washington, D. C., N.A.S.-N.R.C., 1967.
91. Meachim, G.: Age changes in articular cartilage, Clin. Orthop. **64**:33, 1969.
92. Meachim, G., and Collins, D. H.: Cell counts of normal and osteoarthritic articular cartilage in relation to the uptake of sulfate ($^{35}SO_4$) in vitro, Am. Rheum. Dis. **21**:45, 1962.
93. Meachim, G., Ghadially, F. N., and Collins, D. H.: Regressive changes in the superficial layer of human articular cartilage, Ann. Rheum. Dis. **24**: 23, 1965.
94. Meachim, G., and Roy, S.: Intracytoplasmic filaments in the cells of adult human articular cartilage, Ann. Rheum. Dis. **26**:50, 1967.
95. Miles, J. S., and Eichelberger, L.: Biochemical studies of human cartilage during the aging process, J. Amer. Geriat. Soc. **12**:1, 1964.
96. Miller, E. J., Vanderkorst, J. K., and Sokoloff, L.: Collagen of human articular and costal cartilage, Arthritis Rheum. **12**:21, 1969.
97. Muir, H.: Chemistry and metabolism of connective tissue glycosaminoglycans (mucopolysaccharides). In Hall, D. A., editor: International review of connective tissue research, New York, 1964, Academic Press Inc., vol. 2, p. 101.
98. Paget, J.: Healing of injuries in various tissues. In lectures on surgical pathology, London, 1853, vol. 1.

99. Palfrey, A. J., and Davies, D. V.: The fine structure of chondrocytes, J. Anat. **100**:213, 1966.
100. Partridge, S. M., Davis, H. F., and Adair, G. S.: The chemistry of connective tissues. 6. The constitution of the chondroitin sulfate-protein complex in cartilage, Biochem. J. **79**:15, 1961.
101. Pasternak, C. A.: The synthesis of 3′ phosphoadenosine 5′ phosphosulfate by mouse tissues: sulfate activation in vitro and in vivo, J. Biol. Chem. **235**:438, 1960.
102. Perlman, R. L., Telser, A., and Dorfman, A.: The biosynthesis of chondroitin sulfate by a cell free preparation, J. Biol. Chem. **239**:3623, 1964.
103. Quintarelli, G.: Methods for the histochemical identification of acid mucopolysaccharides: a critical evaluation. In Quintarelli, G., editor: The chemical physiology of mucopolysaccharides, Boston, 1968, Little, Brown & Co., p. 199.
104. Rigal, W. M.: The use of tritiated thymidine in studies of chondrogenesis. In McLean, F. C., LaCroix, P., and Budy, A. M., editors: Radioisotopes and bone, Oxford, 1962, Blackwell Scientific Publications, Ltd.
105. Roden, L.: The protein carbohydrate linkages of acid mucopolysaccharides. In Quintarelli, G., editor: The chemical physiology of mucopolysaccharides. Boston, 1968, Little, Brown & Co., p. 17.
106. Rosenberg, L., Johnson, B., and Schubert, M.: Protein polysaccharides from human articular and costal cartilages, J. Clin. Invest. **44**:1647, 1965.
107. Rosenthal, O., Bowie, M. A., and Wagoner, G.: Studies on the metabolism of articular cartilage. II. Respiration and glycolysis of cartilage in relation to its age, J. Cell. Comp. Physiol. **17**:221, 1941.
108. Schubert, M.: Intercellular macromolecules containing polysaccharides. In Connective tissue: intercellular macromolecules, Boston, 1964, Little, Brown & Co., p. 119.
109. Schubert, M., and Hamerman, D.: A primer on connective tissue biochemistry, Philadelphia, 1968, Lea & Febiger.
110. Silberberg, R.: Ultrastructure of articular cartilage in health and disease, Clin. Orthop. **57**:233, 1968.
111. Silberberg, R., Silberberg, M., and Feir, D.: Life cycle of articular cartilage cells: an electronmicroscopic study of the hip joint of the mouse, Amer. J. Anat. **114**:17, 1964.
112. Silberberg, R., Silberberg, M., Vogel, A., and Wettstein, W.: Ultrastructure of articular cartilage of mice of various ages, Amer. J. Anat. **109**:251, 1961.
113. Smith, J. W., Peters, T. J., and Serafini-Fracassini, A.: Observations in the distribution of the protein polysaccharide complex and collagen in bovine articular cartilage, J. Cell. Comp. Physiol. **2**:129, 1967.
114. Sokoloff, L.: Elasticity of articular cartilage: Effect of ions and viscous solutions, Science **141**:1055, 1963.
115. Spicer, S., Horn, R. G., and Leppi, T. J.: Histochemistry of connective tissue mucopolysaccharides. In Wagner, B. M., and Smith, D. E., editors: The connective tissue, Baltimore, 1967, The Williams & Wilkins Co., p. 251.
116. Stockwell, R. A.: The cell density of human articular and costal cartilage, J. Anat. **101**:753, 1967.
117. Stockwell, R. A.: Lipid content of human costal and articular cartilage, Ann. Rheum. Dis. **26**:481, 1967.
118. Stockwell, R. A., and Scott, J. E.: Distribution of acid glycosaminoglycans in human articular cartilage, Nature **215**:1376, 1967.
119. Strangeways, T. S. P.: Observations on the nutrition of articular cartilage, Brit. Med. J. **1**:661, 1920.
120. Strominger, J. L.: Nucleotide intermediates in the biosynthesis of heteropolymeric polysaccharides. In Connective tissue: intercellular macromolecules, Boston, 1964, Little, Brown & Co., p. 139.
121. Thomas, L.: The effects of papain, vitamin A, and cortisone in cartilage matrix in vivo. In Connective tissue: intercellular macromolecules, Boston, 1964, Little, Brown & Co., p. 207.
122. Virchow, R.: Die Krankhaften Geschwülste I, Berlin, 1863. Cited by Ekholm, R.: Articular cartilage nutrition, Acta. Anat., supp. 15, 1951.
123. Wagoner, G., Rosenthal, O., and Bowie, M. A.: Studies of the cells in normal and arthritic bovine cartilage, Amer. J. Med. Sci. **201**:489, 1941.
124. Walker, P. S., Dowson, D., Longfield, M. D., and Wright, V.: Boosted lubrication in synovial joints by fluid enlargement and enrichment, Ann. Rheum. Dis. **27**:512, 1968.
125. Walker, P. S., Sikorski, J., Dowson, D., Longfield, M. D., Wright, V., and Buckley, T.: Behavior of synovial fluid on surfaces of articular cartilage, Ann. Rheum. Dis. **28**:1, 1969.
126. Weiss, C., Rosenberg, L., and Helfet, A. J.: An ultrastructural study of normal young adult human articular cartilage, J. Bone Joint Surg. **50A**:663, 1968.
127. Weissman, G., and Spilberg, I. L.: Breakdown of cartilage protein polysaccharide by lysosomes, Arthritis Rheum. **11**:162, 1968.
128. Woessner, J. F., Jr.: Acid cathepsins of cartilage. In Bassett, C. A. L., editor: Cartilage degradation and repair, Washington, D. C., N.A.S.-N.R.C., 1967.

Author index

Subject index